THE COMPLETE BOOK OF
PREGNANCY
& CHILDBIRTH

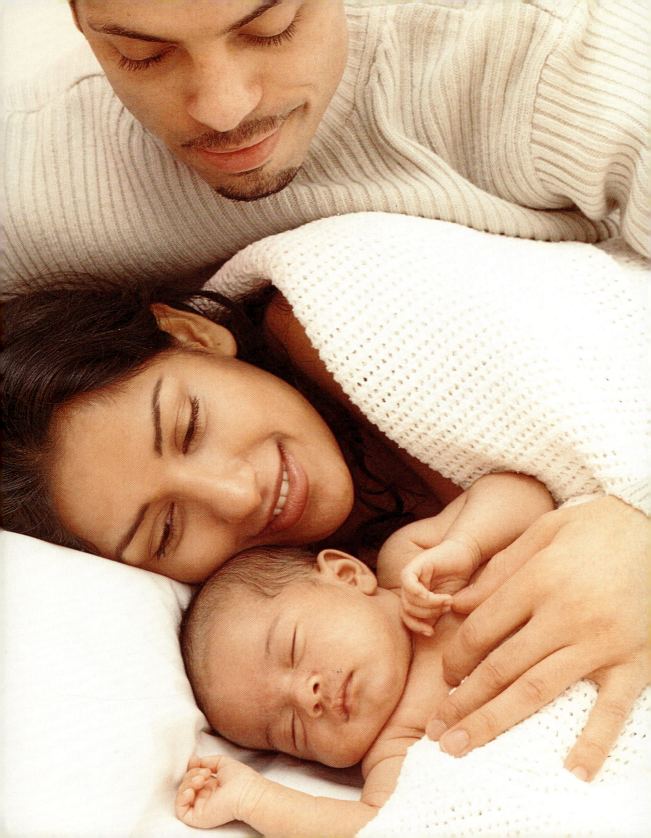

THE COMPLETE BOOK OF
PREGNANCY
&CHILDBIRTH

SHEILA KITZINGER

PHOTOGRAPHY BY MARCIA MAY

FOURTH EDITION

Alfred A. Knopf New York 2004

THIS IS A BORZOI BOOK PUBLISHED BY ALFRED A. KNOPF

Copyright © 1980, 1989, 1996, 2003 by Dorling Kindersley Limited, London
Text copyright © 1980, 1989, 1996, 2003 by Sheila Kitzinger

Library of Congress Cataloging-in-Publication Data
Kitzinger, Sheila.
The complete book of pregnancy and childbirth / Sheila Kitzinger;
photography by Marcia May.—Rev. ed.
p.   cm.
Includes bibliographical references and index.
ISBN 1-4000-4108-2 (hardcover); ISBN 0-375-71047-7 (paperback)
1. Pregnancy—Popular works.   2. Childbirth—Popular works.   I. Title.
RG525.K518 2003
618.2—dc21   2002043433

Published December 8, 1980
Revised Edition, September 10, 1989
Third Edition, November 11, 1996
Fourth Edition, in hardcover and paperback, revised, redesigned, and reset, January 6, 2004
Fourth Edition paperback reprinted August 2004

Printed and bound by R.R. Donnelley & Sons, Crawfordsville, Indiana

CONTENTS

Introduction **7**
Pregnancy week by week **10**

21   PREGNANCY: THE EARLY WEEKS

Finding out you are pregnant **22** • Planning and preparation **36**

67   PREGNANCY: PHYSICAL AND EMOTIONAL CHANGES

Life in the uterus **68** • Forty weeks of life **82** • Expecting twins **88**
Your baby's well-being **96** • Your physical well-being **116**
Emotional challenges in pregnancy **150** • Becoming a father **158**
You and your partner **164** • Pregnant again **172**

179   PREGNANCY: THINKING AHEAD TO BIRTH

In tune with your body for labor **180**
Windows into the uterus **226** • The last few weeks **238**

247   THE EXPERIENCE OF BIRTH

What happens in labor **248** • Different kinds of labor **270**
Giving support in labor **286** • Dealing with pain **304**
Toward the medical control of birth **324** • Gentle birth **356**

369   YOU AND YOUR NEWBORN

The first hours of life **370** • The baby who needs special care **380**
Losing a baby **386** • The first ten days **394**
The challenge of new parenthood **412**

PHOTOGRAPHIC SEQUENCES

A hospital birth **60** • A home birth **264** • A water birth **296**

Useful reading **426** • Useful addresses **427** • Glossary **429**
Research references **435** • Acknowledgments **441** • Index **442**

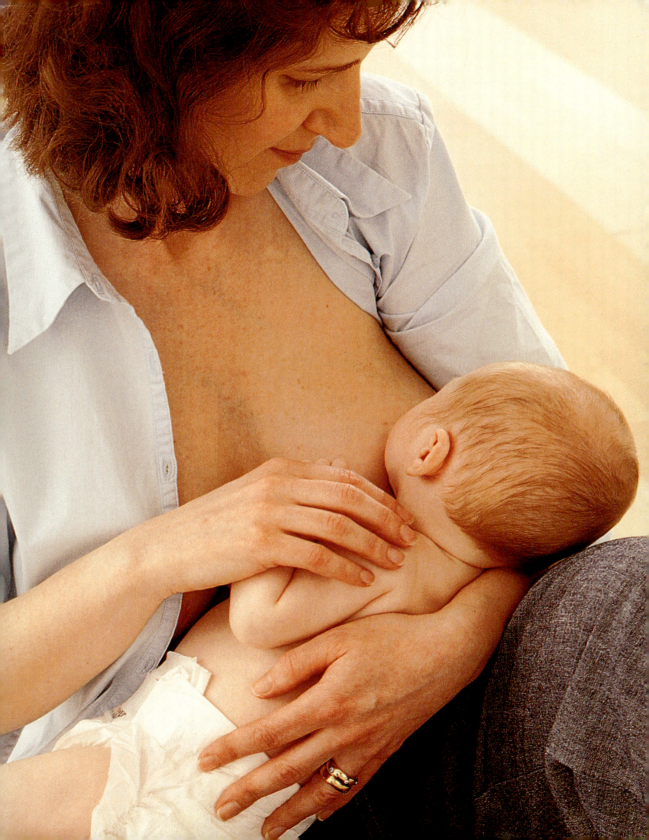

INTRODUCTION

When I first started to teach and counsel pregnant women
in the 1960s, there was little birth education around.
For a small minority of women, there were breathing and
relaxation exercises taught by physiotherapists (who then
had no special training for helping women in childbirth)
and talks by midwives about "what to expect."

There was a handful of books written by the pioneers: Grantly Dick-Read, Kathleen Vaughan, Minnie Randall, Helen Heardman, Velvovsky, and Lamaze. Although some discussed the fear of childbirth, there was nothing about the socially inculcated lack of confidence we felt in our bodies and in ourselves, nor the pressure on women by a powerful medical system to surrender themselves to it as passive patients. It seemed that all we could hope for was to put on a good performance and to be told "well done."

After the birth of my first child, when I started teaching for what is now the National Childbirth Trust, I remember talking to a group of obstetricians from the former Soviet Union who had introduced psychoprophylaxis (a system of training for labor based on breathing techniques) into some of their bigger hospitals and were actually proud because "there is now no noise in the labor ward." It was supposed to be a great achievement—to silence women!

When psychoprophylaxis was first introduced in Britain from France, one woman told me that after a grueling labor involving drugs and the use of forceps, her childbirth teacher had shown up at her bedside and commented: "You didn't do too well!" In those days, if you needed painkilling drugs or help with the birth, you were made to feel that you had failed. The choice was between having doctors take over completely or putting on a solo performance without support from professionals.

Remarkable changes have taken place since then—largely due to women in the childbirth movement who have joined together across continents. It is now acknowledged that women have a right to full and accurate information about their bodies and to participate in all decisions made about them. *The Complete Book of Pregnancy and Childbirth* reflects the many changes that have come about because we refuse to remain ignorant of what doctors are

The birth of a baby
is a biological process.
Yet it is more than that.
Giving birth and caring for
a baby are acts of love.

doing to us. It is an expression of women's courage and growing self-confidence, and of the ways in which we reach out to each other to explore those experiences we have in common.

To take an active part in giving birth, rather than submit passively to delivery, it helps to prepare yourself well in advance, understanding how to adapt to the work of your uterus, using breathing, relaxation techniques, changes of position, massage, and focused concentration to "get in tune with" contractions. There is a good deal of practical material in this book on ways of doing this. It is not just a matter of learning exercises. There is a rhythm about a natural labor: with the wave of each contraction you are swept on toward the birth of your baby in a pattern that transforms birth into a process greater than all its parts, one in which all the techniques you have practiced are submerged by the total amazing experience.

The book describes the choices available to help you decide how you would like to have your baby, in what setting, and how you wish your baby to be welcomed into the world. I include suggestions on talking with your doctor, how to ask about things that worry you and share in the decisions. The book offers a map of the route through pregnancy and labor and out the other side, explaining who does what and why, and what happens when things are not straightforward. I have used some of the words and phrases that you may see written on your medical chart or hear from doctors or midwives, so that you will understand them, but the main focus is on experiential aspects of birth—how it feels.

"I NEVER FELT SCARED OR OUT OF MY DEPTH. THE ATTITUDE WAS, 'IT'S YOUR BIRTH. WE'RE HERE IF YOU NEED US.' THEY KEPT TELLING MY HUSBAND HE WAS DOING A GOOD JOB, TOO."

The book is threaded through with recognition of the father's importance to his partner and baby and suggestions as to how he can help during pregnancy, labor, and the time after birth. A baby is bound to change a couple's way of life, their feelings about each other, and the kind of partnership they have. The man, as well as the woman, faces emotional challenges, and this is rarely acknowledged in our society. So I have focused on the experience of childbirth for him, too.

Through most of this book I assume that there is a man in the picture—but of course this may not be the case. You may, by choice or necessity, be having a baby as a single parent. Or you may be in a relationship with another woman and have conceived with donated sperm. I hope that most of what I write can be adapted to make sense for all of my readers.

Most new parents gain confidence and begin first "conversations" with their baby when there are no rules to be obeyed and no standards to live up to, when they can stroke, hold, and cuddle their newborn as much as they wish. In this book, I show how to create the kind of setting and atmosphere for birth, whether at home or in the hospital, that nurtures relationships.

Pregnancy and childbirth are normal life processes, not illnesses. You feel the surge of life moving inside you, the ripening of your body heavy with fruit, and then the flood of vitality as labor starts and your uterus contracts in wave after wave, bringing your baby into your arms. It is awe-inspiring and deeply satisfying. At the same time, you grow up a little and learn more about yourself and your partner. I hope this book will help you savor the intense reality of childbearing and enjoy it to the fullest.

NOTES TO THE READER

It is always difficult to know whether to use "he" or "she" when writing about babies. I have used a mixture of "he" and "she," since babies have their own budding personalities right from the start. I hope that the reader will not find this too awkward, and if there is a bias toward "she" in the text, note that my five babies were all girls, so it comes naturally.

All references to research papers are marked with an asterisk (*); these are then listed by page number on pages 435–440.

AUTHOR'S ACKNOWLEDGMENTS

Many people have contributed to this book. I want to thank Rick Porter, FRCOG, who read the manuscript and made helpful suggestions, and Georgia Rose, CNM, MS, experienced New York nurse-midwife, with whom it was a pleasure to work. Marcia May took many of the wonderful photographs of birth. Vreni Booth, who teaches movement based on the Feldenkrais method, helped me rethink postnatal exercises.

Nicky Leap, the midwife in some of the birth photographs, is one of the most innovative thinkers and courageous practitioners in midwifery today. I value my discussions with Dr. Michel Odent. They always stimulate lateral thinking, as he raises important questions that need to be answered. I am also grateful to Professor Lesley Page, Director of Midwifery at The Royal Free Hospital, London, for the many times that we have shared our thoughts about the future of midwifery, and its meaning for women and families.

I should also like to thank Sir Iain Chalmers, Director of the Cochrane Institute, for the work he has done to base obstetric practice on scientific evidence rather than on medical "hunches," and to present the benefits and risks so that women can make up their own minds about what they want. I have drawn heavily on the *Cochrane Library* for the material in the book.

My birth activist colleagues in the National Childbirth Trust, especially Mary Newburn, the Trust's Policy Officer, together with Beverley Lawrence Beech of the Association for Improvements in the Maternity Services, and Janet Balaskas, who created the Active Birth Movement, have supported me with their strength and energy.

In the writing of this book, I owe a great deal to my daughter Tess for her clarity of thinking, her understanding, and her skills with the computer. She is designer and mistress of my website, www.sheilakitzinger.com.

PREGNANCY WEEK BY WEEK

This week-by-week guide to what happens to you and your baby during pregnancy starts with the third week—the week of conception. You may not be absolutely certain when that was, so be flexible and read about the week before and the week after, too.

WEEK 3

You have ovulated, and an egg is traveling along one of the two Fallopian tubes toward your uterus. One of the millions of sperm that your partner ejaculated during intercourse has fertilized the egg while it is still inside the Fallopian tube.

Your baby is a cluster of cells that multiply rapidly as they continue on their journey along the Fallopian tube.

WEEK 4

You have probably not noticed anything different, although some women have a strange, metallic taste in their mouths.

The fertilized egg has arrived in your uterus and, after floating in the uterine cavity for about three days, has embedded itself in the uterine lining. It is nourished from blood vessels in the lining of your uterus, and the placenta is beginning to form around it.

WEEK 5

You are beginning to think that you might be pregnant. Your period is late, but you cannot be sure, because you may feel as though it is about to start at any time. Your breasts are slightly enlarged and tender, and you may find you need to pass urine more often than usual.

The embryo is about $1/10$ in (2 mm) long and would be visible to the naked eye by now. Its body has elongated, and a series of tiny bumps has developed along its rounded "back." These will eventually become the spine. The head is becoming distinguishable from the body, and the brain has two lobes. The embryo looks a little like a minute sea horse.

WEEK 6

You may be feeling nauseous first thing in the morning or when you are cooking a meal. Your vagina has become a bluish or violet color. From the sixth day after your period was due, sometimes even earlier, you can find out by a urine test whether or not you are pregnant. Your uterus is now the size of a tangerine.

The baby has developed a head and trunk, and a rudimentary brain has formed. Tiny limb buds are starting to appear. By the end of this week, the baby's circulation is beginning to function. The jaw and mouth are developing and ten dental buds are growing in each jaw.

WEEK 7

You may sometimes feel dizzy or faint when standing for a long time. Your breasts are noticeably larger, and small nodules may have appeared on the areolae, while your nipples may have become more prominent. Pregnancy can be confirmed by a vaginal examination.

The limb buds have developed rapidly and look like tiny arms and legs. At the end of these limbs are small indentations that later become fingers and toes. The spinal cord and brain are almost complete, and the head is assuming a human shape. The baby is about ½ in (1.3 cm) long.

WEEK 8

You may have "gone off" certain foods and like others that were not your favorite foods before. Many pregnant women can no longer drink alcohol, even if they previously enjoyed it, and a dislike of cigarettes and tobacco smoke is common. Your hair may seem less manageable than usual. You may also have a slight vaginal discharge.

The baby has all its main organs in a rudimentary form. The eyes and ears are growing. The face is taking on a human shape, and the baby is just under 1 in (2.5 cm) long.

WEEK 9

You may notice an improvement in your skin; this is due to pregnancy hormones. However, your gums may be softer because of these hormones, and you need to be especially careful about dental hygiene.

The baby's limbs are developing rapidly by this stage, and fingers and toes are beginning to be defined on the hands and feet. The head is starting to look rounded and there is an obvious neck.

The baby is moving about gently to exercise its muscles, although you cannot feel it. At this point it weighs only about as much as a grape.

WEEK 10

Your uterus has expanded to the size of an orange, but is still hidden away within your pelvis. You should be wearing a bra with good support by now. If you buy a bra that fits your breasts but is adjustable to allow for later chest expansion, you may not need to get another size during the rest of your pregnancy.

The placenta, to which the baby is attached, begins to produce progesterone in a process that is completed by the end of the 14th week, when progesterone is sufficient for the placenta to take over the function of the corpus luteum. The baby's ankles and wrists are formed, and fingers and toes are clearly visible. The baby has now grown to about 1¾ in (4.5 cm) long.

WEEK 11

If you have felt nauseated during the last weeks, the sickness may gradually lessen from now onward. The amount of blood circulating through your body has started to increase, and will go on increasing until about the 30th week. You should be discovering what childbirth classes are available, since they often get booked up early.

Your baby's testicles or ovaries have formed at this point, as have all its major organs. These will not develop much further, although they continue to grow inside the uterus. The baby is relatively safe from the risk of developing any congenital abnormalities from the end of this week.

WEEK 12

You may have your first prenatal visit this week. The doctor or midwife may be able to feel the uterus by external examination, as it has risen above your pelvis. Arrangements will be made for future appointments, probably once a month until you are 28 weeks pregnant.

The baby's head is becoming more rounded and its eyelids have formed. Its muscles are developing and it is moving about inside the uterus much more. It is now about 2 in (6.5 cm) long but still weighs only ½ oz (18 g).

WEEK 13

If you have had morning sickness this may be gone by the end of this week. From now on your uterus will be enlarging at a regular and noticeable rate. The bag of water that surrounds the baby cushions it from bumps, keeps it at a constant warm temperature, and enables it to move freely, turn its head, stretch, and bounce around. Your midwife may be able to hear your baby's heartbeat using a small handheld ultrasound device.

WEEK 14

You are less tired than you were at the beginning of pregnancy and probably feel fit and active. You may notice a dark line (the linea nigra) down the center of your abdomen. This will begin to fade after the baby is born. Your nipples and the area around them are also starting to darken. Your uterus is the size of a large grapefruit.

The baby has eyebrows, and a small amount of hair has appeared on its head. Its heart can be heard by ultrasound. The baby drinks some of the amniotic fluid and can pass urine. It is receiving all of its nourishment from the placenta and measures about 3¾ in (8–9 cm) in length.

WEEK 15

Your clothes are getting too tight. Do not try to cram into tight jeans. To cope with the increased amount of blood circulating in your body and the baby's need for oxygen, your enlarged heart has increased its output by 20 percent.

The hair on your baby's head and brows is becoming coarser. If it has a gene for dark hair, the pigment cells of hair follicles are beginning to produce black pigment.

WEEK 16

You feel butterflies in your tummy that might be the baby moving. Your waistline is starting to disappear. If you have not already done so, book childbirth education classes. An "early-bird" class might be available to discuss diet, exercise, posture, emotions, and health.

The baby is completely formed. From now on, its time in the uterus will be spent growing and maturing until it reaches the stage of development where it can survive independently. Lanugo (fine down) is starting to form all over the baby, following the whorled pattern of the skin. The baby is 6¾ in (16 cm) long and weighs nearly 5 oz (135 g).

WEEK 17

You may sweat more than usual (due to the extra blood in your system) and your nose may feel congested, too. Both are common in pregnancy and will return to normal after the birth. You may notice that your vaginal secretions are heavier, too.

The growing baby has by this stage pushed the top of the uterus to halfway between your pubic bone and your navel. From now on, the baby weighs more than its placenta. The baby will be moving around the uterus and touching its toes and face. It may be aware of—and even be temporarily startled by—loud sounds from outside your body.

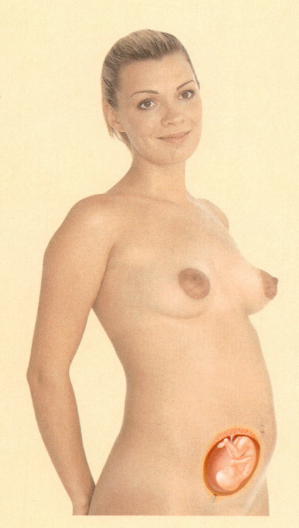

20 WEEKS

Your body at 20 weeks
Finding clothes that accommodate your growing belly may be difficult because your waist has all but disappeared. However, if this is your first pregnancy, it may be some time before you look obviously pregnant.

WEEK 18

If this is your first baby, you may become aware of the first prods and general signs of movement, which are definitely nothing to do with indigestion! At last you know that there really is a baby in there! If you are having trouble sleeping at night, you may be able to make yourself more comfortable with extra pillows.

Measuring about 8 in (20 cm) in length, your baby is now beginning the process of testing its reflexes. Babies often move especially energetically during the evening and bounce around like a cork in water. As well as kicking, the baby is now also grasping and sucking. Some babies find their thumbs while still in the uterus and are confirmed thumb-suckers even before they are born.

WEEK 19

Now is not too early to start practicing deep relaxation, steady, rhythmic breathing, and gentle exercises. Set aside some time each day for this. You may find you are putting on weight on your buttocks as well as your abdomen.

Buds for the baby's milk teeth have formed, and those for the permanent teeth are developing.

WEEK 20

You will notice your baby is more and more active (often in the evenings), and may even be able to see some of its movements. The growing uterus is pushing up against your lungs and pressing your tummy outward. Your navel may pop out and stay that way until after the birth. Your chest (rather than breasts) has expanded and if you do not already have an adjustable bra, now is the time to buy one.

The baby is about 10 in (25 cm) long. Sebum from the sebaceous glands mixes with skin cells and begins to form the protective vernix, which clings to the lanugo all over the baby's skin, especially on the hairier parts and in creases.

WEEK 21

You may have heartburn and bring up small amounts of acid fluid. Ask your doctor or midwife to recommend antacid tablets. If you take antacids, ensure you have a diet rich in iron and vitamin C.

The baby weighs just under 1 lb (450 g), is moving about freely in the amniotic fluid, and is kicking, sometimes high in your tummy, at other times low down.

WEEK 22

Your gums may be swelling because of the pregnancy hormones in your system.

The baby's fingernails are forming. It is settling into a regular pattern of activity and sleep. It is frequently most active while you are resting, and you may feel that you have a jumping bean inside you.

WEEK 23

Different parts of the baby can be felt (palpated) through your abdominal wall. You may feel a stitch-like pain at times down the side of your tummy; this is the uterine muscle stretching, and the pain will probably go away after you have had a rest.

Braxton Hicks "rehearsal" contractions may be more noticeable and more frequent at this stage, gripping and massaging the baby. The baby's fingernails are almost fully formed.

WEEK 24

Another prenatal visit—by now the baby's heart can be heard through a stethoscope or fetal trumpet. The top of your uterus reaches to just above your navel. You may have pain in one or both sides of your lower abdomen, caused by stretching of ligaments attached to your uterus.

The baby is about 13 in (32 cm) long and weighs over 1 lb (0.5 kg). Its vital organs are maturing, but its lungs may not be sufficiently developed for survival outside the uterus.

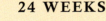

24 WEEKS

Your body at 24 weeks
By now, you will have gained about 10 lb (4.5 kg) in weight, but this varies from one woman to the next. If you are long-waisted, your tummy looks lower than if you are short-waisted.

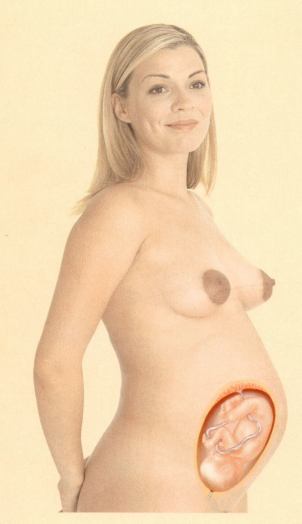

28 WEEKS

Your body at 28 weeks
Now your pregnancy is obvious to everyone. Your uterus is pushing well above your navel, and your breasts will be at least one cup size bigger than they were before you began your pregnancy.

WEEK 25

You may get leg cramps now and later on in your pregnancy. Avoid pointing your toes down. The baby may also press against your bladder, causing you to want to pass urine.

The baby's bone centers are beginning to harden, and tiny veins are visible through the baby's skin.

WEEK 26

You may notice pink streaks in your skin where it has been stretched from underneath. These marks will fade gradually after the birth.

When you speak, your voice goes down into your body, and your baby can hear you. The baby's body is covered with fine, downy hairs, and the skin is beginning to change: instead of being paper-thin and transparent, it is gradually becoming opaque.

WEEK 27

You will be putting on weight fairly consistently now until about the 36th week of pregnancy. Start thinking about what to get for the baby, and buy things before you become so big that shopping becomes an unpleasant chore.

The baby's skin is very wrinkled, but it is protected and nourished by a layer of vernix. Around this time, the baby's eyelids become unfused and it opens its eyes for the first time.

WEEK 28

Colostrum may leak from your breasts. From now on, you may be visiting the doctor or midwife every two weeks. If you are Rh negative, an antibody check is done.

Your baby's heartbeat speeds up when you speak, and he or she can recognize your voice after birth. The baby is about 14 in (38 cm) long, weighs around 2 lb (0.9 kg), and its limbs are beginning to fill out and look more rounded.

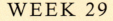

32 WEEKS

Your body at 32 weeks
With your uterus about as high as it can get, your tummy may appear to come straight out beneath your breasts. As the skin over your abdomen stretches, your navel flattens and may pop out like a button.

WEEK 29

You probably feel as if all your internal organs are being crowded out by the baby. There is pressure on your diaphragm, liver, stomach, and intestines.

By now the baby's head is more or less in proportion with the rest of its body.

WEEK 30

It is important to remember to maintain good posture when you are standing or sitting, even though the weight of the baby seems to be dragging you off balance.

WEEK 31

You may find you get very breathless climbing the stairs or with any mild exertion.

However breathless you are, the baby is getting enough oxygen through the placenta. The baby weighs 4 lb (1.8 kg). If the weather is hot or you have had a heavy meal, the baby may be drowsy.

WEEK 32

At each health visit, the doctor or midwife will feel the baby's position. At the same time, they assess the baby's rate of growth and check its heart.

The baby is 16 in (42 cm) long. It is perfectly formed, but the fat reserves beneath its skin are only gradually laid down. If the baby were to be born at this time, it would still need to be cared for in an incubator and might need help breathing.

WEEK 33

You may now be able to distinguish the baby's bottom from, for example, a foot or knee. You feel its movements as prods and kicks—it may be too big now to swoop around in the amniotic fluid.

Your baby has probably adopted the most usual head-down ("vertex" or "cephalic") position, in which it will stay until the birth.

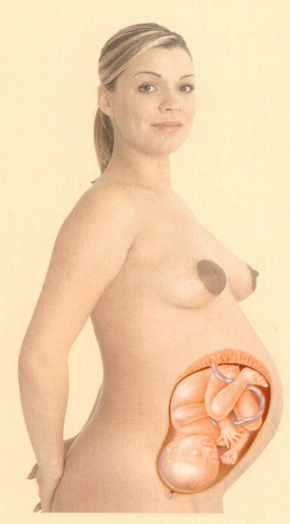

36 WEEKS

Your body at 36 weeks
If the baby's head has engaged, there will now be space between your breasts and the top of your abdomen. You may feel hot most of the time and look flushed as extra blood races around your circulatory system.

WEEK 34

Through the walls of the uterus, the baby can differentiate between dark and light, and is bathed in a red glow when sunlight is on your tummy.

WEEK 35

You may have a backache. This is because ligaments and muscles supporting the joints in the small of your back soften and relax.

The baby's bottom presses against your diaphragm. At this stage of its development, the baby measures approximately 18 in (44 cm) and weighs around 5 lb (2.5 kg).

WEEK 36

Clinic visits may be every week from now on. If this is your first baby, it will probably engage some time this week or soon after, or may have done so already. Your lump will be noticeably lower down, and your breathing will be easier, although you may need to pass urine more often, and your sleep may be interrupted.

The baby is almost fully mature, and any time now the presenting part may drop down into your pelvis ready for birth. It is about 18 in (49 cm) long.

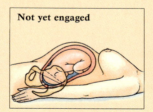
Not yet engaged

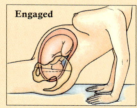
Engaged

Pelvic engagement
A baby may engage in your pelvis at any time from six weeks before the birth. When you lie flat on your back, the baby may not appear to be engaged, but as you sit up, the baby's presenting part slips down into your pelvis.

WEEK 37

If you have chosen a hospital birth, you will have a chance to tour the birth rooms of the hospital.

The baby is rehearsing breathing movements, although there is no air in its lungs. In this way amniotic fluid passes into the baby's trachea, sometimes giving it hiccups!

WEEK 38

There is little space to maneuver, and you may be aware that the baby moves less now. Instead of whole body movements, there are only jabs from the feet and knees, and the strange, buzzing sensation inside your vagina as the baby's head moves against your pelvic floor muscles.

The baby may be putting on as much as 1 oz (28 g) a day at this stage.

WEEK 39

Your cervix is ripening in preparation for labor. You may feel heavy and weary and have strong Braxton Hicks contractions. The amniotic fluid is renewed every three hours.

The baby's bowels are filled with greenish-black meconium, excretions from the baby's alimentary glands mixed with bile pigment, lanugo, and cells from the bowel wall—this will be its first bowel movement after birth.

WEEK 40

The long-awaited day is near, and you probably feel fed up with being pregnant. You may have a mixture of apprehension and excitement. You may notice slight diarrhea.

The baby is about 20 in (55 cm) long. You feel sharp kicks under your ribs at one side or the other. The presenting part presses against the softening cervix. You are very close to the time when you will be able to hold your baby in your arms and see your baby face-to-face.

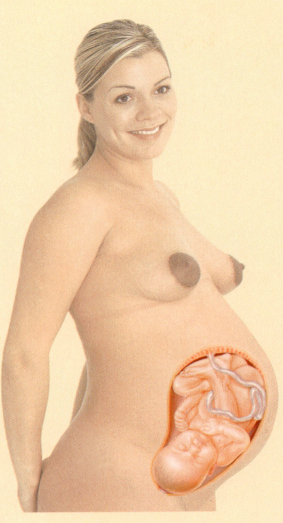

40 WEEKS

Your body at 40 weeks

In the last few weeks, your weight gain may begin to slow down a little. However, you may look more rounded and plump as your body builds up extra fat stores ready for breast-feeding.

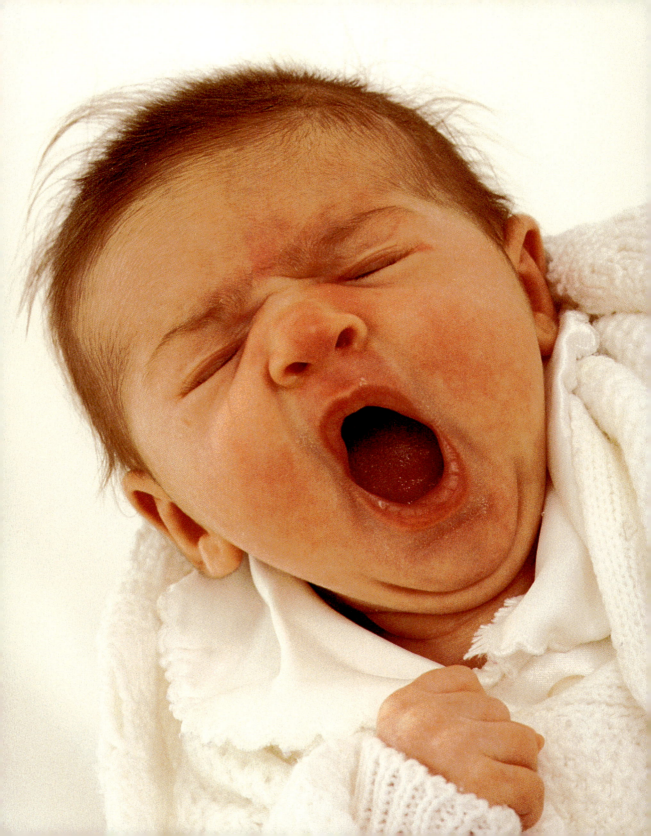

PREGNANCY

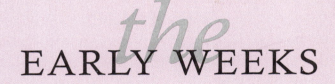 the
EARLY WEEKS

22 | FINDING OUT YOU ARE PREGNANT

36 | PLANNING AND PREPARATION

FINDING OUT YOU ARE PREGNANT

Some women are convinced that they are pregnant from the moment of conception; others have such irregular periods that a long gap in between does not alert them to the possibility of pregnancy. But for most women, the first sign of pregnancy is a missed period.

Perhaps it is five days since the day when you expected it, but then you start wondering if your dates were wrong. Perhaps you usually make a note in your diary, but last time you forgot. You lie in bed, unable to sleep, trying to fix the dates firmly in your mind by finding some useful landmark, like your mother's visit or the end of a particular work assignment. Still another three days go by and the reality gradually dawns: you might be pregnant. You might not be, but it does seem quite possible that you are. When is it sensible to go to the doctor, and how early can you know for certain?

WHEN TO DIAGNOSE

There is a strong case for finding out if you are pregnant before two periods have been missed. It is during these few weeks, while the embryo is still no larger than a hazelnut, that the major organs of the body and the brain itself are being formed; the sooner you know that you are pregnant, the sooner you can start caring for yourself and for the baby.

This is important if you take any medicines. You will want to avoid taking drugs that could harm the developing baby (see page 101). It can also be useful to know early for social reasons—you may be planning to go abroad or to move to a new home at the time the baby is due.

If there is any possibility at all that you may want to terminate the pregnancy, it is essential to diagnose pregnancy in the early weeks: a termination (abortion) at eight weeks is much safer and less upsetting than one after ten weeks.

HOW TO DIAGNOSE

Pregnancy can now be diagnosed about two weeks after conception, on the day your period should have started if you have a regular menstrual cycle, although you are likely to get more accurate results if you wait at least another four days—which can be difficult if you are feeling anxious or excited. When you are pregnant, the embryo releases a hormone called human chorionic gonadotrophin (HCG) into your bloodstream. Minute traces of HCG will be present in your urine approximately six days after conception, but then the level builds up quite rapidly, doubling every two or three days until it reaches a peak about 60 days after conception—approximately 74 days after your last period started—when it begins to decrease. It is possible to detect the presence of this hormone in your urine or blood. Your doctor or midwife will take a urine or blood sample for analysis at a laboratory.

You may prefer to use one of the do-it-yourself pregnancy kits that are widely available (see below). Whichever method you choose, if at all possible, test urine passed first thing in the morning, when you have not drunk anything during the night, since it is at this time that urine contains the highest concentration of pregnancy hormone.

HOME TESTS There are a number of different kits on the market, and most involve mixing a drop or two of urine with the chemicals provided. If you are pregnant, the presence of HCG in your urine will either prevent the mixture from coagulating (ring test) or change the color of the chemical in the test tube or on the dipstick (color test). Depending on the kit, you can use these tests when your period is between one and four days late, but you do need to be sure of when your period was due.

> **"I WANTED TO FIND OUT MYSELF, NOT GET THE NEWS FROM THE DOCTOR. I WASN'T SURE I WANTED THIS BABY AND DIDN'T KNOW HOW I'D REACT."**

Occasionally a woman notices a little spotting (light bleeding) 10–12 days after fertilization. This is not really a period, and the dating of pregnancy can start from your last actual period.

If the result is negative, but your period still has not arrived a few days later, do the test again. It is possible that you conceived later than you thought and that, at the time of the first test, there was not enough HCG in your urine to indicate that you were pregnant. If your periods are irregular or far apart, the chances of a false result are increased. After perhaps one conception in every ten, the fertilized egg does not manage to embed itself in the lining of the uterus. In this case, a pregnancy test will give a positive result, but a second test a few days later will be negative. For this reason, some packs carry the recommendation that you always wait three to five days and then retest, and two tests are included in each pack so that you can do this.

GOING TO THE DOCTOR OR MIDWIFE A doctor or midwife will perform a blood or urine test, and you may also be given an internal examination. He or she introduces two gloved fingers into your vagina as far as they will go, while pressing with the other hand into your abdomen where the top of the uterus lies. If it is more than six weeks since the first day of your last period, they can feel the already softened lower part of the uterus, which is also slightly enlarged. The neck of the uterus, or cervix, which protrudes into the vagina, is felt as firmer than the lower part of the uterus, and it is about the same consistency as the tip of your nose. This internal change is known as "Hegar's sign." The examination may be uncomfortable but will not be painful. As the examining fingers are introduced, give a long, slow breath out through your mouth and continue breathing slowly.

DATING YOUR PREGNANCY

Pregnancy is dated from the first day of your last menstrual period (LMP). If you cannot recollect this with accuracy, the doctor or midwife will probably ask you to guess at it. From then on, the length of pregnancy is estimated in terms of so many weeks, including the weeks from the beginning of your last period to conception. Since ovulation is most common midway between two periods, the usual medical way of dating pregnancy adds an extra two weeks to its length. The length of the average pregnancy is some 266 days from conception. So they arrive at your expected date of delivery (EDD) by adding 280 days, or 40 weeks, to the first day of your last period. You may pay your first visit to the office knowing that it is 10 weeks since you conceived, but emerge from the consultation three months pregnant!

Since not all women ovulate halfway between two periods, the medical convention of adding an extra two weeks is artificial, and an inaccurate method of working out when a baby is due. Think of the EDD as an approximate date rather than the day when you expect to go into labor.

If you have just stopped taking the birth control pill, it is possible that your dates may be completely wrong. The period you have after your last pill may not be followed by ovulation, or you may have a slight spotting of blood that is not really a period. It may take several months to reestablish your natural menstrual cycle, and until then you cannot predict with any certainty when, or whether, you are going to ovulate. You might be a month or more off in your dates. This is obviously important in estimating when the baby is due, especially since it could lead to labor being induced unnecessarily (see page 334). So wait for a clear three months after stopping the pill before trying to conceive. During this time, use some other method of contraception.

Early ultrasound scans are increasingly used to confirm dates, and may reduce uncertainty, but, because no one can be 100 percent sure that ultrasound is safe, especially at this early stage of pregnancy, you may prefer to wait and see.

CONCEIVING WHILE USING CONTRACEPTION

If you conceive with an IUD (intrauterine device or coil) still inside you, your chances of miscarrying are increased. It is important to see your doctor quickly, since the IUD should be removed if possible, and this can only be done early in pregnancy. Sometimes doctors advise termination.

WHEN IS YOUR BABY DUE?

This chart will help you to estimate the date your baby is due. Look along the columns at the figures set in bold type to find the first day of your last period. The date below it is 280 days later and is your estimated date of delivery (EDD). **It is perfectly normal for a baby to arrive two weeks before or two weeks after this date.**

January Oct/Nov	1	2	3	4	5	6	7	8	9	10	11	12	13	14	15	16	17	18	19	20	21	22	23	24	25	26	27	28	29	30	31
	8	9	10	11	12	13	14	15	16	17	18	19	20	21	22	23	24	25	26	27	28	29	30	31	1	2	3	4	5	6	7

February Nov/Dec	1	2	3	4	5	6	7	8	9	10	11	12	13	14	15	16	17	18	19	20	21	22	23	24	25	26	27	28			
	8	9	10	11	12	13	14	15	16	17	18	19	20	21	22	23	24	25	26	27	28	29	30	1	2	3	4	5			

March Dec/Jan	1	2	3	4	5	6	7	8	9	10	11	12	13	14	15	16	17	18	19	20	21	22	23	24	25	26	27	28	29	30	31
	6	7	8	9	10	11	12	13	14	15	16	17	18	19	20	21	22	23	24	25	26	27	28	29	30	31	1	2	3	4	5

April Jan/Feb	1	2	3	4	5	6	7	8	9	10	11	12	13	14	15	16	17	18	19	20	21	22	23	24	25	26	27	28	29	30	
	6	7	8	9	10	11	12	13	14	15	16	17	18	19	20	21	22	23	24	25	26	27	28	29	30	31	1	2	3	4	

May Feb/March	1	2	3	4	5	6	7	8	9	10	11	12	13	14	15	16	17	18	19	20	21	22	23	24	25	26	27	28	29	30	31
	5	6	7	8	9	10	11	12	13	14	15	16	17	18	19	20	21	22	23	24	25	26	27	28	1	2	3	4	5	6	7

June March/April	1	2	3	4	5	6	7	8	9	10	11	12	13	14	15	16	17	18	19	20	21	22	23	24	25	26	27	28	29	30	
	8	9	10	11	12	13	14	15	16	17	18	19	20	21	22	23	24	25	26	27	28	29	30	31	1	2	3	4	5	6	

July April/May	1	2	3	4	5	6	7	8	9	10	11	12	13	14	15	16	17	18	19	20	21	22	23	24	25	26	27	28	29	30	31
	7	8	9	10	11	12	13	14	15	16	17	18	19	20	21	22	23	24	25	26	27	28	29	30	1	2	3	4	5	6	7

August May/June	1	2	3	4	5	6	7	8	9	10	11	12	13	14	15	16	17	18	19	20	21	22	23	24	25	26	27	28	29	30	31
	8	9	10	11	12	13	14	15	16	17	18	19	20	21	22	23	24	25	26	27	28	29	30	31	1	2	3	4	5	6	7

September June/July	1	2	3	4	5	6	7	8	9	10	11	12	13	14	15	16	17	18	19	20	21	22	23	24	25	26	27	28	29	30	
	8	9	10	11	12	13	14	15	16	17	18	19	20	21	22	23	24	25	26	27	28	29	30	1	2	3	4	5	6	7	

October July/Aug	1	2	3	4	5	6	7	8	9	10	11	12	13	14	15	16	17	18	19	20	21	22	23	24	25	26	27	28	29	30	31
	8	9	10	11	12	13	14	15	16	17	18	19	20	21	22	23	24	25	26	27	28	29	30	31	1	2	3	4	5	6	7

November Aug/Sept	1	2	3	4	5	6	7	8	9	10	11	12	13	14	15	16	17	18	19	20	21	22	23	24	25	26	27	28	29	30	
	8	9	10	11	12	13	14	15	16	17	18	19	20	21	22	23	24	25	26	27	28	29	30	31	1	2	3	4	5	6	

December Sept/Oct	1	2	3	4	5	6	7	8	9	10	11	12	13	14	15	16	17	18	19	20	21	22	23	24	25	26	27	28	29	30	31
	7	8	9	10	11	12	13	14	15	16	17	18	19	20	21	22	23	24	25	26	27	28	29	30	1	2	3	4	5	6	7

This is certainly not necessary if you want the baby. Even if it is too late to remove it, many women deliver the IUD with the placenta after an uneventful pregnancy and birth.

You can conceive while taking the pill if you miss one or more days when you should have been taking it, if you have an upset stomach with vomiting so that you fail to absorb the hormones, or if you are on antibiotics. If you conceive but continue to take the pill for several months while pregnant, there is a slightly increased risk to the baby of congenital abnormalities, though the vast majority of women who have taken the pill while pregnant give birth to babies who are healthy and normal.

PREGNANCY AND HIV INFECTION

If you live in the U.S. you will be offered a blood test early in pregnancy for the HIV antibody. Anyone who has these antibodies is infected with the virus. You are not compelled to have this test. Be sure to ask for counseling, since deciding to be tested has social and emotional implications. As one woman who found that she was carrying the virus said: "The only difference between now and before is this piece of knowledge. And it's such depressing, unhappy knowledge, I find it quite paralyzing."*

A pregnant woman can infect her unborn baby, though 85 percent of babies of HIV-positive mothers are born healthy. Babies born to HIV-positive mothers almost always test positive to HIV because the test picks up the mother's antibodies, which readily cross the placenta into the baby's blood. Over time these maternal antibodies are cleared, and testing a baby after 6 to 18 months will more accurately tell if a baby has become infected.

The safety measures usually proposed to help avoid transmission include not breast-feeding; having a Cesarean section, because babies often pick up the infection as they come down the birth canal; and being treated with antiviral medications during the last six months of pregnancy. With these precautions, the transmission rate can be reduced to 2 percent.

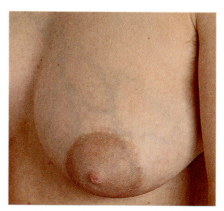

The first physical changes of which you become aware may occur in your breasts. Veins may become more prominent and the areolae darker.

EARLY SIGNS OF PREGNANCY

Even before your pregnancy has been confirmed by a test result, there may be subtle indications, apart from a missed period, that make you think you are pregnant.

BREAST CHANGES You will begin to notice breast changes in preparation for milk production in the first weeks of pregnancy. The brownish circles around the nipples (the areolae) become darker and the little bumps on them more prominent. If you are pink-skinned you may notice that the lacy network of blood vessels in your breasts has become much more obvious. Blue veins run over the breasts like rivers on a map. Your breasts may also feel tender and heavy. Women with small breasts may note an obvious increase in size very early on. If you have large breasts already, you may not notice any size change at this stage.

TIREDNESS Enormous metabolic changes take place in pregnancy, and your whole body has to adjust to the process of growing a baby. It is not surprising that you may feel tired and that you cannot carry on as you did before. Many women complain of extreme tiredness during the first eight or ten weeks. But as your body adjusts to the pregnancy, the fatigue vanishes and the middle months are often easy. If you are feeling tired, go to bed early; take a rest at midday if you can or an early-evening rest when you get home from work.

If this is your second (or third) pregnancy, you may feel constantly tired. Women who thoroughly enjoyed their first pregnancy say that the second one is much harder to cope with because of the nonstop pace of their first child's daily life. The only solution is to try to have at least a short time every day when you are free from domestic responsibilities. Even half an hour every evening, while your partner attends to the child and the dishes, can be relaxing if you are able to enjoy it to the full. (See pages 172–177 for more about second and later pregnancies.)

> "I CAME IN FROM WORK AND FELL ASLEEP IN A CHAIR BEFORE I COULD START TO GET A MEAL. I WONDERED HOW I WOULD GET THROUGH THE REST OF PREGNANCY FEELING LIKE A ZOMBIE—BUT THEN AT ABOUT 12 WEEKS I CAME ALIVE AGAIN!"

NAUSEA Another common sign of pregnancy is nausea. These waves of sickness often happen early in the morning, when your blood-sugar level is low, but they may also occur in the early evening or at other times of the day. Some women just feel very sick. Others actually vomit. Tiredness contributes to nausea, but so does an empty stomach. Frequent small snacks of bland foods like dry crackers or a banana may relieve the feeling. If you suffer from morning sickness, a cup of tea and a few crackers or dry toast immediately on waking may prevent it, or crackers alone may be better. A late-night snack, ginger in a tea or capsule, and acupressure bands for the wrists may help, too. As a general rule, cut out all greasy fried foods, tobacco, and alcohol. Avoid strong odors, especially cooking smells, exhaust fumes, and perfume, and if nausea and vomiting are still bad, speak to your doctor.

Some women become really ill with vomiting (see page 137), although most stop feeling sick during the fourth month. Women who experience pregnancy nausea are less likely than others to have miscarriages. This can be a cheering thought. But nausea is not associated with pregnancy in all cultures; many societies have other illnesses and disabilities, or special dreams, that they connect with pregnancy. Margaret Mead points out that in some societies of New Guinea, boils are considered a typical symptom of pregnancy. Some Jamaicans do not acknowledge pregnancy until they have had a special fertility dream of ripe fruit bursting with seed. Dreams of this kind are characteristic of early pregnancy. It is as if all women need definite signs to link with pregnancy so that they can say, "I feel this, therefore I must be expecting a baby."

You may suffer from nausea for the first time in your second or third pregnancy. This is almost certainly the result of tiredness, and you may not be able to relieve the nausea within three months unless you can somehow arrange to have more rest.

EMOTIONAL REACTIONS TO PREGNANCY

However much you want a baby, finding out that you really are pregnant can produce a flood of conflicting emotions: triumph ("We've done it!"), a sense of being trapped ("There's no going back—now what?"), fear ("Mom had an awful time having me—will I be able to stand the pain?"), apprehension ("Will we still love each other in the same way?"), and doubt ("Will he still want me once my waist starts getting thicker?"). It is surprising how many women respond to their first pregnancy with shock and feel that it has happened "too soon," even though they very much want a baby and have considered the matter carefully before stopping contraception. Confronted with the reality and the physical changes of pregnancy, they want to say: "Stop! I haven't prepared myself for this. Let's go back and start again."

If you discover that you are pregnant when you did not plan to be, you may also feel trapped. Yet, perversely, many women (for whom pregnancy is not a disaster) are aware of an odd pleasure that their fertility has triumphed over their conscious wish. Your partner may suspect that you wanted a baby all along and have not been "playing fair." Starting a baby under such circumstances can lead to conflict between you, because he may feel that you have not been open with him. Talk about it together: you need to understand each other.

FEELINGS ABOUT MOTHERHOOD When you find out that you are pregnant, you may have a crisis of self-confidence, feeling that you will be no good as a mother and have no maternal instincts. But mothering is a learned activity, and there is not much of it that is purely instinctive. Moreover, for the first-time mother, who may never have handled a newborn baby, most of the learning goes on after the baby is born. The teacher is the baby. Even though you may not start as an expert, your baby will turn you into one.

The realization that you are responsible for creating a new person may be awesome and sometimes overwhelming.

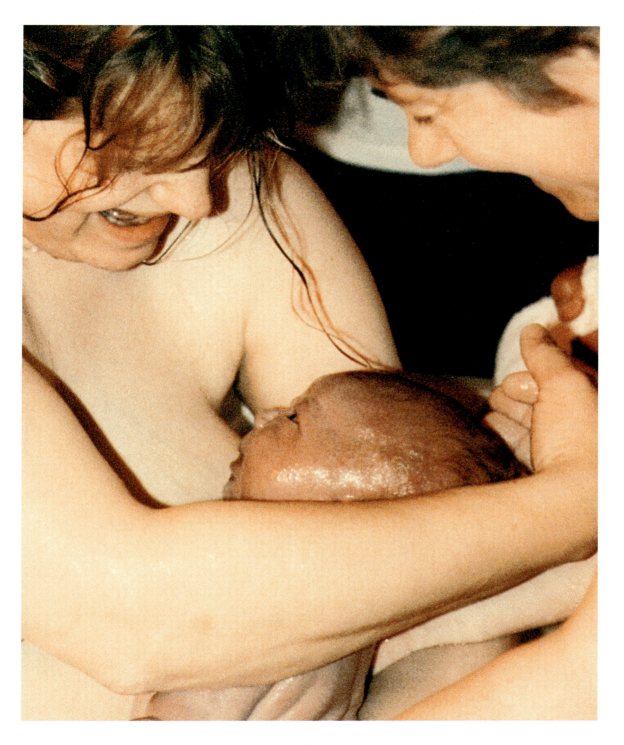

FEELINGS ABOUT BEING ON SHOW You may feel suddenly that your most intimate relationship with the man you love is being publicly displayed, not just because you are pregnant and everybody knows, but because of the physical examinations and exposure at the doctor's office and the advice that people keep giving you. This sense of becoming public property may also be intensified by the obvious pleasure of your parents, who may have long been waiting for you to become pregnant.

Yet your body holds life. The wonder of that cannot really be understood by anyone else. You stand naked in front of the mirror and look for the first signs of change. You rest your hand on your tummy and wonder if you can feel the tiny seed of a baby beginning to grow inside you. You think back to the occasions when you made love and wonder which time it was that you conceived.

FEELINGS ABOUT YOUR BODY If you feel on bad terms with your body as it starts out on the work of early pregnancy, arrange to attend some pregnancy exercise or dance classes if these are available in your area. Organizations that can help you are on pages 427–428. If these classes are not specially for pregnant women, let your teacher know that you are pregnant. Get out in the fresh air and walk. Swim regularly. Start doing the movements suggested on pages 122–124 a few times each day to pep up your circulation and increase vitality. In some countries, massage is an anticipated and very pleasant part of being pregnant, so you could go to a masseuse, or your partner could find out how to massage you (see pages 192–200). This can be particularly useful if you are tense and find it difficult to release your muscles at will.

YOUR PARTNER'S FEELINGS You are not the only person who has to adjust in pregnancy. Your partner does not have to cope with physical changes, but the passage into fatherhood is a major transition in his life. For a man, this process is often delayed until several things have happened: the pregnancy has been officially confirmed; your figure has obviously changed; the baby has moved and he has felt it fluttering.

Emotions of joy, pride, and wonder may be in conflict with other emotions of a more disturbing nature. There may be financial problems, which can cause a man to feel a sense of deep and burdensome responsibility for the new life that is coming.

A man, too, may feel trapped by pregnancy. Perhaps he imagined that his relationship with his partner would remain free and unencumbered by babies (especially if the couple have not discussed pregnancy and planned it together). His job may now assume importance, not only in its own right, but because he feels an urgent need to be successful before the baby comes. It is as if this new development threatens his own powers of achievement. A man, too, may be anxious about his partner's well-being and frightened of the birth itself. Even his partner's pregnant body can seem dangerous and not to be touched in case the baby is dislodged. He may feel that his own sexual desire is a terrible threat to the baby.

DISCUSSING YOUR EMOTIONS TOGETHER

It does not help to bottle up these emotions. If you pretend they are not there, they become destructive. Anxiety has a positive function. It prods you to examine options, develop coping strategies, plan ahead, prepare yourselves emotionally and practically for the future. For example, you could avoid certain relatives until you feel you can cope with them. You may be able to arrange prenatal appointments together, so that your partner can meet the doctor or midwife and be present during the physical examination. Reading together about pregnancy and birth helps to replace ignorance with knowledge about the role a man can actively play in childbirth. Lying together in bed, cuddling and exploring each other's bodies is a way of communicating through loving touch and tenderness.

Pregnancy is not merely a waiting time. It is a time for working out together what you value in your relationship and what kind of world you both want to create for your child. This is not a question of making a nursery and buying things for the baby, but of helping each other to change from people who are responsible just for themselves into a mother and a father, with the new responsibility that parenthood brings. A man and a woman need to grow into parents. Then not only a baby but a new family is born.

THE WOMAN ALONE

Pregnancy and childbirth are not easy when you have no partner to give you love and care. The challenge of taking complete responsibility may seem overwhelming. Yet many women have coped with pregnancy and birth alone and have brought up happy, healthy children.

Talking about the single mother and the challenges she faces is misleading, because women on their own bearing babies do not fall into one category any more than women with partners. The reasons single women embark on pregnancy, and decide to go on with it, vary widely. Some continue with a pregnancy because they are unwilling or unable to face up to it and drift on hoping that it may go away. Others are bearing a much-wanted child "before it is too late." Others again loved the father of the child and hoped that the relationship would continue, but then found themselves rejected and bearing a child alone. There are also women

"HAVING JANE THERE WAS WONDERFUL.
SHE HAD THREE CHILDREN AND KNEW EXACTLY WHAT I WAS FEELING. SHE TOLD ME TO THINK OF MY CERVIX OPENING DURING CONTRACTIONS AND BREATHED WITH ME WHEN THE GOING GOT DIFFICULT."

whose partners die while they are pregnant. Whatever your reasons for having a child on your own, financial problems may loom large. Trying to combine a job with rearing a child, knowing that there is no one else to take over in time of need, is difficult. It is important to anticipate and share the problems you will be coping with, and to seek counseling from people who understand and who can put you in touch with other sources of help. Contact the organizations listed on pages 427–428 before you have your baby and see what they have to offer. They can help you cope with practical difficulties such as housing and sorting out which benefits you are entitled to. Book childbirth education classes (see page 180) as early as the third month. Many women delay until the last minute and find that classes are full. The International Childbirth Education Association can tell you about classes, postnatal support, and breast-feeding counseling available in your area.

Sometimes a man who is not a permanent partner is still willing to accept some responsibilities of fatherhood, though the couple do not plan to stay together. Be frank with your prenatal teacher so that she has a chance to get to know you. It may be possible for you to arrange to see her privately for a session.

EMOTIONAL SUPPORT IN LABOR

Think ahead to the birth and decide whether you would like to have a companion with you. Childbirth can feel very solitary if you do not have someone to encourage you and provide continuous emotional support. It could be a woman friend, a childbirth educator, a doula (a birth partner who is experienced in supporting laboring women), a sister or your mother, or even a man friend who knows what birth is about and can give the right kind of help. Most hospitals allow companions in labor, although some restrict you to one person. Discuss the matter with your nurse and your prenatal teacher, and, if necessary, state your request in writing to the Director of Obstetrics or Nursing.

If there is no one who can be with you, discuss the subject with your nurse. Say that you want someone with you throughout labor. Ask whether there is anyone—preferably someone you could meet beforehand—who could be with you. She may say that you will have a labor nurse and will not be left alone. But a birth companion is different and is simply there as a friend to give emotional support and to remind you of your relaxation and breathing. If you are having your baby in the hospital, there may be a student midwife who can fill that role.

Suppose that you have to be without a companion in labor. Make the labor nurse your friend and ask her for help. Unfortunately, there is still little continuity of care in many hospitals, and you may have to get to know two or three nurses, one after another—a lot to ask of someone in labor. On the other hand, sometimes one will stay on duty so that she can be with you until after the birth.

MANAGING ALONE

If a man has been unwilling to accept responsibility or perhaps even acknowledge your pregnancy, you probably feel angry and resentful. One woman, who had been told she could never have a baby but who found herself pregnant, said, "I hadn't realized just how much his marriage was a going concern. Just when I most needed him I had to come to terms with the fact that he didn't want to break up his marriage and was devoted to his kids. My pregnancy was terribly embarrassing for him! I felt dread on my own. I didn't hear from him through a large part of the pregnancy because it was the summer vacation period and he went abroad with his family."

> "THE FATHER OF THE BABY WAS INSISTENT THAT HE DIDN'T WANT A RELATIONSHIP WITH HER. I DECIDED I DIDN'T WANT HIM AT THE BIRTH, BECAUSE I COULDN'T HANDLE HIS EMOTIONS. MY SISTER WAS WITH ME, AND THAT WORKED WELL."

Another woman's husband left her when she was four months pregnant because he said he could not stand the idea of a third child. He had left her before for short periods, and the baby was conceived during a reconciliation. Her great fear was that she would find him on the doorstep again, since she had been through so much emotional turmoil that she did not feel she could cope mentally with any more scenes. This led to a strained and difficult pregnancy followed by a prolonged labor and forceps delivery.

A university professor who had decided that she wanted a baby but not a man said that her colleagues accepted this, but she found it difficult to tell her family: "Mother thought I was crazy and said how could she ever let her friends know. I thought about them all at their coffee mornings and thought, 'Oh my God, I don't suppose she can.' I thought it would be hardest explaining to my eighty-year-old grandmother, but it turned out that she was the one who understood best." In fact, the woman's parents adjusted after the baby was born, and they became very proud grandparents.

Some women are rejected by parents, but one woman said: "In a way I rejected them and their values, by going ahead and having the baby." Even so, however free of your parents you may feel and however you delight in being independent of them, cutting roots like this can be extremely painful. You may feel guilty, even if you do not accept the social conventions that thrust feelings of guilt upon you. You may worry about imposing your views on your child, who will learn that in friends' houses there is likely to be a father as well as a mother.

The media tend to present single motherhood as a choice that many actresses and pop stars in their 30s or 40s are making. Glamorous photographs accompany feature articles that give the impression that, like any other fashion accessory, a baby is the flavor of the moment. These women are not likely to be short of money and can employ nannies and other help. The decision to go it alone with a baby may result in many more practical difficulties for most of us.

Single mothers all stress that you need help and must have the grace to accept it, for your child's sake as well as your own. There are the all-important questions of where you are going to live, what you are going to live on, and when you can go back to work. You must also consider how you are going to retain mobility with a baby, how you will deal with the relationships between sex, motherhood, and the other things you want to do, and how you are going to feel when things are difficult or impossible because of the baby. Many difficulties confronted by single women are the same as those faced by those with partners, but intensified because they are alone and unsupported.

CO-MOTHERING

Consider building a support network of friends to help you through the stressful times and to be there when you need them—women whom you can help in turn. These will be friends who know what pregnancy and birth are like, and who will be able to talk through your priorities, prepare you emotionally for what is a deeply moving life experience, and help you feel more confident about the birth.

After the baby is born, it helps to be part of a circle of co-mothers. Bearing total responsibility for a small baby, especially one who cries a lot, can be very tough and you may get to the point where you begin to hate yourself and blame the baby for the way you feel. You need to make sure that you are not socially isolated. This is much less likely to happen in traditional cultures, where a first-time mother can usually take it for granted that there will be co-mothers—willing hands to help and a pool of women's wisdom and experience to dip into. Her

"MY SISTER LIVES NEARBY AND HAD HER BABY TWO WEEKS BEFORE ME. WE SPENT THE FIRST THREE MONTHS FINDING OUT ABOUT BABIES TOGETHER. IT WAS ABSOLUTELY LOVELY!"

baby is not totally dependent on her as an individual in the way that a baby usually is in most industrialized countries. Other laps, other comforting arms, even other lactating breasts, are available if need be.

In such cultures, co-mothering is easy because women tend to mother in a similar way. The concept is more difficult in urban cultures where we do not live in tight communities, where some of us work and some stay at home, and where we may not always trust each other. But don't let this deter you from forming your own group of like-minded women who can support each other emotionally and in practical ways. You may want to explore some of these possibilities in your childbirth class or with close friends, particularly those who are in a situation similar to your own.

A SURROGATE MOTHER

A woman who decides to be a surrogate mother may have to work out carefully how she is going to describe this pregnancy, the parting with the baby, and her reasons for being a surrogate mother, possibly to her other children, and deal with questions and concerns. There may be times, too, when she feels anxious about the eventual outcome. As her pregnancy becomes obvious, she has to decide just how much she is going to tell other people, and how she will respond to any hostile comments and perhaps ill-advised warnings.

However, a recent report suggests that women who contract to serve as surrogate mothers cope well with the emotions aroused when parting with the baby and are not usually swamped by remorse. What is more, babies born as a result of egg donation and surrogate pregnancies turn out to be generally well adjusted and emotionally stable, and adoptive mothers of surrogate babies tend to be especially loving. The report concludes, "The surrogacy family seems to be characterized by warm relationships and high quality of parenting."*

In my own experience, arrangements appear to work best between women who become friends and who keep in touch with each other, and when the child knows the birth mother as a very special "auntie." There needs to be open discussion and clear agreement about what happens during and immediately following the birth, and the doctors or midwives should be involved in this. The surrogate mother should be confident that the baby she is having is going to loving parents.

> "I ACTUALLY CUT THE CORD AND, APART FROM THE MIDWIFE, I WAS THE VERY FIRST PERSON TO HOLD HIM. IT JUST FELT SO NATURAL AND SO NORMAL TO HAVE THIS BABY IN MY ARMS, LOOKING AT ME AND PUTTING ALL OF ITS TRUST IN ME."*

PLANNING AND PREPARATION

Throughout history, most babies were born at home. Maternity hospitals were first started for homeless women and were extensions of the poorhouses. Many babies born in these hospitals were put in orphanages.

The first maternity hospitals were convenient centers for medical students to learn and practice obstetrics, but infection was rampant, as doctors conveyed bacteria on their hands from one patient to another, and many babies and mothers died. They were the most dangerous places in which women could give birth. Today, modern hospitals are no longer dangerous. Yet, despite the tendency for most doctors to recommend hospitals, many women still feel a home birth would be best for them.

WHERE WOULD YOU LIKE TO HAVE YOUR BABY?

Even before you are pregnant, or as early in pregnancy as you can, think about where you would like to have your baby: at home, in a hospital, or in a birth center, and find out which of these options are available in your area. You may have decided, for example, that you want to have your baby at home, yet discover that there is no doctor or midwife willing or able to attend you, so home birth is not an option for you. Or partway through your pregnancy you may discover a midwife or doctor who does attend home births. If there are no specific medical reasons against planning a home birth, you will probably want to switch to their care. You can do this at any stage of pregnancy, but it is sometimes difficult to make different arrangements once wheels have been set in motion. Make a list of things that are important to you about your birth and the time after, and decide which environment best meets your requirements.

> "I'M CONSIDERING THE OPTIONS OPEN TO ME AND AM FINDING OUT ABOUT HOME BIRTH BECAUSE I'D LIKE IT TO BE AS NATURAL AS POSSIBLE."

FINANCIAL PLANNING

In the U.S., health care is not directly funded by the national government, so one of the first issues faced by a family planning a baby is financial. It is possible to pay directly for health care (fee-for-service), but the cost is very high and unpredictable since complications may make estimates inaccurate. Many women have "private insurance" that is paid for by their employer or their husband's employer. This pays most or all costs but will probably restrict the choices somewhat. Some insurance pays only for certain hospitals or doctors. It may or may not cover care from a midwife or in a birthing center or home birth.

You should contact your insurance plan as soon as you are contemplating a pregnancy

For some women *a one-to-one relationship with a midwife is an important element in choosing where to give birth.*

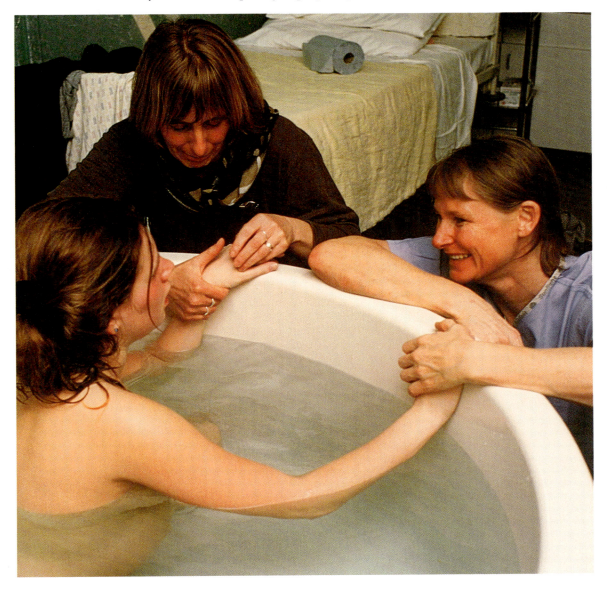

and find out what care will or will not be paid for, and any restrictions on your choice of the provider of that care and the place of birth.

Not all employers cover health insurance, so even if you are employed you may not be insured. Most states have some form of public health care for pregnant women who lack private insurance. These plans vary enormously depending on the individual state, but in general there are even more restrictions on a mother's choices because many doctors and some midwives will not accept the low rates of reimbursement these plans offer. Prenatal care may be at a clinic with different providers at every visit and little personal attention. Hospital birth is always covered, but delivery in a birth center may not be available. Home birth is not usually an option.

HOSPITAL BIRTH

Most women who decide to have their babies in the hospital do so primarily because they are convinced it is the safest place. They want to be sure that all the skills and equipment of modern obstetrics are at hand for their baby's sake. For some women, especially those having their first child, giving birth is a frightening experience, a step in the dark, and they feel more secure in the knowledge that they are in the hands of a team trained to cope with any emergencies that might arise. Often, a woman who fears that her labor will be painful opts for a hospital delivery, knowing that some painkillers are available only at the hospital and not wanting to take the chance of finding herself in labor at home without any relief from pain when it is far too late to do anything about it.

Sometimes a woman may know and trust a particular obstetrician and want to be cared for by this person, while another woman wants to go to the hospital because she feels she would benefit from a short period of release from the pressures of home and family. Occasionally, a woman's partner would prefer her to go to the hospital because he is very concerned about birth at home. He may just be frightened of being involved, but more frequently he is afraid that he might have to deliver the baby himself.

"THE OBSTETRICIAN WAS VERY PLEASANT. HE TOLD ME HIS WIFE HAD HAD A BABY THREE MONTHS AGO. THAT MADE A LOT OF DIFFERENCE."

HOSPITAL BIRTH AND SAFETY

You may be planning the birth in the hospital for medical reasons. It is wise to consider hospital care if you have diabetes or a heart or kidney condition. You will be admitted to the hospital if you get preeclampsia (see page 141) or if you go into labor three weeks or more before your baby is due; you will probably be advised against home birth if your baby is breech, since the baby may need some help with breathing immediately after birth (see page 380). There are no absolutes, but there are certain factors that contribute to making childbirth a little more risky.

For instance, if you are over 40 and a first-time mother, your labor may be longer than if you were younger, and many doctors would advise you to be in the hospital so that you can have labor speeded up or get help with the delivery. You may decide that this is not what you want, and still go ahead and plan a home birth. Some doctors believe that all first-time mothers (primigravidas) should give birth in a hospital because, they say, a labor is only normal in retrospect and there is always a small chance that, even after a normal pregnancy, you may have complications during the birth that will entail your being moved to the hospital at the last minute for specialist care.

If you have had a previous Cesarean section, most doctors will advise a hospital birth in case the labor is complicated, and the scar in the uterus becomes at risk of tearing. If you have had a hemorrhage with a previous labor, either before or after the birth, you might want to choose a hospital birth because you may need a quick blood transfusion if it happens again. (On the other hand, did you bleed because of aggressive intervention, and are you less likely to bleed if the labor progresses naturally?) The same goes for a retained placenta in a previous labor. Sometimes hospital interventions themselves contribute to the likelihood of birth complications. If you are very short, under 5 ft 2 in (1.55 m), your pelvis may be a tight fit for the baby to get through, although many short women can and do give birth easily. Any other indications of disproportion, because of the way the baby is lying, for example, could also lead you to consider a hospital birth. Three or more miscarriages are another reason for having the baby in the hospital, because previous problems of this kind may mean that labor will present problems (although often everything is straightforward). If you have lost a baby because of a previous difficult birth, you will want to know that, if the baby should need it, intensive care is available at the hospital where you are giving birth. Doctors also advise mothers of twins to give birth in the hospital, partly because they may come early and be of low birth weight, and partly because the second twin sometimes gets stuck. But if both babies are head down and full term, you may decide that home is the best place for the birth because you want to avoid any unnecessary intervention and know that you have the support of experienced and skilled midwives.

CHOICES IN HOSPITAL CARE

Many hospitals now offer a certified nurse midwife program. The Director of Maternity Nursing (a registered nurse) and the Director of Obstetrics (an obstetrician/gynecologist) are responsible for policies and routines that a particular hospital follows. One hospital may expect women to have continuous electronic fetal monitoring and an intravenous drip and move the mother to a delivery room for the actual delivery. Another hospital a few blocks away may offer a birth pool and homelike birthing rooms. There are tertiary major medical centers with the capability of handling high-risk complications of pregnancy and there are community hospitals, which are geared to normal labor and birth. The differences among various hospitals are also highlighted by the wide variation in the rate of Cesarean section, episiotomy, the number of mothers who breast-feed, and types of anesthesia available.

If you have a choice of hospitals available to you, you will want to investigate each one. You will also need to think about the alternatives available to you within the hospital system.

THE PRIVATE OBSTETRICIAN OR FAMILY PHYSICIAN

The vast majority of women expect to have an obstetrician provide prenatal care in his or her own office. There are some family practice physicians and a few general practitioners offering prenatal care in some areas of the country. Each individual practitioner is affiliated with one or more hospitals. If you have already decided where you would like to give birth, you will need to choose a provider that uses that facility. This is something you should ask about ahead of time. Sometimes the hospital closest to your doctor's office is not the one where you want to give birth.

THE OBSTETRICAL CLINIC Most obstetrical clinics are located within large metropolitan teaching hospitals. In exchange for low-cost or free care, the patient serves as "teaching material" for the medical students and resident physicians. Teaching hospitals tend to have a great deal of technologically advanced machinery and may be justified for the mother and baby "at risk," when there is a higher than average chance of something going wrong during the labor. These hospitals often have neonatal intensive care units where sophisticated technology and a specially skilled staff will be available to treat the high-risk baby immediately after birth. Those teaching hospitals with family practice residency or nurse-midwifery training programs may provide lower intervention care.

CERTIFIED NURSE MIDWIFE CARE Some midwives are employed by physicians and work in their offices. There are also midwives who practice independently (they are more likely to offer home birth). In the public health-care sector there are midwives working in many clinics that target low-income women.

The typical hospital nurse midwife practices in a group, backed by one or more obstetricians. The certified nurse midwife has been specifically trained to deal with normal pregnancy, normal birth, and normal postpartum. She cares for the well woman at all stages but if any abnormality develops will refer the patient to an obstetrician. Even if this happens, the nurse midwife usually stays with her client, offering her emotional support.

LOOKING OVER THE HOSPITAL

No matter what type of hospital care you choose, be sure to tour the hospital before you make a definite decision. If this is not the usual practice in the hospital, get in touch with the prenatal outpatient department and ask if you can talk to whoever runs childbirth classes. There is probably a visit by the prenatal class to the labor and delivery room, and you may be able to go, too (see page 185). Contact the Director of Nursing or Obstetrics to ask about the things that matter most to you.

THE BIRTH ROOM

Until recently, birth rooms were organized exclusively for the comfort and convenience of doctors and nurses, instead of the woman having the baby. In many hospitals that has changed, and there are birth beds and other equipment that enable the woman to sit upright, kneel, squat, and stand with something solid to grip onto. This is fine in principle, but obstetric practice still limits women's opportunities to move about and get into different positions. If you have an intravenous drip and are tethered to an electronic fetal monitor, it may be almost impossible to move.

Women who can remain upright in the first stage of labor have less pain, so need fewer pain-relieving drugs, and dilate faster than those women who are lying down. Their babies' heart rates are also more likely to fall within the normal range.*

In the second stage, being upright also results in less pain, fewer drugs, easier pushing, fewer tears, more normal vaginal births, and a more positive birth experience.* When you look around the hospital, take special note of how you could use ledges at different heights and furniture in the birth room to give you support and move your pelvis. Ask for a beanbag or "birth ball" to flop over or lean against, or take one into the hospital if it is not provided.

"I GOT STUCK FLAT ON MY BACK LAST TIME I WAS IN LABOR AND FELT TRAPPED. THIS TIME IT WAS MUCH BETTER SINCE I WAS ABLE TO MOVE AROUND; I FELT IN CONTROL, AND IT WAS SO MUCH EASIER TO HANDLE THE PAIN."

Hospitals may now offer a rocking chair for the first stage and a birth stool and squatting bar to grasp in the second stage. Some have elaborate birth beds or chairs that can be switched to almost any position. These may look impressive, but the important thing is to have the equipment under your own control, not someone else's, and to be free to move your pelvis.

Whatever happens, the equipment is less important than you. It should not be allowed to dominate or restrict what you do during birth. Look critically at what is available and think how you may want to use it, if at all. One problem with sitting on a rigid chair or stool for a long time, especially one with back support that limits pelvic movements, is that you may develop swelling around your vulva, and the circulation of blood may

UNDERSTANDING YOUR MEDICAL RECORD

It can be confusing to try to decipher your medical record, and some abbreviations may suggest alarming abnormalities. Here are the abbreviations most likely to be used. Ask your doctor or midwife to explain any that you do not understand. Two-way communication is vital in a working partnership.

ABBR/TERM	FULL TITLE/NAME	MEANING OF ABBREVIATION
Para 0		The mother has had no previous birth.
Para 1 (or 2)		The mother has had one (or two) previous births.
Para 2 + 1		The mother has had two previous births plus a miscarriage (or termination) before 28 weeks.
LMP	Last menstrual period	Date of first day of last menstrual period.
EDD/EDC	Expected date of delivery	Expected date of delivery or expected date of confinement.
Proteinuria	Protein in urine	Your urine is analyzed for the presence of sugar, which may be a sign of diabetes; and protein, which may be a sign of preeclampsia. When either is present, it is noted by + signs from + to ++++. Ideally, protein should not be present at all. However, there are occasional traces of sugar and protein in a normal pregnancy.
Hb	Hemoglobin	Hemoglobin is an oxygen-carrying substance present in red blood cells. If your hemoglobin level is lower than 10.5 percent, or your hematocrit (see below) is below 32 percent, you may be considered anemic and be prescribed iron, but attitudes vary widely about when this is necessary. Because of the greater quantity of circulating blood, most healthy pregnant women have reduced hemoglobin.
Hct	Hematocrit	Hematocrit is the percentage of red blood cells in the blood.
Fe	Iron	This means that you have been prescribed iron.
BP	Blood pressure	This is the pressure inside the arteries as blood is pumped from the heart. The pressure built up every time the heart beats is systolic pressure. Between beats, the heart muscle relaxes and the pressure drops. This lower level is diastolic pressure. Systolic pressure is the upper figure on your card, diastolic pressure the lower. The lower figure is more significant than the upper one. A woman is considered to have moderately high blood pressure (hypertension) if it exceeds 140/90 when measured on more than one occasion.

Abbr/term	Full title/Name	Meaning of abbreviation
FHR	Fetal heart rate	The number of fetal heartbeats per minute.
H/NH	Heard/not heard	This refers to the fetal heart.
Edema	Swelling	Part of your weight gain is due to water retention, causing puffiness in the feet and ankles, hands, and vulva. Having a great deal of fluid may be a sign of preeclampsia, but there is usually no need to be concerned. It is just a fact of pregnancy.
Fundus	The top of the uterus	As the baby grows, the fundus is pushed up to just above your navel at 22 weeks and under your ribs at 36 weeks. But when the baby drops down into the bony pelvis ready for birth, the fundus is lower again. You can find your own fundus and chart its position week by week through your pregnancy. Lie on your back with your tummy bare and, with the sides and palms of your hands, feel around the hard top of your uterus, pressing against what feels like a wall of muscle.
Cx	Cervix	The neck of the uterus, which softens, shortens, and opens during birth.
PP	The presenting part of the baby	This is the part that is down at the bottom of the uterus and likely to be the first to press through the opening cervix if you are at the end of pregnancy. In the last few weeks, the doctor or midwife may note the presentation precisely, so that you can get an idea of exactly what part of the baby is in the cervix.
Vx/Vtx	Vertex	This indicates the baby is head down, as it should be.
Ceph	Cephalic	This also indicates that the baby is head down.
Long L	Longitudinal lie	The baby is lying parallel to your spine.
LOA **LOP** **ROA** **ROP**	Left Occipito Anterior Left Occipito Posterior Right Occipito Anterior Right Occipito Posterior	These refer to the position (anterior or posterior) of the crown of the baby's head (occiput) in relation to your body (right or left). ROP means that the baby's crown is to your right and back.
RSA	Right sacrum anterior	This is the most common breech presentation.
Eng/E	Engaged	This is written on your chart when the baby's head has dropped down into your pelvis, which can happen any time from about six weeks before you go into labor until after you have started.
T	Term	The doctor or midwife writes this on your chart when it is estimated that you are 40 weeks into your pregnancy, which is at your estimated date of delivery.

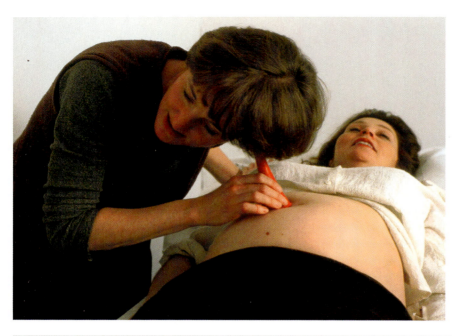

A midwife gets to know her client during the pregnancy, and routine checks are part of an ongoing relationship (left).

Your blood pressure is less likely to be raised when you are happy and relaxed (below).

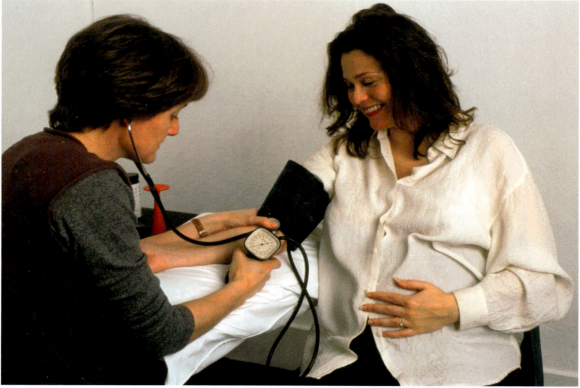

be impeded, so that you bleed more heavily.* The best physical support may come from other human beings holding you while you do whatever you want to do at the time. Some hospitals have a birthing pool or jacuzzi, although in many they are used for labor rather than birth. Seize the opportunity to use one of these, if only during the first stage of labor. They give extraordinary relief from pain and a more private, personal environment for your labor. In larger pools you can move freely, and there is plenty of room for you to give birth in the water.

If a pool is not available in your hospital, it is possible to rent a portable pool and take it with you into the hospital. Discuss this arrangement with the midwife at the prenatal clinic. Details of places from which you can rent pools are given on pages 427–428.

A BIRTH CENTER

Birth centers usually offer a package that includes prenatal care and delivery at the same location. They are run by midwives whom you will get to know well. Although many women may not have the choice of a

"WHEN I TOLD THE MIDWIFE I WANTED AN ACTIVE BIRTH, THE BED WAS REMOVED FROM THE ROOM AND REPLACED BY A MATTRESS, PILLOWS, AND A BEANBAG."

birth center in their area, if the choice exists, it is well worth considering. It offers the opportunity to give birth in a relaxed, low-tech environment, with freedom to do whatever you feel like doing, and to be cared for by midwives who see birth as a normal process—and know how to keep it normal.

A study of the experiences of 12,000 women who gave birth in 84 birth centers in the U.S. revealed that they had far fewer obstetric interventions of all kinds than women in a hospital, while birth was equally safe.* In one English birth center, women have a 37 percent reduced risk of an emergency Cesarean compared with women giving birth in hospitals in the same area and are four times less likely to have an episiotomy.*

HOME BIRTH

It is often claimed that, because far fewer mothers and babies die than, say, 60 years ago when most women had their babies at home, hospital birth must be the cause of this. But, of course, the fact that two things happen at the same time does not mean that one causes the other. Nor should we use statistics of home births from the past, or in developing countries. Many other things are different, including our health, our access to contraceptives and abortion, and our socioeconomic conditions. These have a profound effect on perinatal mortality. As the standard of living rises, fewer babies die at birth in every country, whether or not they are born in a hospital.

Unplanned births outside the hospital are often included in the statistics for home births, too, and this gives a completely wrong impression of the comparative risks of home and hospital births.

Nowadays, around 35,000 American women give birth each year at home or in a freestanding birth center. Many more would do so if there were the midwives to attend them, but midwives are few and far between. In Canada, following the legalization of midwifery in some provinces, it is easier to get midwife care than in the U.S., and midwives both work in hospitals and attend home births.

In the Netherlands 38 percent of babies are still born at home. Women there may be cared for either by a midwife or a family practitioner, and if they give birth in a hospital, they may be attended by midwives or doctors. If you look at baby deaths in terms of both where the birth took place and who attended the birth, research reveals that care given by a midwife at home is safer than care from midwives in the hospital, and home birth with a midwife is safest of all.*

A meta-analysis, research based on the most reliable studies into planned home births in different countries, shows that home birth is a valid alternative if you are not at special risk of difficulties in childbirth, and also reveals that if you give birth at home you will have fewer medical interventions. That research covered 24,092 home births, matched with births to low-risk women who were planning birth in the hospital.*

"I KNOW THAT I CAN TRUST MY BODY AND WORK WITH IT MOST EASILY IN MY OWN PLACE. I'D ONLY GO INTO HOSPITAL IF SOMETHING WAS WRONG."

Significantly fewer women who planned a home birth had their labors induced, received an episiotomy, or ended up with an operative vaginal delivery or Cesarean section. They were less likely to have a bad perineal tear. Moreover, the babies were in better condition at birth. The conclusion is: "Home birth is an acceptable alternative to hospital confinement for selected pregnant women, and leads to reduced medical interventions."

While hospital birth remains the standard way to have a baby, there is a small but steady increase in the number of women who decide to have their babies at home. Most women who have a baby at home after a previous hospital birth say that they enjoyed it much more and feel that it must have been much pleasanter for the baby. Some opt for home because they want to give birth in a familiar, comfortable, nonmedical environment. They want to make their own decisions, give birth in their own way, and behave spontaneously, without being forced into the role of patient and having to conform to hospital rules.

Women who opt for home birth also want to avoid having to change rooms and move from a bed to a delivery room, and to be able to move freely. In your own home you are in charge, and the midwife and doctor and his or her assistant are familiar and welcome guests. This continuous relationship with a limited number of helpers may be extremely important.

Some women say that since birth is an act of love, personal and intimate, it should take place in your own environment, without unnecessary observers, among friends in a loving atmosphere. They want to know that the father of the baby or close friends can be present, to take an active part and give emotional support through the labor. Some would like him to "catch" the baby himself. Most hospitals allow fathers to be present, but they are sometimes sent out just when the woman feels she needs her partner most. Often a woman would like to ensure that her baby has a "gentle birth," is welcomed into the world with tenderness, without the machinery and bright lights that are often inevitable in hospitals.

> **"MY EIGHT-YEAR-OLD DAUGHTER MADE A BIRTHDAY CAKE FOR THE BABY WHILE I WAS IN THE FIRST STAGE OF LABOR, AND WE CELEBRATED AFTERWARD WITH THE CAKE, CHAMPAGNE, AND LEMONADE."**

"BONDING" OCCURS NATURALLY

Research on "bonding" between mother, father, and baby points toward the importance of the time immediately following birth for the couple to get to know their baby and feel it belongs to them and that they belong to it. In some hospitals, separation immediately after the child is born is still arbitrarily imposed on new parents. Time for cuddling is restricted or denied, and routines take precedence over the emotional unfolding that heralds the birth of a family.

Many women suspect that medical intervention is often unnecessary and that they will have a better chance of giving birth naturally and without drugs at home. They believe that full awareness of what is happening is a valuable experience and that drugs can harm their unborn babies. After a previous difficult hospital birth, one pregnant woman said: "I was determined to have a natural birth this time. Last time I had the whole works, and finished up with an epidural and a forceps delivery. I can't help thinking that if I let things take their own time and keep walking around, and can relax and use my breathing and feel comfortable in my own home, with the people I love around me, my body will know what to do."

If you already have other children, you may want them to see birth as a normal, happy part of life, not a surgical operation that entails going to the hospital. Birth is a family affair, and the baby should belong to the whole family. Some women hope that the other child or children can be involved in the labor, and some would like them present at the birth. This is difficult or impossible to arrange in most hospitals. Some mothers who have never left their toddlers worry that separation will lead to emotional and behavioral problems in the older child. There are also mothers who just find it impossible to get someone to look after their family while they are in the hospital. It is sometimes stated that women having their fourth or subsequent babies should always give birth in the hospital, but if all your previous pregnancies and labors have been straightforward, there is no additional risk with a fourth or fifth birth, and some definite advantage in giving birth at home where the other children can be involved.

Some doctors are reluctant to give their approval to home birth once you are pregnant, even though they have seemed flexible earlier. For example, one woman said that her doctor had agreed to a home birth for her third child "in principle" before she was pregnant but then "did her best to change our minds. She did not really seem to understand that there was absolutely no one who could come to look after our other children, and that I would not be able to have my husband with me if the baby was not born at home. There were many occasions when I was reduced to tears on my arrival home. If I had been less determined, or if my husband had not been so supportive, I might have given in." If you are concerned that this might happen to you, arm yourself with information. You can find out more in my book on home birth* and by contacting the organizations on pages 427–428.

"I HATED GOING TO THE DOCTOR'S OFFICE. IT SEEMED TO TURN A MIRACLE INTO A MEDICAL ROUTINE. SO I SWITCHED FROM STANDARD HOSPITAL TO ONE-TO-ONE MIDWIFE CARE. I FELT I HAD RECLAIMED MY PREGNANCY."

PRENATAL CARE

One ingredient of a happy birth is good prenatal care, checking that you are healthy and the baby starts life under the best possible conditions. But the care you give yourself is probably more important than the care you receive from professionals. It includes learning how to cope with stress and understanding how to work with your body. You do not need to attend classes until you are five or more months pregnant, but it is worth thinking about the different classes available, and perhaps beginning a few exercises earlier than this.

Prenatal care has progressed piecemeal since the 19th century, and we do not know which elements in the package are valuable for all women, which are best kept for those at special risk, and which might be discarded altogether. It is common for confusion to occur about whether a baby is growing well inside the uterus, for example, and many women are told that there is intrauterine growth restriction when, in fact, it turns out that everything is fine. In spite of this, good medical care every now and then can make all the difference between life and death for the baby—and even, very occasionally, for the mother, too.*

In the prenatal clinic, a long wait is usually a fact of life. Take a magazine or a book or some needlework, or make friends with other expectant mothers attending the same office. Many offices encourage fathers to be there, but sometimes they are asked to remain in the waiting room. If it is important to you that you both talk to the doctor or midwife, it is worthwhile being quietly but firmly persistent to get what you want. Think through beforehand any questions or worries that you may have. Write down questions so that you will not forget to ask in the rush. If there is anything you hope for concerning the way in which you have your baby, ask the doctor or midwife to note it on your records.

Many tests in pregnancy, the value of which has been taken for granted in the past, are now being questioned. Multi-center research is taking place to determine whether they do what they are assumed to do, or if they do more harm than good. This is the only way to discover which are useful and which should be discarded. If there is uncertainty about a screening procedure or other intervention, you may be invited to take part in a randomized controlled trial. Consider all the implications: you have the right to be fully informed about any research in which you are taking part; you can consent or refuse; and you can leave the study if and when you wish.

ROUTINE TESTS

Most women see their doctor or midwife once a month until they are 28 weeks pregnant. At this stage you will be seen every two weeks; in your final month you will be given weekly appointments. However, there is a trend to reduce the number of visits if all is well, particularly if this is your second or subsequent pregnancy.

HAVING A VAGINAL EXAMINATION

You may be examined vaginally early in your pregnancy. If you are more than six weeks pregnant, the midwife or doctor will be able to detect a slight enlargement and softening of the uterus. The embryo is well protected and cannot be dislodged by the examination.

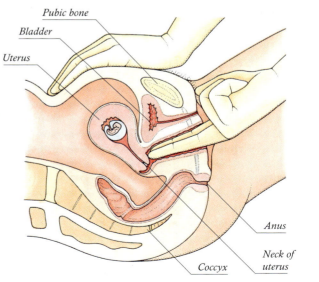

Pubic bone

Bladder

Uterus

Anus

Neck of uterus

Coccyx

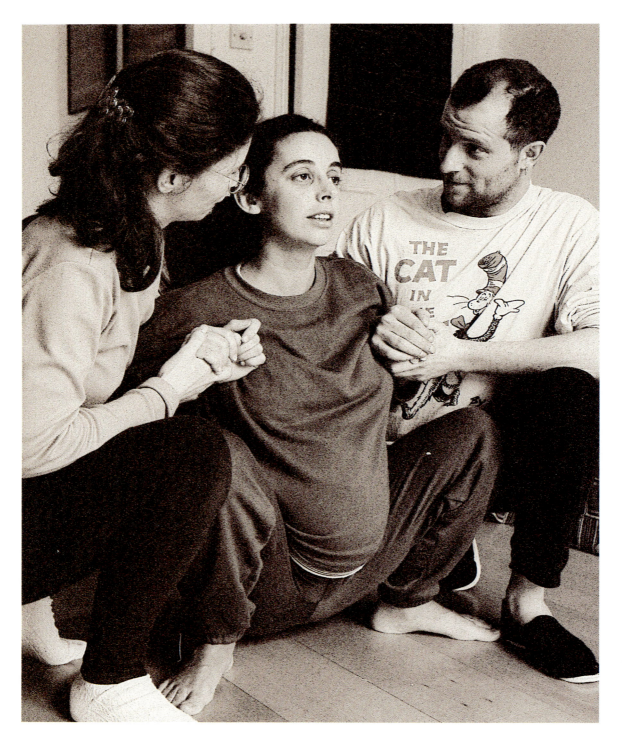

At the first prenatal visit, the midwife or doctor may listen to your heart. Heart sounds change during pregnancy, and a heart murmur may be detected. This is usually perfectly normal.

Your blood group is determined, and a test is done to check whether the baby might develop Rh disease (see page 113). Your blood is automatically tested for syphilis and for hepatitis B. You will also be offered testing for HIV. At each visit your blood pressure and urine will be tested, and your weight, the height of the fundus, and the fetal heartbeat (as soon as it is audible) will also be checked. You may be offered screening for spina bifida and Down's syndrome (see pages 226–227). Depending on your ethnic and family background, you may be offered one or more blood tests to determine if you carry certain genetic disorders that could cause disease in your baby.

Regular blood tests are done for anemia (see page 144). But what was once treated in pregnancy as "anemia" is usually a normal drop in hemoglobin due to plasma volume expansion. A pregnant woman has about 40 percent more blood flowing in her body. It used to be thought that women's hemoglobin levels must be kept high during pregnancy with iron supplementation. But women whose hemoglobin concentration does fall are more likely to go to full term and to have babies of good birth weight. If hemoglobin concentration fails to fall, there is a marked increase in the incidence of low birth weight and preterm birth.* In fact, a woman who is pregnant is better able to absorb iron from food. If you drink orange juice instead of tea or coffee (both of which inhibit absorption of iron), your body will make good use of the iron that is naturally present in the food you eat.*

An ultrasound scan (see page 229) may be suggested at any time during pregnancy. Ultrasound at around 18–20 weeks is routine in most practices. You can refuse if you do not want one. If you have a series of scans, an estimate can be made of the baby's rate of growth and expected date of delivery.

At the first prenatal visit, you may have a vaginal examination. At most later visits, the uterus and baby are felt by abdominal palpation. As this is done, give a long breath out and release your tummy completely. Then go on breathing slowly, releasing on each breath out. This makes it easier to find out how the baby is lying and is more comfortable for you than when you are tense.

The examining hands feel first for the distance between your pubic bone and the baby and then the top of the uterus. This process is called fundal palpation. The hands move down the sides of the baby so that by late pregnancy the back and limbs can be felt. The part of the baby that is over the cervix is said to be "presenting." The doctor or midwife turns to face your feet and presses his or her hands downward and from side to side to discover whether the baby's head, buttocks, or any other part, is presenting. The next maneuver tends to be uncomfortable

In childbirth classes you learn different positions and movements to help you give birth actively.

51

MAKING YOUR BIRTH PLAN

Here are some questions to consider in constructing your birth plan. Some may not be relevant to you, and you will probably want to include others, but this should get you off to a good start. Read the section on "The Experience of Birth" before you come to any definite decision.

Q Whom would you like to have with you during labor and at the birth? Do you want to place a limit on the number of people caring for you?

Q What is your top priority while in labor? Is there anything that matters to you apart from the safety of your baby and yourself?

Q Do you want to put yourself unreservedly in your caregivers' hands and leave them to get on with it, or to be kept fully informed of all developments and to share in any discussions and decisions made?

Q How do you plan to cope with the pain you are likely to experience during labor?

Q Are there any things you would like to have in the birth room with you, for example, pictures, familiar objects, music, candles, aromatherapy essences, or equipment to give you physical support and enable you to get into comfortable positions?

Q Do you have any special requests about the birth itself, such as having the lights in the birth room dimmed, being given or avoiding having an episiotomy, and the way in which the baby is delivered?

Q Is there anything that is important for you to be able to do during labor, such as using a shower, tub, or birth pool, being able to adopt upright positions and move your pelvis, using alternative methods of pain relief, or being free to make a lot of noise?

Q What are your thoughts about common medical procedures that may be used during labor, such as artificial rupture of the membranes, hormone stimulation of the uterus, electronic fetal monitoring, an intravenous drip, pain-relieving drugs, restriction of positions and movements, and the active management of labor?

Q Do you want the third stage to be speeded up with a hormone injection and controlled cord traction immediately after the birth, or would you prefer the afterbirth to be delivered physiologically?

Q Do you have any special requests about the hour following birth, for example, keeping your baby in bed with you and in skin-to-skin contact, and being left alone with your partner and your baby? Would you like the baby to be examined in your presence?

Q In the 24 hours after birth, how much time would you like to spend with your baby? For example, would you like to keep her in bed with you, in a crib beside your bed, or in the nursery for some or most of the time? Are you happy to be woken up at night to feed your baby, or would you rather be left to sleep?

Q How do you intend to feed your baby? If you plan to breast-feed, are you willing for your baby to be given supplementary formula, dextrose, or water, or do you want her to have breast milk only?

Q How soon would you like to go home after the birth?

but is quickly performed. Facing you again, one hand is spread wide and presses in above your pubic bone to feel the exact position of the presenting part in relation to the pelvis.

Throughout pregnancy, prenatal checks are a chance to find out more about your baby and discuss your concerns, so think through the questions you want to ask, and explore all the options. In late pregnancy, for example, you will want to know how your baby is lying, whether it can still change its position, and if not, whether its position has implications for the birth. Be aware of fetal movements, and tell your caregivers about any change in their frequency or how they feel.

TALKING TO DOCTORS

Some people have doctors with whom they quickly feel at ease and experience little difficulty discussing what they want. However, you and your doctor are more likely to meet in a system in which time is at a premium, and you may find it difficult to avoid a formal relationship, with all that this implies in terms of authority and subordination.

Being pregnant involves a kind of emotional journey into being a patient. And it propels you into new kinds of social relationships. Some of these are with the professionals you encounter during your pregnancy. So, as well as having to understand the changes taking place in your body and your emo-

"I REMEMBERED HOW YOU SAID, 'IF IT'S REALLY DIFFICULT, THINK OF YOUR DOCTOR IN HIS PAJAMAS,' AND PLUCKED UP THE COURAGE TO SAY WHAT I WANTED."

tions, you may have to develop new social skills to create a satisfactory dialogue with those who care for you. This is especially the case when you meet different doctors and midwives at each clinic visit and others again when in labor. The lack of continuity in care is one of the main criticisms that women make about childbirth in hospitals.*

Women who have had an assisted conception already see themselves as patients, and are likely to be on a medical conveyor belt that they never jump off of. It is difficult to trust your body to work well if you had to start a pregnancy by IVF. Yet those nine months are an important time to learn the self-confidence that you are going to need not only for childbirth, but when you become a mother.

Some women feel very vulnerable emotionally when they are pregnant, and cannot help crying under pressure, even though (or perhaps because) it is the last thing they want to do. You are not abnormal if you feel intense surges of emotion that are difficult or impossible to control, but you may feel at a disadvantage in an interview with a doctor when you want to ask for something or talk about the kind of birth you are hoping for. So have your partner or a close friend or relative with you. It is important to discuss your wishes thoroughly with this person first. You may find it useful for him or her to play "the devil's advocate" and act out an imagined encounter so that you have some practice in discussing the subject and can develop a strategy. Stay calm as you present your case. Do not make the mistake of anticipating opposition from hospital staff. You may be pleasantly surprised.

See that you are well briefed about matters you want to discuss. Read any literature available which contains up-to-date information. Make sure your partner reads it, too, and then decide together the key issues that are important to you.

PREPARING YOUR QUESTIONS

Since questions may go out of your head when you have a chance to ask them (pregnancy amnesia is a well-known phenomenon), and because some doctors seem to concentrate on the lower end of your body to the exclusion of you as a person, jot down subjects on paper. Hospitals vary in their routine interventions. You may not want some or all of them, so state your preferences as early as possible. On the other hand, you may want an intervention that would not usually be given but is probably available if you make a special request. Your list could include questions about ultrasound. You can find more about that on page 229. You may also want to explore policy on induction and augmentation of labor, intravenous drips, electronic fetal monitoring, episiotomy, forceps (see page 346), and Cesarean section. You could ask about the policy concerning drugs for pain relief and epidurals (see page 319) and inquire whether you will be able to keep your baby with you day and night. It may also be important for you to know whether there will be a lactation specialist to help with breast-feeding, and to know her name in advance. Be specific in your requests, to avoid any misunderstandings later on.

Sometimes the doctor's office is so crowded that you feel reluctant to take up time with questions. Even so, it is worth saying that you have made a note of things you would like to discuss and ask whether it is convenient that day, or, if not, whether you can have time to talk at the next visit. There is no need to be apologetic about wanting further information or asking for help to achieve the kind of birth you would like. You are not just a baby-producing machine!

During the interview, make sure you sit in a relaxed way, check that fingers and toes are unclenched, and breathe out just before speaking for the first time. Make eye contact and address the doctor by name or ask his or her name if you do not know it.

When a woman is feeling nervous, she tends to pitch her voice too high. Modulate it so that it does not sound too demanding. You may also smile nervously without realizing it. This is confusing for a caregiver, who thinks that you are happy about something when you are not. Or the doctor may smile because he or she is concerned to get you to accept another point of view and is sugaring the pill; your spontaneous reaction may then be to smile back, giving the impression that you are content when you are not.

Avoid aggression and state your requests clearly and concisely. If you lose your temper, you may be classified as difficult or neurotic. If you encounter opposition or are made to feel that you cannot know what is in your best interests, restate your wishes firmly and give the reasons for them. It is a good idea to include requests that are not top priority, so that there is a possibility of compromise on some matters. Belligerence provokes further opposition. Say instead how happy or disappointed you are. Always try to give "I" messages rather than "you" messages. Say "I prefer . . ." or "I'm unhappy about . . ." Be assertive in a pleasant way. You may not have any medical knowledge about your body, but you know a great deal about it, since it is you who lives in it. If a woman acts as if she expects to be bossed around, it is more likely that she will be. Some doctors think it is enough to have a chat with you when you are lying flat on your back with your panties off. Say that you would like to talk clothed and face-to-face. If a test or intervention is proposed that you do not want, either now or during childbirth, simply say "No, thank you," and repeat it if necessary.

"I'M NOT USED TO BEING ASSERTIVE BUT MY DOCTOR WAS OKAY ABOUT IT AND WE'VE HAD SOME LIVELY DISCUSSIONS."

If this seems too difficult, practice speaking out in less threatening situations, perhaps with colleagues at work or with family members. Complain in a store that has sold you shoddy goods, tell guests who are still hanging around at midnight that it is time you went to bed, or send back bad food in a restaurant.

You may want to take notes of the conversation you have with your doctor, and can always say: "I'd like to think more about that; may I just make a note of it?" But do not imply that you are cross-examining the doctor and writing down answers in preparation for a later attack. Make it clear that you are listening closely by "playing back" the important statements: "Do you mean . . . ?" "So you are saying that . . . ?" and rephrase whatever has been said as accurately as you can. You can sometimes add to your remark the implications that you think such a statement entails. By clarifying a point in this way you may be working toward modifying it. For example, if the doctor says, "I never allow husbands to remain if I have to do a forceps delivery because they only get in the way," you might ask: "Are you saying that it is dangerous for him to stay because he might affect your judgment?" Few experienced obstetricians would say that the presence of a woman's partner could affect their professional judgment, but the doctor might reply by telling you a story about men who have fainted. In response to this you could say:

"I take it you feel happier about a man who stays calm and who can give emotional support?"

If your interview has gone badly, consider changing your doctor, or, if there is more than one in your area, the hospital where you are to have the baby. But it is best to give yourself a couple of days to simmer down and think it over calmly before finally deciding. Write a letter explaining your reasons for seeking other care. Send copies to the manager if it concerns a hospital. But such drastic measures are usually unnecessary, and you will find that you can open up the possibility of getting the kind of childbirth you want by other means. There is always a price to pay for being submissive. A woman avoids conflict, but afterward she is likely to feel that birth was something done to her, not something she did herself. Women who have suffered a sense of complete powerlessness in birth may go on feeling this long after the baby is born. It often leads to their feeling incompetent with the baby, too.

Good communication means that if you do not get all you had hoped for, you still take an active part in decision making. And it may be that you will improve conditions for other women.

"EVERYONE HAD READ MY NOTES AND TOOK A GREAT DEAL OF TROUBLE DOING THE THINGS I HAD REQUESTED."

CHOICES

Being handed leaflets about choices does not mean that you actually have them. Printed information is sometimes used to obtain "informed compliance" and to avoid discussion about alternatives, instead of providing genuine choice.* Some interventions—ultrasound and electronic fetal monitoring in labor, for example—have become so routine that many midwives and doctors no longer consider them as optional. Even if a midwife or junior doctor is positive about the choices you want to make, it may be tricky if they run counter to routine clinical practice. Many doctors limit choice because they are anxious about the risk of litigation if they have not used every test and every type of monitoring available, even when the use of this technology is contradicted by research evidence.

Many of us are too well behaved for our own good. As one study revealed: "Childbearing women generally complied with expected norms in their encounters with staff, whom they perceived as busy people with many demands on their time."* Another problem is that you may never see the same midwife twice, and this makes it difficult to ask searching questions and have any ongoing discussion about possible options. Choice is eradicated when there is no continuity of care. Women speak and no one hears them, or, like children's whispering games, what they say gets passed on but is distorted. Women are denied choice when nurses are rushed off their feet trying to care for three or four patients in labor simultaneously. They are denied choice when their self-confidence is destroyed.

Getting information may be hard enough. If you want to go on from there to make active choices, you need courage to think through what you want—and then go all out for it. After they have given birth, women who do this usually say that it was well worth it.

YOUR BIRTH PLAN

A birth plan is a list of your priorities and wishes for the birth and the time immediately afterward. It is best constructed after you have met your caregivers and discussed your options with them, but early enough for you to negotiate modifications in hospital protocols or a midwife's standard practice. One copy is clipped to the notes and you keep another copy yourself. Some notes have dedicated pages for birth plans.

If you have had a baby before, you will be pretty clear what is most important to you. If you work in the health services yourself, or have listened to other women's accounts of birth, you may also have a clear idea of exactly what you want and do not want. This may include the kind of setting in which you wish to give birth, and the general style of birth you prefer—high-tech, epidural or drug-free, and mobile, for instance.

Some people think the idea of a birth plan is ridiculous because no one knows in advance how birth is going to be. That is true. But if you were setting off on safari, or even on a picnic when you were not sure how the weather would turn out, you would plan for alternatives. It is the same with birth. You know what you want, and you also know what you want if things do not turn out exactly as expected.

Doctors and midwives do not have to be burdened with patients' trusting reverence. Increasingly they prefer women to think through what they want and to make choices. There are still caregivers who feel threatened by birth plans and see them as undermining their authority and expertise, like the obstetrician who said he could not stand "backseat drivers." Yet when women become utterly dependent on those caring for them,

"FROM THE MOMENT I WAS WELCOMED UNTIL I LEFT, MY WISHES ABOUT HOW THE BIRTH SHOULD BE CONDUCTED AND HOW I CARED FOR MY BABY WERE GIVEN PRIORITY."

it can be more threatening than open confrontation, for if things go wrong and a baby is damaged or dies, total faith then often turns to litigation. It is almost invariably those who put their unquestioning trust in an obstetrician who sue for malpractice—not women who accept responsibility, weigh the pros and cons, and make decisions for themselves. It is also sometimes suggested that making a birth plan shows lack of trust in the doctor or midwife. But at best it is something you do together. It enables your caregiver to learn about you at the same time that you learn about him or her. It can be a positive part of your developing relationship and contribute a lot to it. Those who oppose the idea of birth plans often urge women to be nice to their doctors to get what they want. But being nice is often not enough. The kind of doctor who brushes aside a request for "natural childbirth" by saying, "Of course you can give birth naturally. All birth is natural," or who tells you, "You can hang from a chandelier as far as I'm concerned," is likely to want you harpooned to a fetal monitor, and may be knife-happy, too. Stating your wishes in writing and confidently affirming expectations gives you a greater chance of having what you want than playing the part of the obedient patient. Birth plans are a vital part of an active approach to labor, which sees birth as a spontaneous process in which a woman's body knows how to act without anyone having to "manage" it. Yet they can be equally well used if a woman is certain that she wants an epidural or is convinced that induction is a good thing to have if she goes a week "overdue."

WHAT TO INCLUDE IN YOUR BIRTH PLAN Some things will be simple and straightforward: for example, "I would like to hold the baby immediately, skin to skin," or "I would like to be helped to lift the baby out of my own body." These may already be standard practices for your midwife or doctor. Other choices may be more complicated and entail further discussion. As an example, if the early stages of labor are long-drawn-out, what, if any, interventions might be proposed and which would you prefer? With active management of labor, increasingly popular in hospitals all over the world, every woman whose cervix fails to dilate one centimeter every hour has her uterus stimulated artificially by hormones introduced through an intravenous drip. The principle behind this is that no labor should be allowed to exceed 12 hours. The Irish obstetricians who devised this system of management say it is what women want, that women like to know that the baby will be born by 11 a.m., or 6 p.m., or whatever. They also say that it reduces the need for Cesarean section, a claim that research has been unable to substantiate.*

> "WORKING ON A BIRTH PLAN HELPED ME AND MY PARTNER SORT OUT WHAT WAS MOST IMPORTANT AND DISCUSS IT WITH THE MIDWIFE."

In the hospital in Dublin where this method was first introduced, each woman has her own special midwife who stays with her. Meta-analysis of clinical data and randomized control of trials of active management show that it is not hormone stimulation but the presence of someone who gives one-to-one care and stays with the mother throughout labor and birth that makes Cesarean section less likely.* You may welcome the whole package of active management. Or you may want only specific elements, to be sure, for instance, that you have a midwife who does not disappear at the end of a shift, but stays with you until you have given birth. And you may want to add that you would like to get to know the midwives before you go into labor, so that you have a chance to talk to whoever your personal caregiver might be. You may also want to have a doula. This is a woman who is experienced in providing encouragement, reassurance, nonmedical advice, and physical comfort throughout labor and birth. She also gives support to the father or woman's partner. You can find out about the possibility of having a doula if you contact a doula organization (address on page 427).

There may be interventions you want to avoid entirely, if possible. For many women, episiotomy, the cut to enlarge the vaginal opening as the baby is being born, is one of these. There is ample research now to show that a woman is most comfortable afterward when she has been helped to give birth gently without a cut or tear. So you may want to find out the episiotomy rate and to ask specifically for help from someone who is good at delivering without damage to the perineum. Research also shows that most tears are small ones—first or second degree—and that they heal better than episiotomies. So you can state in your birth plan that you would like to avoid an episiotomy, would prefer a tear if an intact perineum proves impossible, and that, whatever happens, you do not wish an episiotomy to be performed without giving your consent first. On the other hand, you may not care very much either way, and just want whoever is assisting with the birth to get on with it.

When you are constructing your birth plan, it helps to have an idea of normal practice in the hospital and with the caregivers you have chosen. In the U.S. there are wide variations in what is routine practice between different areas of the country.

Keep your birth plan concise, no longer than two pages. Retain one copy yourself and have it ready with the other things you need to take to the hospital with you when labor starts. Make sure that your birth companion also knows what is in it. Birth plans are not set in stone. Think of your plan as an expression of your individuality—a way of describing the sort of person you are, so that if a doctor or midwife meets you for the first time in labor, he or she will get an idea of how you want to be treated and the things that matter most to you. Use your birth plan as part of a developing dialogue with the people caring for you.

A HOSPITAL BIRTH

Louise's first labor was long, and she was worried that her second labor would be similar. But birth is usually quicker the second time around if the baby is in a good position.

This labor lasts four and a half hours, and Louise has not felt the need for drugs or any form of pain relief. She is wired to an electronic fetal monitor. Electrodes strapped to her abdomen record the strength of uterine contractions and her baby's heart rate, and these are registered on the chart emerging from the monitor.

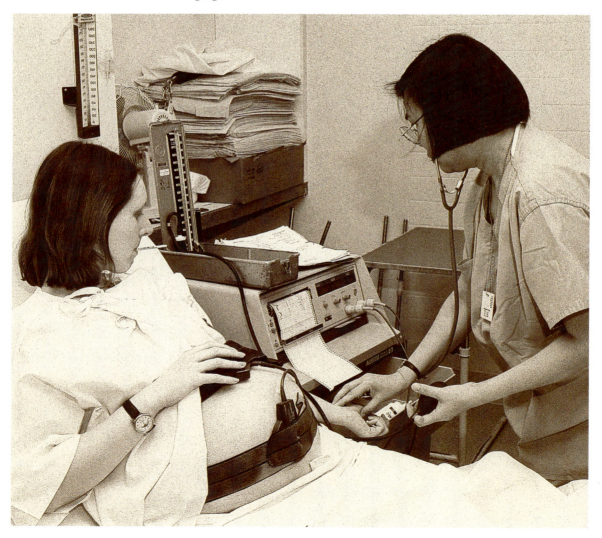

There has been a shift change and another midwife is caring for
Louise now. The delivery room is not suitable for a more active birth, so
Louise is sitting on a standard delivery table instead, supported by foam-
rubber wedges and pillows. She is entering the second stage of labor now
and is getting hot, so the midwife has turned on an electric fan. However,
Louise continues to wear socks, because she finds, like many women,
that her feet get cold during labor.

Well into the second stage, Louise has an overwhelming urge to push
with each strong contraction. She is making some progress but is finding
it difficult to push effectively with her knees up and sitting on her coccyx.
She tells the midwife that she wants to change her position.

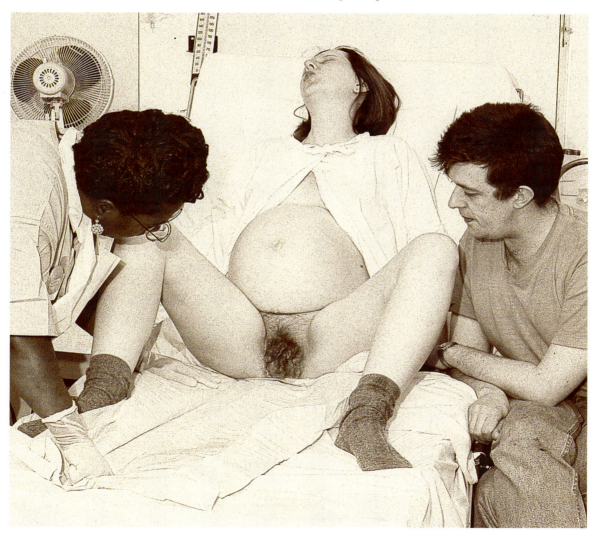

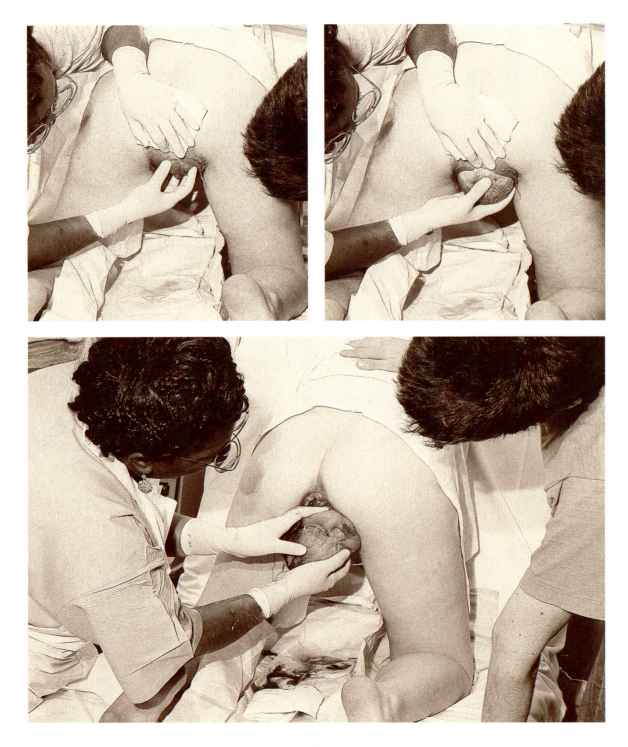

Louise decides to turn onto her hands and knees, which she finds much more comfortable. After a while she adopts a forward-leaning position with her head resting on her arms. Her perineal tissues fan out easily as the baby's head presses through. The midwife supports the head, then holds the baby under the shoulders as she lifts her out.

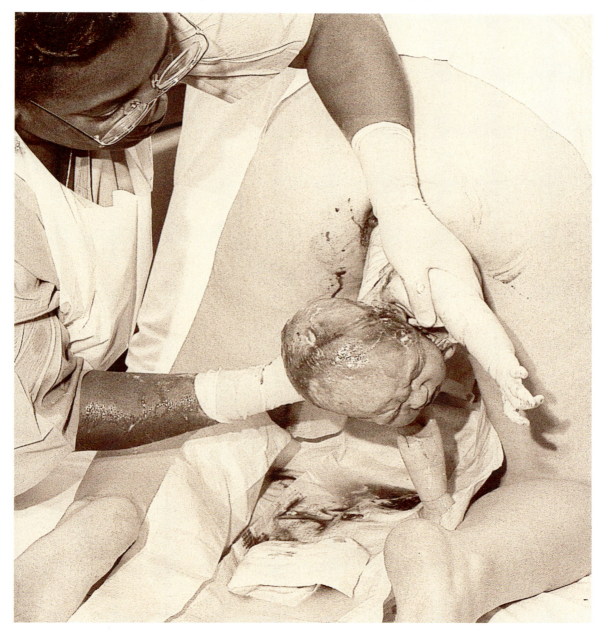

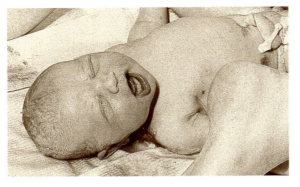

The midwife clamps and cuts the cord, and then places the baby in her mother's arms. She has no episiotomy, and only a small labial tear, which the midwife sutures immediately. Her baby weighs over 9 lb (4 kg)—much heavier than the first.

Afterward the midwife says: "She coped brilliantly with her breathing, and her partner was there to rub her back and encourage her. Louise knew exactly what to do and when to do it. She chose her positions, including kneeling, and they helped the baby's descent and birth."

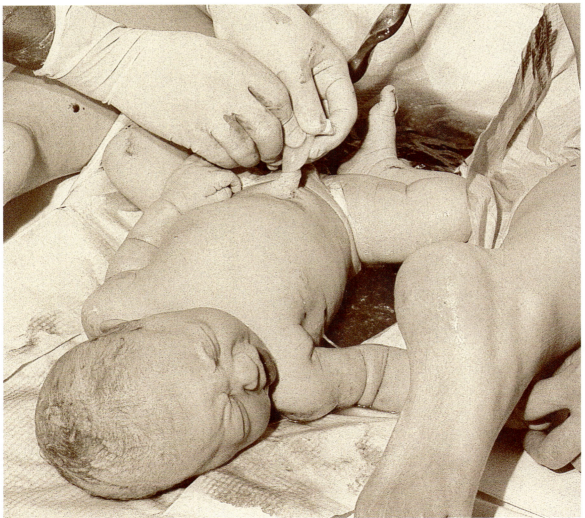

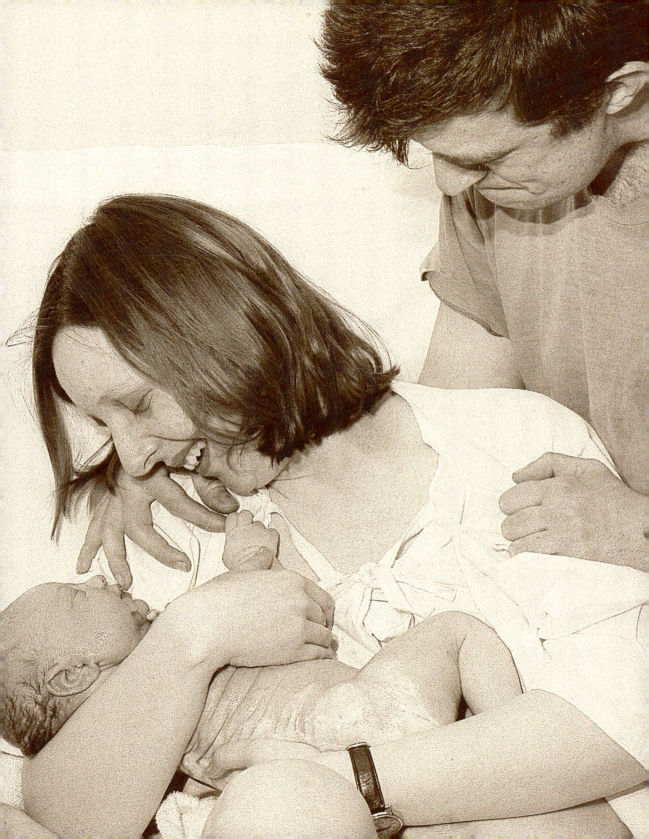

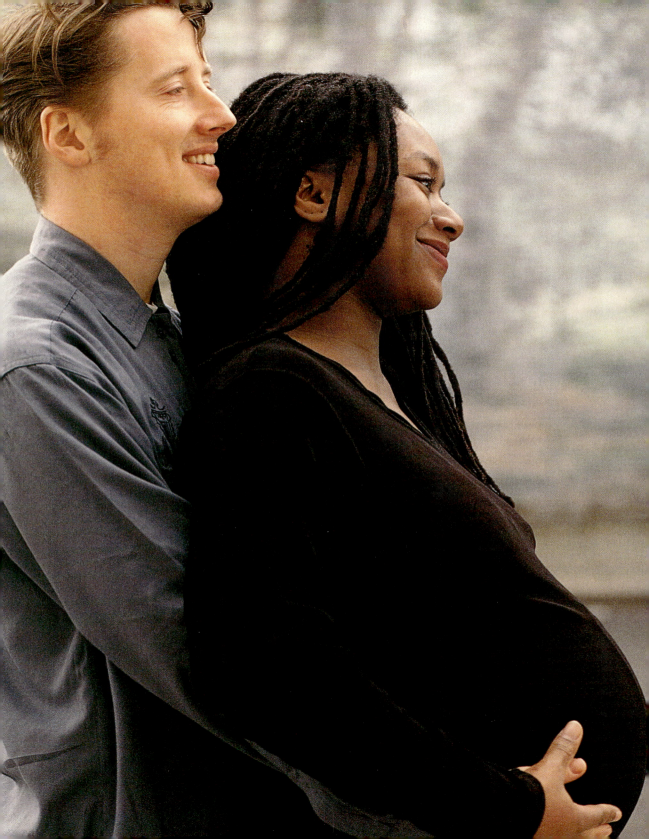

PREGNANCY

PHYSICAL & EMOTIONAL CHANGES

68 LIFE IN THE UTERUS

82 FORTY WEEKS OF LIFE

88 EXPECTING TWINS

96 YOUR BABY'S WELL-BEING

116 YOUR PHYSICAL WELL-BEING

150 EMOTIONAL CHALLENGES IN PREGNANCY

158 BECOMING A FATHER

164 YOU AND YOUR PARTNER

172 PREGNANT AGAIN

LIFE IN THE UTERUS

In the first days of pregnancy, life is budding in cells far smaller than a pinhead. Because everything is happening on such a minute scale, it can be difficult to accept the reality of a baby growing deep inside you. Even when you begin to believe in your pregnancy, other people remain unaware of it.

It can seem as if an explosion has taken place without anybody noticing, or as if all the colors have become more brilliant but everyone else is carrying on as usual. The chance meeting of one out of four hundred million sperm with a ripe and vibrant egg has resulted in a dramatic series of events, conducted on a scale so minute that you cannot feel the astonishing life process unfolding inside you, even though you know it is happening.

FERTILIZATION

At birth, the ovaries of every baby girl contain almost 500,000 potential single-cell eggs, but they do not ripen until the menstrual periods begin. Each cell that ripens into an egg is nourished by nearly 5,000 other eggs that will never themselves ripen. From your first period until menopause, when your periods stop, you may carry up to 4,000 ripe eggs; each month,

THE FEMALE REPRODUCTIVE ORGANS

Thousands of eggs are stored in a woman's two ovaries, but usually only one egg matures and is released each month. This egg is drawn into a Fallopian tube, where it may be fertilized by a sperm that has made the journey up the vagina after intercourse. If a fertilized egg embeds in the lining of the uterus, a pregnancy begins.

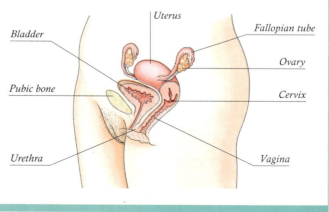

Bladder

Pubic bone

Urethra

Uterus

Fallopian tube

Ovary

Cervix

Vagina

between 100 and 150 begin to ripen, but usually only one a month reaches maturity and is capable of being fertilized. The frequency with which eggs are produced and released is determined by hormones, which interact regularly in the menstrual cycle.

This cycle lasts for about a month, and begins when a hormone released by the pituitary gland stimulates an ovary to start ripening an egg. As the egg matures, the ovary releases estrogen into the bloodstream. This

THE MENSTRUAL CYCLE

Every month between puberty and menopause, a woman's body prepares for conception. First, hormones stimulate an egg follicle to form in an ovary, and an egg matures inside. Meanwhile, the lining of the uterus thickens. Around mid-cycle the ripe egg is released. If it is not fertilized, it is shed with the lining of the uterus (menstruation).

OVULATION CYCLE

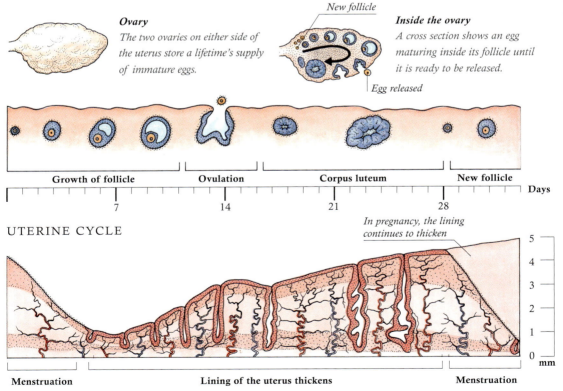

Ovary
The two ovaries on either side of the uterus store a lifetime's supply of immature eggs.

New follicle

Inside the ovary
A cross section shows an egg maturing inside its follicle until it is ready to be released.

Egg released

| Growth of follicle | Ovulation | Corpus luteum | New follicle |

Days

7   14   21   28

UTERINE CYCLE

In pregnancy, the lining continues to thicken

5
4
3
2
1
0
mm

| Menstruation | Lining of the uterus thickens | Menstruation |

stops the pituitary gland's production of hormone, so no more eggs ripen. It also makes the uterine lining change and thicken in anticipation of the egg, which bursts out of the follicle (a capsule bulging on the surface of the ovary) about midway through each cycle. It is then drawn by the fingered tentacles of the Fallopian tube into its long canal, which is about the thickness of a ballpoint refill.

The egg itself is a minute speck. It is barely visible to the naked eye, yet when it meets with a still more minuscule sperm it has the potential to develop into a human being. The follicle (also known as the corpus luteum) that held the egg begins to produce progesterone, which carries on the work that the estrogen has been doing. If the egg is not fertilized within a few days, the follicle dries up and the progesterone level falls dramatically. As a result of this drop in progesterone level, the uterine lining decomposes, and a menstrual period occurs. Even while bleeding is going on, the menstrual cycle renews itself: the pituitary gland is stimulating the ovary into ripening a new egg.

However, if the egg is fertilized, the follicle does not shrivel up, the progesterone level does not drop, and the uterine lining continues to thicken, so that you do not have a period.

The usual pattern is that the ovary on one side releases an egg one month, the one on the other side the next. Sometimes one ovary becomes especially active for a few months. Occasionally, only one ovary is functioning. If part of a Fallopian tube or an ovary has been surgically removed, the other one usually takes on the work of both.

Sperm are so tiny that 30,000 of them placed side by side would just stretch across a bottle top. A man ejaculates hundreds of millions of sperm every time he has an orgasm. After intercourse, a mere 2,000 of these survive the journey up the vagina to the Fallopian tubes, and only one can fertilize a ripe egg, which immediately puts up a chemical barrier to keep all others out. Each sperm is shaped like a tadpole with a long, lashing tail; a healthy sperm is highly mobile. The head is rounded and holds the gene-carrying nucleus. When a sperm meets the egg it burrows its way deep into it, and its nucleus fuses with the nucleus of the egg. It is at this moment that the parents' genes, or units of inheritance, first meet.

Sperm

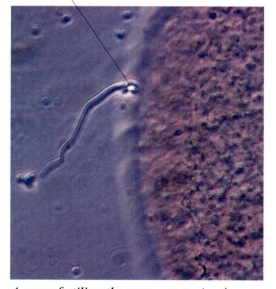

A sperm fertilizes the ovum, *penetrating the outer membrane; the ovum sucks it in.*

GENETICS

Inside the nucleus of every body cell—with two exceptions—there are 46 chromosomes, making 23 pairs. The two exceptions are the egg cell and the sperm cell, which have 23 chromosomes each, instead of 46. Chromosomes are rodlike structures, each containing thousands of genes.

When the nucleus of the sperm cell fuses with the nucleus of the egg, each chromosome—and each gene inside each chromosome—unites with its opposite number. The newly fertilized cell now contains 46 chromosomes, like every other human cell. The physical characteristics of the future person are determined, and the cell can start to develop into a human being.

BOY OR GIRL?

Out of the 23 pairs of chromosomes in every human cell, one pair determines the person's sex. The two sex chromosomes in a female cell are known as XX, and the two in a male cell as XY. Since the egg and the sperm cell contain half the usual number of chromosomes, every egg cell contains 22 chromosomes plus one sex chromosome, which is an X. Every sperm cell contains 22 chromosomes plus one sex chromosome, which can be either an X or a Y.

The sex of the baby depends on these differences between sperm cells. If a sperm with an X chromosome fertilizes the egg, the union of the two sex chromosomes will result in XX: a girl. If the egg is fertilized by a sperm with a Y chromosome, the union of the two sex chromosomes will result in XY: a boy. There is usually a 50/50 chance that a boy or a girl will be conceived; but statistically it appears that as women grow older, and also as they bear more children, the chance of having a girl is slightly increased.

Although the sex of the baby is determined by the sperm, it is also partly a consequence of the environment into which that

YOUR BABY'S SEX

An egg cell and a sperm cell each contain 23 single chromosomes. These pair up when the cells meet. One of the 23 chromosomes is a sex chromosome. An egg always has an X (female) chromosome, but a sperm may carry an X or a Y (male) chromosome.

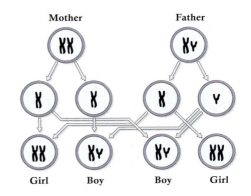

Sex chromosomes
If an egg is fertilized by a sperm carrying a Y chromosome, the result is a boy. An egg fertilized by a sperm carrying an X chromosome develops into a girl.

sperm is received. Natural alkalinity or acidity of the secretions in your reproductive tract makes it easier for some sperm to survive their long journey than for others. Traditionally, an acid medium has been thought to increase the chances of having a male child, and an alkaline medium a female child; because of this people have douched with acid or alkaline solutions before intercourse, but there is little evidence that this significantly affects your chances of producing one sex or the other.

DOMINANT AND RECESSIVE GENES

When a Y chromosome meets an X chromosome, the Y chromosome dominates to produce a boy. Similarly, when a gene encounters its opposite number, one always takes precedence. A baby receives half of its genes from each parent. If a gene for brown eyes from one parent meets a gene for blue eyes from the other, the gene for brown eyes will always prevail. This does not mean that a child of one brown-eyed and one blue-eyed parent will always have brown eyes. But the gene for brown eyes is known as dominant, the one for blue eyes as recessive. So someone with brown eyes who has received a gene for blue eyes from one parent retains the blue-eye gene as a recessive gene. If he or she should have a child by another brown-eyed person also with a recessive gene for blue eyes, there is a one in four chance that both parents will pass on their recessive genes for blue eyes to produce a blue-eyed child.

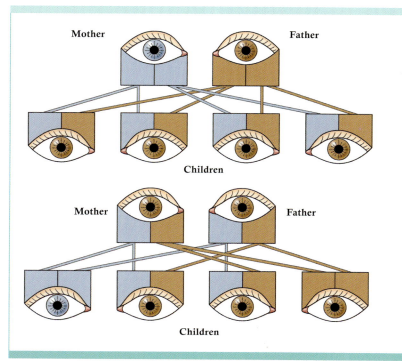

Mother   Father

Children

Mother   Father

Children

Dominant and recessive genes
When several different genes are found on a pair of chromosomes, the cell takes instructions from only one, the dominant gene. This masks those of the other, the recessive gene. For a recessive gene to succeed, a child must inherit from its parents two copies of the recessive gene.

Blue or brown eyes?
If both parents have one gene for brown eyes and one for blue, each of their children has a three in four chance of having brown eyes.

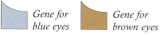

Gene for blue eyes   Gene for brown eyes

DEFECTIVE GENES

Occasionally genes are defective. But healthy genes are usually dominant over faulty ones. Some defective genes are carried by the sex chromosomes, and then the children of one sex only are affected. Color-blindness, for instance, is carried by some women on one of their two X chromosomes; since the normal gene on their other X chromosome is dominant over the faulty one, they are not color-blind. But if a boy inherits an X chromosome with a faulty gene, he has no other X chromosome with a healthy gene to dominate it, so he is color-blind. Hemophilia is passed on in the same way.

If you are anxious about the possibility of your children inheriting any diseases or disabilities from your family or your partner's, tell your doctor before you become pregnant, if possible. Failing that, as soon as your pregnancy is confirmed, ask to talk to a genetic counselor. All hospitals have access to a genetic counselor who can tell you the mathematical chances of bearing a child with a disability and the tests that can be carried out (see pages 226–237). If you are carrying an abnormal child, your pregnancy can be terminated if you wish. Nobody has to agree to termination of pregnancy.

THE BEGINNING OF PREGNANCY

The genetic makeup of the future child is decided at the moment of fertilization. But conception is a process, not a split-second event. Immediately after it has been penetrated, the egg starts to divide. It divides repeatedly as it is swept along the Fallopian tube to the uterus, which it reaches seven days after leaving the ovary. By then it is a ball of cells, called a blastocyst, like a tiny blackberry but hollow in the center. The blastocyst floats in the cavity of the uterus until about the tenth day, when it embeds itself into the uterine lining. Some blastocysts do not manage to root themselves into the wall of the uterus, and are swept out with the next menstrual period. Conception is complete only when the blastocyst has nested in the wall of the uterus. You have not yet missed a period.

IMPLANTATION

The cells now number hundreds. The blastocyst releases enzymes that penetrate the lining of the uterus, causing tissues to break down and blood and cells—on which the blastocyst feeds—to seep out. It is a kind of nourishing soup. The quality depends on the state of the lining of the uterus. Sometimes this is not as rich as it needs to be and as a result there is a miscarriage, which resembles a late and heavy period, without your ever realizing you have been pregnant. An inadequately nourishing uterine lining is one cause of infertility.

EARLY DEVELOPMENT

During the second week of the fertilized egg's life, the cells become differentiated. One set becomes the amniotic sac, an envelope of salty fluid in which the baby will later grow. Another cluster develops into the yolk sac, from which the embryo can make blood corpuscles. Yet another group becomes the placenta (see page 76). In between these are other rapidly developing cells that will form the baby. These cells are at first just an embryonic disc, but they grow lengthwise in the third week until there is a head and a tail end, with the yolk sac attached by a stalk to the middle of the disc.

At this point you are only about one week past the date when you expected your period to come. Although you cannot be sure, perhaps you suspect that you are pregnant.

SIX WEEKS PREGNANT It is three or four weeks after the meeting of sperm and egg, two weeks since you missed your period. According to the medical method of dating pregnancy (see page 24), you are five or six weeks pregnant. The cluster of living cells has developed into an embryo. There is a neck and a head with rudimentary eyes and ears, a brain, and a heart that is already beating, though it has only two chambers instead of the four that will develop shortly. There is a bloodstream and a digestive system, kidneys, and a liver, and tiny buds that will become arms and legs.

A rod of cells develops—the notochord—which later becomes the spine. The embryo develops from the head end down, so that at this stage the lower part of its back is barely formed and looks more like a tail. In fact, while now the size of a coffee bean, it looks like a miniature sea horse.

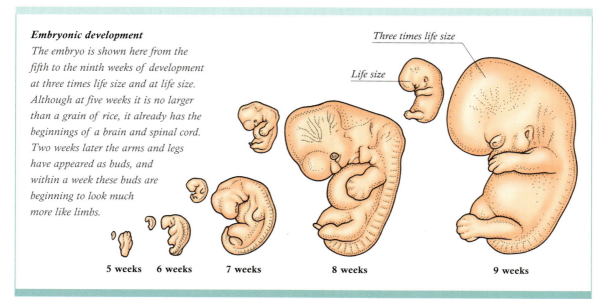

Embryonic development
The embryo is shown here from the fifth to the ninth weeks of development at three times life size and at life size. Although at five weeks it is no larger than a grain of rice, it already has the beginnings of a brain and spinal cord. Two weeks later the arms and legs have appeared as buds, and within a week these buds are beginning to look much more like limbs.

Three times life size

Life size

5 weeks   6 weeks   7 weeks   8 weeks   9 weeks

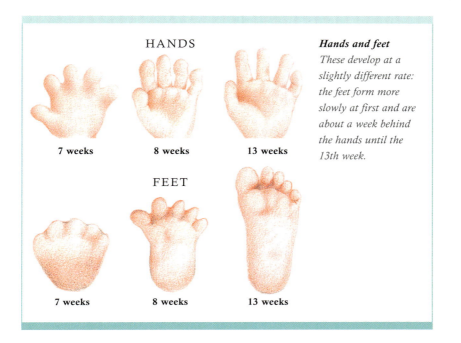

HANDS

Hands and feet
These develop at a
slightly different rate:
the feet form more
slowly at first and are
about a week behind
the hands until the
13th week.

7 weeks   8 weeks   13 weeks

FEET

7 weeks   8 weeks   13 weeks

SEVEN WEEKS PREGNANT A week later the embryo is about the size of a baby broad bean. Its body has plumped out into a baby shape, although the head is at a strange angle in relation to the body. It has nostrils, lips, and a tongue, and even the buds of its first teeth. Four chambers have developed in the heart. The limb buds have grown into arms and legs, although the hands and feet are just ridges.

EIGHT WEEKS PREGNANT The baby is still smaller than your little toe. It floats in the amniotic sac like an astronaut in space, attached to its life-support system. The heart has started the vigorous pumping of blood that will continue for a lifetime. The brain shows through skin as thin as wax paper, revealing every tiny branching blood vessel beneath. The jaw is not yet fully formed, and the ears are slung low and have not been molded into their correct position. The eyes are covered by an intact skin, which will eventually split to become eyelids. The head of the embryo is huge in relation to its body. The limbs elongate; elbows and knees begin to appear. Even now the baby is trying out some gentle kicking, although you cannot feel any movement.

All the organs and features of the embryo are completed in the next month. The face grows from the top, and as the lower parts form, the neck is elongated and a chin develops. The nose and outer ears are completely constructed. Fingers and toes are visible, although webbing stretches between them. By the time you are 12 weeks pregnant (see page 77), the basic physical equipment of your baby is in working order. The head is still big for the body and the limbs small; few muscles are working yet. All the internal organs have formed and some of them are functioning. The genitals have developed, but it is not yet easy to tell what sex the baby is. The umbilical cord has started to circulate blood between the baby and membranes attached to the wall of the uterus. At this stage, the baby begins to rely on these membranes for nourishment and the placenta starts to function. From now on, the developing baby is known as a fetus, and the rest of its time in the uterus is spent on growth and maturation.

THE PLACENTA

In the early weeks, one cluster of cells begins to develop into the placenta, an organ grown especially to nourish the baby and to excrete its waste products. The outside layer grows into a membrane with hundreds of tiny roots that penetrate the uterine tissues.

Your blood does not flow directly into the baby. It passes across tissues on the maternal side of the placenta, and the baby's blood passes back across tissues on the other side. The two bloodstreams are separated by the membrane. Chemical substances are diffused from one bloodstream to the other, but the bloodstreams themselves normally never mix. (Some fetal

FETAL CIRCULATION

This diagram shows blood that has received oxygen through the placenta traveling along the umbilical cord toward the fetus. Before it reaches the fetal heart, it mixes with deoxygenated blood that has already circulated through the fetus. This travels through the heart and is pumped up into the head and around the body, becoming less oxygenated. The blood then returns to the placenta via the heart again, most of it bypassing the lungs. At birth, the blood vessels around the baby's navel are sealed off, and the lungs take over the vital function of oxygenating the blood.

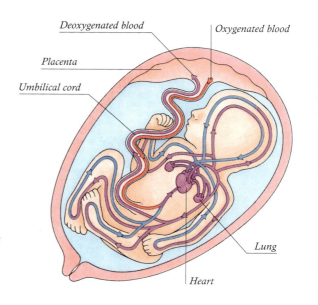

Deoxygenated blood

Oxygenated blood

Placenta

Umbilical cord

Lung

Heart

blood cells do cross the placenta, but usually without any significant effect.) The baby can thus have a different blood group from yours, while still taking nourishment from your blood. In the same way, the baby's waste products are passed back through the placenta into your bloodstream, to be filtered and excreted by your kidneys.

Although the baby makes breathing movements, it does not really breathe inside you: it takes its oxygen from your blood and passes back carbon dioxide. The oxygen diffuses through the membrane in the same way that oxygen from air passes through the lining of your lungs. The placenta works rather like a coffee filter: the coffee grains never enter the pot, but substances from them filter into it.

Changes in your blood as a result of stress, illness, or toxic substances will affect the quality of the substances that flow through the membrane. Blood takes only half a minute to flow from the baby's heart to the placenta and back again to the baby's heart. The flow of blood through the placenta in the fourth month of pregnancy is about 7.5 gallons (27.5 liters) a day, and by the end of pregnancy 87 gallons (330 liters) of blood are passing through the placenta each day.

As the placenta starts to function, it gradually takes over production of a range of hormones, including estrogen and progesterone, from the glands that normally secrete these hormones. Estrogen and progesterone control most changes in your body during pregnancy. Estrogen stimulates the growth of the uterus and the development of new uterine blood vessels, and causes the milk glands in your breasts to develop so that you can feed the baby. Progesterone prevents the uterus from contracting strongly and endangering the baby, and holds off the start of labor until the baby is at term. When the baby is ready to be born, the progesterone level drops. By this time the uterus has become exquisitely sensitive to the level of hormones in the blood, so that when the placenta reduces its output of progesterone, estrogen takes over, initiates labor, and ensures that the uterus begins to contract strongly.

THE GROWING BABY

It is a moving experience to picture how your baby is developing inside you as you share the nine-month journey to birth. If you already have other children, they will probably be excited by this, too.

AT 12 WEEKS The fetus has a large head and small, rounded rump; the sex organs are distinguishable though incomplete. Eyes are closed, the retina dark and round through translucent skin. Toes and fingers are formed. Arms are the right length in proportion to the body, and nails are beginning to grow. The ribs and spine are starting to harden into bone, and the fetus is moving. You cannot feel these movements, but it is kicking, curling its toes up and down, rotating ankles and wrists, clenching and unclenching its fists, pressing its lips together, frowning, and making other facial expressions. The fetus is also swallowing amniotic fluid, gurgling it from its mouth or passing it out through its bladder. There is still plenty of room in the uterus, so it can swoop and undulate in its own enclosed sea.

AT 16 WEEKS Although the fetus is growing rapidly, it could still nestle easily into a teacup. Its face is developing specifically human features, although the chin is still small and the mouth wide. The eyes are huge, closed, and spaced far apart. The baby is covered with a fine down, called lanugo. This is the earliest stage at which you may first become aware of movements. At first these feel like butterflies or little fish zigzagging around in bursts of activity, but soon they are unmistakably the kicking and lunging movements of a live being deep inside your body.

AT 20 WEEKS The baby is half as long as it will be at birth and about as heavy as a medium-sized Spanish onion (8 oz or 225 g). You could still hold it in the palm of your hand. The closed eyes are bulbous, because the face has not yet plumped out. Hair on the head is starting to grow and there are delicate eyebrows. The movements are becoming more complex and the baby may suck its thumb.

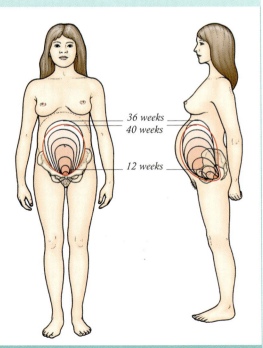

The changing uterus
The uterus expands throughout pregnancy, but the increase in size is not usually visible until the fourth month. From the 12th week it enlarges until the 36th week, when the fundus (the top of the uterus) is just below the breastbone. In women having their first child, the baby sometimes engages in the pelvis at about this date, so the fundus descends slightly, even though the uterus has not shrunk.

36 weeks
40 weeks

12 weeks

There are times when your baby is asleep and times when it moves actively (often when you have just settled down to go to sleep yourself). This seems to be partly because when you lie down it is easier for the baby to move. When moving around, you automatically rock the baby in your pelvis, so when you are busiest the baby is often asleep.

AT 24 WEEKS The baby is about 13 in (33 cm) in length. It is covered with vernix, a creamy substance that protects its skin inside the uterus and prevents it from becoming waterlogged. The vernix sticks to hairy parts, and many babies are born coated with it. Your baby may respond to loud noises and to music, especially to the brass section of an orchestra or a rock concert, and leap around. The sound-wave patterns of babies' cries and of adult speech can be recorded by spectographs. The spectograph of a baby's first cry can be matched with that of its mother's speech. This is the case even if the baby is born in the seventh month. The baby has been listening to its mother's voice and has learned her speech characteristics. Your baby is now considered legally viable. If it is born, it must be registered as a birth. If the baby dies, it is now a stillbirth rather than a miscarriage.

AT 28 WEEKS If born at this stage, a baby has a 60 to 70 percent chance of survival with modern intensive care—higher in some hospitals. The main problem is that the baby's lungs have not yet developed bubbles of surfactant, the substance that prevents complete collapse of the lungs between each breath. Another problem is that there is very little fat under the baby's skin, so its temperature control mechanisms cannot yet work efficiently.

The baby has filled all the available space in the uterus. Most babies turn upside-down at some point during the seventh month and then seem to fit more comfortably.

By now you may be able to distinguish the baby's bottom from a foot or a knee. When you lie in the bathtub you can enjoy watching the baby swivel from one side of your abdomen to the other. Foot and knee movements are more jerky than whole-body movements. At this stage, other people may be able to feel the baby kicking when they place a hand on your abdomen. Throughout later pregnancy, you can often anticipate periods of most hectic movement; many babies are at their most energetic between eight and eleven in the evening.

AT 32 WEEKS By the eighth month, the baby lacks only some lung surfactant and a good layer of insulating fat before it is ready to be born. Movements are vigorous: the prods coming from the feet are so energetic that they may make you catch your breath. Every now and again the baby may jerk spasmodically in what can be an alarming manner; some women worry that their babies are having seizures. But it is usually an attack of hiccups, brought on perhaps because the baby has been gulping amniotic fluid.

AT 36 WEEKS At some point between 36 weeks and term (which is around 40 weeks from the first day of your last period), the baby will probably descend into the pelvis with its head firmly fixed like an egg in an egg cup. It is then said to be "engaged"; this is a good sign and one indication that the baby can pass through the pelvic cavity without difficulty. Once your baby has engaged, you can often feel the head like a coconut hanging between your legs. It is not comfortable to sit down suddenly on a hard chair, and you may also feel sensations in your vagina like mild electric shocks (see page 238).

When you are examined lying flat on your back, the baby's head may not seem to be engaged. But if you sit up, the head engages.

After the baby has engaged, its larger body movements tend to be more limited. You probably feel only the kicking of legs and feet, the action of the head as it uses the pelvic floor as a trampoline, and the fainter movements of the arms. However, no day should pass without some lively indications from the baby of its presence (see page 245).

The last weeks may be tiring and tedious. The baby is three times as heavy at birth as at 28 weeks. It now weighs from 5½ to 11 lb (2.5 to 5 kg), and is between 18 and 22 in (45 and 55 cm) long. It is ready for its journey to life.

PATTERNS OF GROWTH

Babies do not all grow at exactly the same rate. One baby may weigh nearly twice as much as another, yet both are normal. A steady increase in your weight during pregnancy is reassuring because it suggests that the baby is growing well. Many women, however, experience a plateau in weight gain at some stage of their pregnancy, only to put on more weight again by the next prenatal checkup.

QUICKENING

The moment when a woman first becomes aware of her baby's movements is very important, and has been throughout history. It even has a special name—quickening. Italian paintings celebrated the meeting between Elizabeth, who was pregnant with John, and her sister Mary, pregnant with Jesus. When the two women reached out to each other, Mary's baby "leapt within her."

For centuries pregnancy had little social acknowledgment before quickening occurred. Only after quickening was the baby considered to be a "life." And only a woman knew when it had taken place. It was her personal experience. Neither medicine, church, nor state controlled that.

Today, doctors claim "bonding" can be achieved via ultrasound, and after the scan at 16 to 18 weeks many women are handed a photograph of a spotted image of the baby. There have been studies of the effect on pregnant smokers who see their babies on the ultrasound screen, and it did not reduce their smoking. Whether ultrasound promotes bonding probably depends on the quality of communication during the scan.* A woman should have a chance to discuss what she sees with the obstetrician or radiologist, and what the baby looks like and what it is doing.

You may treasure a photograph of the ultrasound image. It is proof that there really is a baby, that it has tiny limbs, feet and hands, and is even sucking its fingers. On the other hand, it may not feel quite right. It may seem like an intrusion. Women somehow bonded with their unborn babies long before ultrasound was invented. They did not need the external image because they cherished the internal reality—the bumps, twists, turns, and kicks that assured the mother that she was cradling life within her, and were part of the continuing communication between her and her baby.

"I LOOKED FORWARD TO REST TIMES NOT JUST BECAUSE I COULD RELAX, BUT BECAUSE THOSE WERE SPECIAL TIMES FOR ME AND THE BABY TOGETHER, AND I COULD STROKE MY BELLY AND TALK TO HER."

It is thrilling when you first feel your baby move. But it is more than that. It is the start of a journey shared by a pregnant woman and her unborn child in which they are—quite literally—in touch with each other. You carry on an intimate conversation. Sometimes you press your hand firmly over the baby's back and the rapid movements are stilled. You have soothed your baby. You massage around where the baby lies and it is as if you are playing together—the baby rolls, dips, and dances in response. You exercise on all fours and the baby drops away from your spine, cradled by the muscles of your abdominal wall. It seems that it is joining in the exercises. As the weeks pass, your baby can hear the rumblings of your digestive system, the steady beat of your heart, and noises from the outside world—the vacuum cleaner, the bark of a dog, and the zoom of an aircraft, music, television, and radio programs, the chattering of children, and your voice with its modulations of mood and intensity, changing rhythms and pitch, speaking, singing, whispering, and humming. By the 24th week, the baby is starting to listen to and learn the sounds of language. A woman who listens to her baby, knowing that her baby is listening to her, is already bonding with her baby months before she holds her newborn in her arms.

FORTY WEEKS OF LIFE

The next six pages show stages of development of a baby from the moment of conception to its last week in the uterus. The illustration below shows the five-day journey of the egg along the Fallopian tube, where it is fertilized, to the uterus.

THE UTERUS AND FALLOPIAN TUBES

Nestling deep inside the pelvis between the bladder in front and the intestines at the back, the uterus is cupped by springy pelvic floor muscles (see page 118). The Fallopian tubes branch out at either side, ending in fronds—like those of a sea anemone—that hold the ovaries.

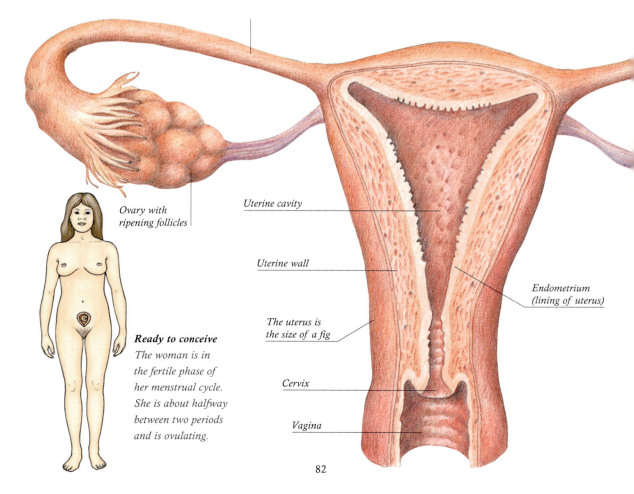

Ovary with ripening follicles

Uterine cavity

Uterine wall

Endometrium (lining of uterus)

The uterus is the size of a fig

Ready to conceive
The woman is in the fertile phase of her menstrual cycle. She is about halfway between two periods and is ovulating.

Cervix

Vagina

A RIPE EGG IS RELEASED FROM THE OVARY

The egg is ready for fertilization for only 12–24 hours. A sperm burrows its head into the egg. The sperm's tail drops off. The egg absorbs the sperm. In three days there is already a cluster of 32 cells, and within five days a cluster of 90 cells.

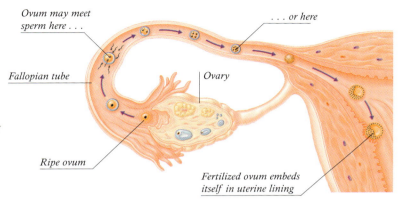

Ovum may meet sperm here . . .

. . . or here

Fallopian tube

Ovary

Ripe ovum

Fertilized ovum embeds itself in uterine lining

THE GROWTH OF THE CELL CLUSTER

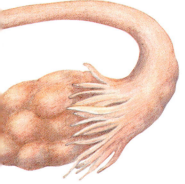

Each Fallopian tube ends in fronds

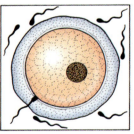

1 One of the sperm that has arrived in the Fallopian tube penetrates the ripe egg.

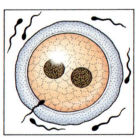

2 The head of the sperm separates from the tail and approaches the egg's nucleus.

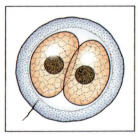

3 The chromosomes of the two nuclei pair off to create a two-celled egg.

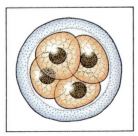

4 The two cells divide as the egg continues its journey along the Fallopian tube.

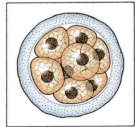

5 As the cells continue to divide they gradually get smaller and smaller.

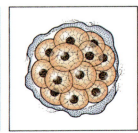

6 On about the fifth day the egg reaches the uterus and loses its jellylike coating.

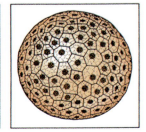

7 Six or seven days after fertilization the egg embeds itself in the uterine lining.

DEVELOPING FETUS

It is exciting to think how your baby is growing and changing. You don't have to rely on diagrams in a book or an ultrasound picture to know the baby inside you. For thousands of years, and all over the world, pregnant women have been in touch with their babies inside them through being aware of fetal movements. You can feel the kicks, twists, and turns that tell you that your baby's limbs are strong and growing fast.

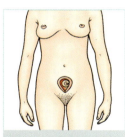

Pregnant!
The uterus is still hidden inside the pelvis. The pregnancy is dated from the first day of the woman's last period— before she conceived.

EIGHT WEEKS PREGNANT

The baby is just under 1 in (2.5 cm) long. The bones of its arms and legs start to harden and it makes slight movements, still too feather-light for the mother to notice. The face is developing. Sometime during this week the baby starts to open its mouth and the upper palate forms. The lower jaw is taking shape, with muscles that will enable the baby to suck and chew. The sound-perceiving mechanism of the ear has now developed.

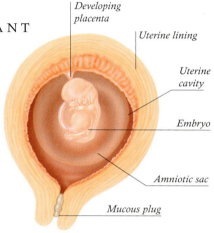

Developing placenta

Uterine lining

Uterine cavity

Embryo

Amniotic sac

Mucous plug

The embryo in the uterus

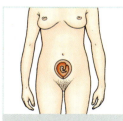

The metabolism adjusts
The growing uterus can now be felt through the abdominal wall. The woman may be feeling tired as her body adapts to pregnancy.

TWELVE WEEKS PREGNANT

The baby is now just over 2 in (5 cm) long. It has developed sexual organs that later will show whether it is male or female. Its head is more rounded and it is no longer so top-heavy: it is about two-thirds the size of the body. The eyes are widely separated in a broad face. The jaws have 32 permanent tooth buds and the baby is starting to suck. It is already exercising the muscles that will be used in breathing after birth.

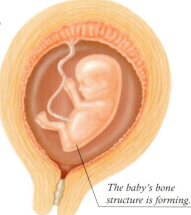

The baby's bone structure is forming.

From embryo to fetus

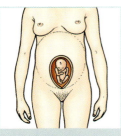

Your baby is kicking
The top of the uterus reaches to just below the navel. The mother can feel the baby's movements, especially when she rests.

TWENTY WEEKS PREGNANT

The baby's rapid rate of growth slows down a little at this stage. It is about 10 in (25 cm) long from head to toe. The legs are the right length in proportion to the body, and there are miniature toenails and fingernails. The baby kicks, twists, jumps, and somersaults. Hair on the baby's head and delicately etched eyebrows have appeared, and there is fine, downy hair called lanugo over much of the body.

The baby swallows amniotic fluid and may sometimes have hiccups.

The skin becomes smoother as fat is laid down.

The fetus in the uterus

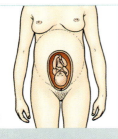

Mid-pregnancy
The fundus is in line with the top of the hips and the mother may be gaining ½ lb–1 lb (225 g–450 g) a week.

TWENTY-FOUR WEEKS PREGNANT

The baby is thin and its skin is wrinkled. A network of veins and arteries shows through the translucent skin. The face is now fully formed and the eyes are rather prominent because fat pads have not yet built up in the cheeks.

The network of blood vessels in the placenta supplies everything the baby needs for rapid growth.

A rich cream called vernix covers the skin and protects it.

The fetus and the uterus are growing

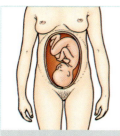

Four weeks to go

The top of the uterus reaches its highest point, just below the breast-bone. The mother may feel heavy with her pregnancy. The ligaments below her abdomen may ache, and standing for any length of time is uncomfortable.

THIRTY-SIX WEEKS PREGNANT

There is no longer enough room in the uterus for the baby to move around freely. It has settled into one position and the main movements the mother feels are jabs from the arms and legs. By now the skin is smooth and peachlike and the body has plumped out. When the baby is awake, the eyes are open, and it is aware of strong light flowing through the tissues of its mother's abdominal wall. If it is born at this time, the baby has an excellent chance of survival.

In comparison to the rest of the baby's body, the arms and legs are thin and have yet to fill out.

Fine hairs (lanugo) and creamy vernix begin to disappear from the skin, although some may remain at birth.

By this time, most babies have moved into a head-down (cephalic) position ready for birth.

The baby turns head down in the uterus

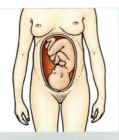

Impatient for the great day

The uterus has moved down a little into the pelvis, so the fundus has dropped slightly. The mother may feel very warm most of the time because her circulation is at maximum efficiency.

FORTY WEEKS PREGNANT

The baby is now about eight times bigger than it was at three months, when all its vital organs were formed, and has increased in weight approximately 600 times. Most of the lanugo has dropped off, although there may still be some down the center of the back, in front of the ears, and low on the forehead. The fingernails extend beyond the fingers and may need cutting at birth so that the baby does not scratch its face.

The baby almost fills the uterus, and there is less amniotic fluid than there was a few weeks ago.

The arms and legs are now plump and well rounded—the baby is fully formed.

In a first pregnancy, the head may be engaged in the pelvis. In subsequent pregnancies, this may not happen until labor begins.

The baby is ready to be born

EXPECTING TWINS

Finding out that you are going to have twins usually comes as a shock. Some women suspect quite early in their pregnancy that this will be the case, especially if they have had a singleton pregnancy with which they can compare this one.

If you are a fraternal (nonidentical) twin (see right), you are about twice as likely to give birth to twins yourself as are other women. The chances of having fraternal twins depend on heredity, age, race, and the number of children you have already had. Although fraternal twins often skip a generation, the chances of their occurring in successive generations are high. The frequency of identical twins seems independent of these variables.

MIXED FEELINGS

However, if nothing has led you to suspect that you are carrying more than one baby, it can be very upsetting to be told, after an ultrasound scan or a prenatal visit (see page 48), that suddenly all your expectations of birth and the time afterward need readjusting. If you are to be a mother for the first time, the natural apprehension you originally felt about the labor and how you would cope with a new baby may be even greater. Added to this, you wonder how you will manage two babies at the same time in all their noisy reality—two mouths to feed, two diapers to change each time, two babies to bathe, two loads of clothes to wash, two budding personalities who will need your love and attention.

"THE CONSULTANT HAD FAITH IN ME AND DIDN'T INTERVENE. HE SAID THE AIM WAS FOR ME TO HAVE THESE THREE BABIES MYSELF. BY TELLING ME HOW WONDERFUL I WAS, HE GAVE ME COMPLETE CONFIDENCE IN MY OWN ABILITY."

One woman, who was dismayed on hearing that she was expecting twins, said that she never really veered from this attitude throughout her pregnancy. During a hospital stay in her eighth month of pregnancy, she took the opportunity to watch mothers who had just given birth to twins, and felt that all her worries were justified, since they seemed to have such trouble in managing two babies. However, shortly after her twins were born, she told me eagerly about the totally unexpected delight of being able to breast-feed both of her babies, often simultaneously. She did admit, though, that it was hard work at first and said that "the intense joy and delight the babies now give has only come as we have gotten to know them."

HOW TWINS ARE CONCEIVED

Normally, conception occurs when one egg released from a woman's ovary is fertilized by one sperm from a man's testes. Seven out of ten pairs of twins are the result of the woman releasing two eggs, which are then fertilized independently by two different sperm (fraternal twins). Usually, the two eggs then implant and develop separately in the uterus. Less commonly, one egg fertilized by one sperm divides, resulting in two developing babies with the same inherited characteristics (identical twins). Often this division occurs after implantation in the uterus.

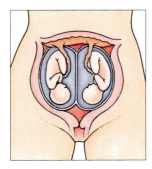

Identical twins

Monozygotic or identical twinning takes place after, rather than at, fertilization, and it often occurs after implantation in the uterus. As a result, twins almost always share a placenta, although each has its own cord and bag of water.

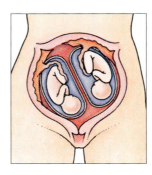

Fraternal twins

Dizygotic or fraternal twins have separate water bags, cords, and separate placentas. Occasionally, the two eggs implant close together in the uterus, so that the placentas become fused and it looks as if there is only one.

Monozygotic (one-egg) or identical twins

Dizygotic (two-egg) or fraternal twins

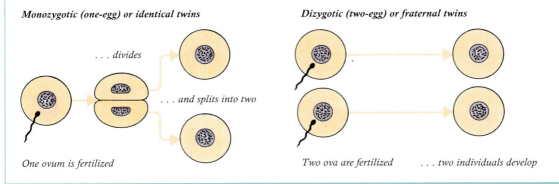

... divides

... and splits into two

One ovum is fertilized

Two ova are fertilized

... two individuals develop

Sometimes a woman is unhappy to discover that she is expecting twins because she has been planning a home birth and this may no longer be possible. Doctors and midwives nearly always advise hospital birth for twins, since the chances of a complicated delivery, especially for the second twin, are increased and the babies may be preterm and underweight. If you go to term, however, and both babies have grown well and are head down, you may decide on a home birth after all.

POSITIONS OF TWINS IN THE UTERUS

Twins fill the available space in the uterus more quickly than a single baby,
so they may adopt the positions in which they will be born at an earlier stage.
The pictures below show fraternal twins (with two placentas), but the
same positions apply to identical twins (with a single placenta).

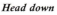

Head down

*This presentation, with both twins in the
cephalic or head-down position, is the most
common. It is also the most straightforward:
birth should present no special complications.*

Head down / breech

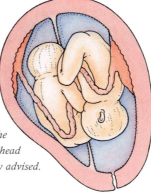

*When one twin is head down
and the other is head up, the
breech baby is often born
second. The first baby opens up
the birth canal so that the
breech baby can usually be born
vaginally without difficulty. If the
first twin is breech and the second head
down, Cesarean section is usually advised.*

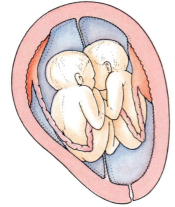

Both breech

*If both babies are breech, the risk
of complications will be evaluated
in advance. Cesarean section may
be performed in preference to a
vaginal delivery.*

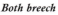

One transverse

*When one baby is lying
transversely and the babies are large,
a Cesarean section will be carried out. If
the babies are not large, it is usually possible
to turn the second baby after delivery of the first.*

On the other hand, a woman may be overjoyed to find that she is going to have twins. Perhaps she had wanted more than one child, but was not particularly enjoying her pregnancy and certainly not looking forward to another. Suddenly she discovers that she can have two children for the price of one pregnancy and labor!

GETTING ENOUGH REST

The first thing to accept is that a pregnancy with two babies tumbling around inside can be more of a strain than an ordinary pregnancy. The risk of developing preeclampsia (see page 141) is higher; the babies are more likely to be born preterm, and they may not be very strong. Because they have to share the space in the uterus and the nutrition available through sometimes only one placenta, twins are often of low birth weight. You will feel better if you have regular rest times and frequently go to bed early. You need help with housework and cooking and someone who will, at least occasionally, bring a delicious meal to your bed. If you already have other children, it is worth making an effort to find some motherly (or fatherly) person who can look after them for an hour or so each day so that you can relax without feeling that you will be needed in a minute. Many obstetricians advise women pregnant with twins to get more rest. However, there is no evidence to support the value of total bed rest in twin pregnancies.* Plan ahead and see if you can reorganize your life to allow you to get enough rest at home.

Plan the things you can do in bed: read, write, sew, learn a new language, take up a craft you have always wanted to try your hand at. If you think for a moment about the extra demands made on your body by a multiple pregnancy, you will realize that your whole system has to adjust to the babies' needs. This adjustment involves widespread metabolic changes. Extra pressure is put on your digestive organs and on your diaphragm and lungs, as well as stress on bones (on your lower ribs, which tend to splay out, and your spine, for example). Your muscles, too, have to cope with much of the stress of a twin pregnancy, especially your tummy muscles, your pelvic floor, and the muscles of legs, feet, arms, shoulders, and back, which have to support the extra weight and do the work of lifting and coping with your body mechanics. Above all, there is a general crowding out that may make you feel very full and heavy.

So rest will help your body adapt to the increased demands made on it by a multiple pregnancy. And the rest that helps most is rest that you decide to take before you become exhausted and irritable and before you feel that you cannot carry on a minute longer.

"WITH THREE UNDER TWO I KNEW I WOULD BE STRETCHED. SO BEFORE THE BIRTH I RESTED ON THE BED SO THAT THE OLDER ONE GOT USED TO PICTURE BOOK, MUSIC, AND CUDDLE TIMES, AND ANDY TOOK OVER IN THE EVENINGS."

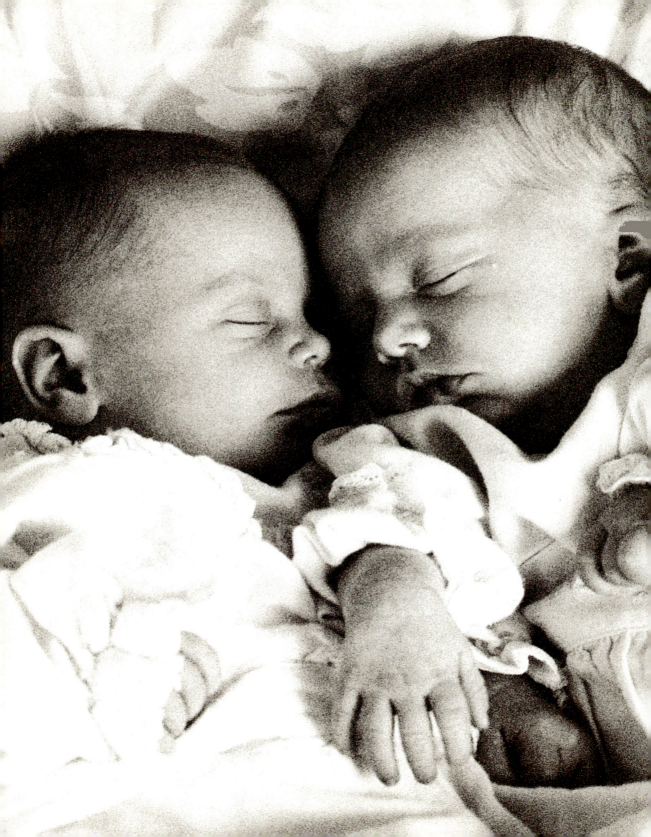

LYING COMFORTABLY

You may find it very uncomfortable to lie flat. Your heavy uterus is pressing on major blood vessels in that position, too, so, both for your own comfort and for the blood supply to the babies, lie either well propped up or in the "three-quarters-over" position. Prop your breasts with one pillow and put two under your upper knee if this feels good. Even more than with a singleton pregnancy, special back supports may be needed. A large bean-bag may feel comfortable; and so might a contour pillow used with other pillows, two firm foam wedges, or the kind of cushion that is sold for making it comfortable to read in bed. Whatever you choose, get something solid that will support the exaggerated curve of your lower spine.

POSTURE AND EXERCISE

Sensible body mechanics are also more important when you are expecting more than one baby (see pages 122–129). Learn how to counteract the effect of the enlarged and heavy uterus by standing straight and tall, with tail tucked in. Aim to balance on the balls of your feet rather than going flatfooted and waddling like a duck, which is only too easy to do when you are overtired.

Above all, learn how to get up from a lying-down position by rolling over, if necessary kicking off with your foot and hand against solid objects, and then rising onto all fours.

"I'VE NEVER BEEN CRAZY ABOUT EXERCISES, BUT I LIKE THE IDEA OF KEEPING MUSCLES TONED ACTIVELY, HAVING A BODY THAT'S ALIVE."

Pelvic floor toning activity (see pages 120–121) is very important, whether you are carrying one baby or two; with twins it will be especially vital after the birth, as the muscles around the vagina have been stretched by the extra weight of two babies. It is a good idea in any case to do these movements from early pregnancy, before there is any appreciable change in weight, as muscle tone is really best built up before there is any particular stress on the muscles. If your pelvic floor muscles are under a great deal of strain, you can do these movements while lying on the floor with your lower legs raised on a chair. In this position weight is not pressing on the pelvic muscles, and it is easier to feel what is happening there. In advanced pregnancy, however, when the babies are low down, it may be impossible to use this position. Try letting your pelvic muscles "dance" when sitting propped up with pillows.

You will probably be aware of the babies moving a great deal inside you. Your abdomen feels like a basket full of puppies. It can be difficult to sleep and you are often awakened by all the internal activity. Practicing release from tension and letting muscles relax all over your body can help enormously. Some mothers worry that with all this movement the babies are in danger of harming each other.

Your babies may look like two peas in a pod, but they already have distinct personalities.

They can certainly shuffle each other up a bit, but each one is sealed off in its own bag of waters. Fluid cushions the babies from shock and allows free movement until the very last weeks of pregnancy, when the pelvic girdle cradles the babies so closely that you may feel only small movements.

NUTRITION

For a discussion of diet in pregnancy, see pages 96–101. The demands made on your body by a twin pregnancy require even more careful attention to diet than in a singleton pregnancy.

The more tired you get, the more you may feel that you cannot be bothered to prepare nutritious meals and shop for food. But your health depends on your having a good diet and not skimping on protein, vitamins, and minerals. To save laboring over a hot stove, have at least one raw food meal a day, which will give you a good supply of vitamins. Is there any chance of getting help with a supermarket run? It is important that you do not lift boxes and bags into the trunk yourself or attempt to unload them! A growing number of supermarkets will now arrange home delivery. Or, you might find this is the best possible time to get to grips with shopping online.

Twins may seem a bit daunting at first, but you will be surprised by your remarkable ability to cherish them both.

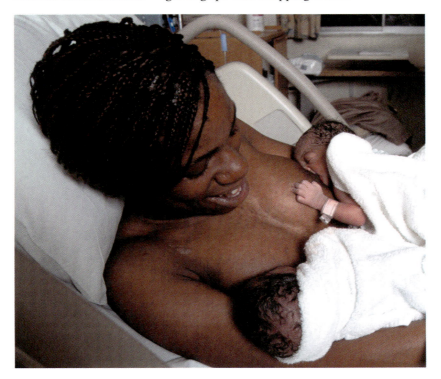

YOUR BABIES, YOUR BODY

When a woman is pregnant with more than one baby she tends to become "an interesting case." You are much more likely to have interventions of all kinds with a multiple pregnancy and be led to doubt your body's ability to give birth. I remember when I had my own twins I was warned about the possibility of "locked twins" (when the head of one baby is twisted around the head of the other), but discovered from searching through obstetric textbooks that this is an extremely rare condition.

You may be particularly lacking in confidence about the birth if your babies were conceived by IVF because of fertility problems. It may feel as if other people are making all the decisions for you. Think through what you really want.

Certainly you don't need a Cesarean section simply because you are having twins or even triplets. If you have had a Cesarean before, your obstetrician may suggest that the babies should be delivered this way, but if you prefer to give birth vaginally, make your wishes clear. There is no evidence that birth is more dangerous for the babies if you go into labor naturally and see how things go. And you are much more likely to avoid infection and hemorrhage if you give birth vaginally.

"ALTHOUGH THEY WERE IVF BABIES, I DIDN'T SEE WHY THE BIRTH SHOULD BE HIGH-TECH. I WANTED TO GIVE MY BODY A CHANCE TO WORK AND TO TRUST MY INSTINCTS."

Bear in mind that a multiple pregnancy may increase your blood pressure, cause aches and pains and varicose veins, and put stress on your pelvis, simply because there are two or more babies bouncing around in there and being nurtured by your body. Yet there is no reason that the whole experience of pregnancy should be medicalized. It can be an exciting and happy experience in which you are in charge. Examine the evidence, weigh the advice the professionals give you, and come to your own decisions about the birth.

YOUR BABY'S WELL-BEING

Looking after yourself in pregnancy, from the very first weeks, is probably more important for the welfare of your baby than anything else you can do. It ensures that you provide the best possible environment for the developing baby—and, equally important, it gives you the best chance of being healthy and full of vitality, ready for the birth day and the first stages of motherhood.

NUTRITION

If a woman is nutritionally deprived, her baby is deprived, too. She is more likely to have a miscarriage, and her baby is more likely either to be born prematurely or to be of low birth weight. Research studies also show that poor nutrition in late pregnancy can affect a child's brain development.* It may have a long-term effect on health. A baby who was deprived in the uterus tends to become an obese adult and to develop type 2 diabetes.

Food intolerance is common in the first weeks of pregnancy. If you are suffering from nausea and vomiting, you may be anxious that you are depriving your baby of essential foods. In many traditional cultures, it is believed that the baby asks for the foods it wants and rejects others. So it is important to give a pregnant woman exactly what she craves because it is her baby speaking through her.

When you vomit, your body is refusing food with which it cannot cope. Trust your feelings and eat what you want. Do not worry that you are not getting a "balanced diet." In a few weeks you will enjoy a wider range of foods. Metabolic changes that take place in pregnancy mean that you make better use of the food you eat, and this increased efficiency extends into the period of breast-feeding, too.*

WOMEN AT RISK

Some women are "at nutritional risk" and need to pay special attention to diet. They include teenagers who are still growing themselves, women who are very overweight or underweight, and those who eat from a very restricted range

Take time to enjoy food during pregnancy and eat plenty of fresh fruits and vegetables.

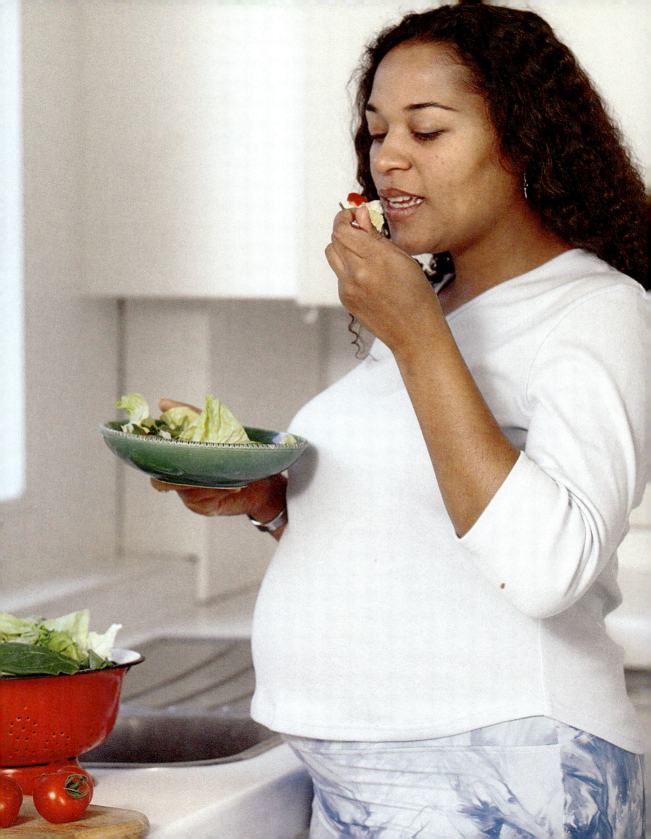

of foods (a macrobiotic diet, for instance). Women who have lost a baby from miscarriage or stillbirth or have had three pregnancies within two years are also at risk. Then vitamin and mineral supplements may be a good idea.

YOUR WEIGHT

It is normal to put on between 24 and 32 lb (11–14.5 kg) during pregnancy. Some women put on more with no ill effects. Do not assume that because your baby will weigh only 6¼–8½ lb (3 to 4 kg) at birth, the rest is fat. Consider the weight of the placenta, membranes, and amniotic fluid, and the increase in size of the uterus and breasts and in the volume of your blood. Fluid retention also accounts for a substantial weight gain in some women. All these things return to normal after the birth.

It is impossible to be dogmatic about how much weight you should put on, because different women gain weight at different rates. Medical opinion is that "arbitrary weight restriction is potentially harmful to both mother and baby."* If you start pregnancy underweight, you and your baby may benefit from a bigger weight gain than a woman who starts pregnancy overweight. However, if you start pregnancy overweight, you are likely to put on more weight than a woman who is of average weight at the onset of pregnancy, and are also more susceptible to conditions such as high blood pressure and urinary tract infection.*

One way of checking to see whether you are putting on superfluous fat that may be hard to lose in the months after the birth is to measure your upper thighs each week. The measurement should stay about the same throughout your pregnancy.

WEIGHT GAIN IN PREGNANCY

Since most women gain weight at different rates, it is impossible to say how much weight you should put on. However, if you are seriously overweight or underweight this may lead to complications during pregnancy and labor.

Proportions of weight gain	
Your total weight gain in pregnancy is made up as follows:	
Weight of baby	38%
Weight of placenta	9%
Weight of amniotic fluid	11%
Increase in weight of uterus and breasts	20%
Increase in weight of blood	22%
Total weight gain	**100%**

Timing of weight gain	
0–12 weeks	5%
12–20 weeks	20%
20–30 weeks	50%
30–36 weeks	25%
36–40 weeks	0%

So you can assume that if, for instance, you are 30 weeks pregnant, the weight you have gained in pregnancy will be about 75% of your total weight gain.

PROTEIN

Every day have one dish from each of the following categories: (a) meat or fish, two eggs, a cup of peanuts or cashew nuts; (b) 4 oz (100 g) of hard cheese, 8 oz (200 g) cottage cheese, or 1 pint (500 ml) of milk (or soy products or tofu); (c) four slices of whole-wheat bread, some brown rice, or whole-wheat pasta, or one large potato baked in its jacket. If you are vegan, have a good helping of legumes instead.

CARBOHYDRATES

You need to eat carbohydrates for energy. Whole-wheat bread provides B vitamins, iron, and the fiber that helps to prevent constipation. If you are already overweight, or are putting on a lot of superfluous fat, try to cut out white flour and sugar and products containing them.

MILK AND DAIRY PRODUCTS

Milk is usually recommended, but you do not need more than 1 pint (500 ml) a day. If you fill yourself up with milk, you are likely to dampen your appetite for other foods that you and your baby need. Some women who do not like milk or are allergic to it never drink it, and their babies are fine.

VITAMINS

Most vitamins should come from food, not supplements. A varied diet that includes vegetables, fruits, and nuts will supply all the vitamins necessary for you and your developing baby. Research suggests that vitamin E, found in fresh fruits and vegetables and oily fish such as herring and sardines, is of particular value because it boosts the baby's immune response to allergens and may reduce the risk of asthma.

FOLIC ACID

From conception and through the crucial early weeks, the baby's spinal cord is being formed. If the spine does not close up properly, the baby is born with spina bifida, which can result in paralysis and incontinence. If the brain and skull do not develop properly, the baby is anencephalic and is unable to survive. Taking folic acid supplements (0.4 mg) in the first 12 weeks of pregnancy cuts the risk of having a baby with spina bifida or other neural tube defects by up to 70 percent. Folic acid supplements also reduce the risk of cleft palate.

When women who have previously given birth to a baby with a neural tube defect take folic acid supplementation (4 mg daily) for a month before conception and up to the second missed period, they are much less likely to have another baby with a disability. All women are now advised to take folic acid supplements (0.4 mg daily) as soon as they try to become pregnant.

MINERALS

If you are eating plenty of foods rich in protein and vitamins, you are unlikely to suffer from any mineral deficiency.

IRON is necessary for the formation of red blood cells. If blood contains insufficient hemoglobin, not enough oxygen is carried to your baby and you get very tired. Vitamin C helps your body to absorb iron, whereas antacid medicines stop you from benefiting fully from it. Good sources of iron include dark molasses, egg yolk, whole grains, dried peas and beans, all dark green leafy vegetables, raisins, prunes, brewer's yeast, and nuts.

Extra iron is often prescribed in pregnancy, but if you eat foods rich in iron, you should have good reserves stored in your liver and should not need to take iron supplements. The fetus draws on these reserves, so that it can store enough in its liver to last several months after birth. If you were anemic before pregnancy, a supplement is a good idea. Iron supplementation is not necessary for the normal drop in hemoglobin that occurs from mid-pregnancy onward. It is a sign that plasma volume is rising and that the placenta is providing good nutrition for the baby (see page 76).

CALCIUM is necessary for the formation of strong bones and teeth. It enables blood to clot and muscles to work smoothly, and may protect against high blood pressure and preeclampsia. Oxalic acid in spinach and cocoa reduces absorption of calcium. You baby's teeth start to bud very early in pregnancy, so your calcium intake in the first four months matters a great deal. Milk and dairy foods are useful sources. Calcium is also found in leafy vegetables, seaweed, whole grains, legumes, nuts, and carrot juice.

MAGNESIUM levels in pregnant women are often low. This may be one cause of muscle cramp. Magnesium may also help prevent preeclampsia. Good sources are cereals, nuts, soybeans, milk, fish, and meat.

ZINC deficiency may result in miscarriage, growth restriction in the uterus, stillbirth, or congenital handicap.* Zinc is necessary for muscles to contract well, and, although it is difficult to measure zinc in human tissues, shortage is a cause of long labor.* Iron supplements can interfere with the absorption of zinc. High-fiber foods—especially bran—contain zinc, as do Brazil nuts, Parmesan and other hard cheeses, seeds, herring, and meat.

SALT AND FLUID RETENTION

It used to be thought that salt was dangerous in pregnancy and a cause of preeclampsia (see page 141), but when a group of expectant mothers were given no-salt diets, they had more preeclampsia than a control group who had as much salt as they wished.* Cutting out salt can also cause cramps in hot weather.

Occasionally, special diets are prescribed to reduce fluid retention, but these can harm the unborn baby. Women with mild fluid retention (edema) usually produce babies in just as good a condition as those who have no signs of it at all. Ankle, foot, and leg swelling on very hot days, or after standing for a long time, is nothing to worry about. If your skin is looking puffy, check that you are eating enough protein (see page 99). If your fingers and face get swollen, mention it to the doctor or midwife, since it may be a sign that your kidneys are not coping well with the excretion of waste products and that the placenta is not working well.

"MY FEET SWELLED UNCOMFORTABLY IN THE HEAT WHILE I WAS PREGNANT, SO I SHOWERED MY LEGS WITH COLD WATER AND RESTED WITH MY FEET UP."

Cutting down on your intake of fluids will not prevent edema. So drink as much liquid as you want. Four or five glasses of water a day will help your kidneys to function well.

DRUGS

Around 25 percent of all birth defects are genetic in their origin. Around 65 percent have an unknown cause. Only 2 to 3 percent are caused by drugs. This is partly because the total amount of water in a woman's body goes up by 17 pints (8 liters) in pregnancy, so drugs are more diluted.* On the other hand, the range of substances to which the embryo may be vulnerable is not yet known. So it is wise to take the fewest possible medicines during pregnancy, especially in the first few weeks when the embryo is forming and when the placenta is only just starting to be active. (Be careful during the second half of the menstrual cycle if there is any chance that you might be pregnant.) It used to be thought that the placenta acted as an effective barrier to poisons present in the maternal bloodstream, but it is now known that drugs can cross the placenta and may affect the baby.*

If you think of how the fertilized egg has to segment, travel along the Fallopian tube, embed itself into the lining of the uterus, and develop into a baby, you can imagine how such delicate and complex processes can be interfered with by poisons in your bloodstream.

The liver and the kidneys are the organs of your body that deal with drugs and turn them into material that can be excreted in the urine. In an unborn—and even a newborn—baby, these organs are still immature. The fetus is therefore not able to excrete many of the drugs that may reach it through the placenta. Instead, such drugs can accumulate in its tissues in toxic quantities. It is vital to remember, when taking any drug, that a dosage that may be right for you is far in excess of that which is suitable for your tiny baby. There was, for example, the thalidomide disaster, when a sedative that was thought to be mild and safe was prescribed for women in early pregnancy. As a result, more than 5,000 babies were born with badly deformed limbs or none at all. Thalidomide is an extreme example of the effect that a drug can have on the development of an unborn baby. But all drugs, including prescribed drugs, medicines bought over the counter such as laxatives and painkillers, and nicotine and alcohol, are potentially harmful if misused. Think carefully before taking any drug when pregnant, especially in the early weeks.

Drugs known to cause abnormalities are said to be "teratogenic." In the first few days of a pregnancy, any toxic or teratogenic drugs would probably prevent the egg from ever settling firmly in the uterus, so that you would not even realize that you were pregnant but would just have a delayed period. If you were to take the same drug slightly later, you would probably miscarry. At a later stage still, the pregnancy might continue, but there would be a risk of the baby's being damaged by the drug.

If the cell cluster is damaged some time between conception and 17 days, either it dies and there is a very early miscarriage, it is reabsorbed into the mother's tissues, or the embryo survives intact because cells multiply to replace those that have been lost. Organogenesis, the development of the different parts of the baby's body, takes place during the period 18 to 55 days from conception. After 56 days, drugs do not cause major disabilities, although they may reduce growth and cause loss of function.

WEIGHING THE RISKS

Some pregnant women need drugs and may be very ill without them. Illness in the mother can also affect the developing baby. For instance, running a very high temperature (see page 111) seems to be teratogenic at certain phases of pregnancy, so it may be safer to take acetaminophen to get your temperature down than to try to cope without taking any medicines. It is always a question of balancing the risks to the baby against your need and the stress that may be caused to you by not having drug treatment.

Since the thalidomide disaster, there has been acute awareness of the need to screen all new drugs before they are prescribed. However, drugs that have been in use a long time remain on the market without being tested. It is difficult to be certain about any drug, because safety testing is often done using animals; what is safe for one species may not be safe for another.

People are often ignorant about the chemicals they introduce into their bodies. Antacids for the relief of indigestion, cough medicines, sleeping pills (barbiturates), antihistamines used in the treatment of hay fever, and antibiotics are commonly used drugs that alter the body's chemical balance. Many pregnant women take over-the-counter drugs, homeopathic and herbal remedies, and prescribed drugs in the first weeks of pregnancy, and no one is sure of the risks. There are other substances that you may not think of as being drugs, including cigarettes and alcohol. Even tea and coffee have been researched for possible harmful effects, although normal use (up to half a dozen cups a day) seems to be fine.*

SMOKING

Whether or not you inhale, nicotine passes into your bloodstream and into the baby's bloodstream. It makes the fetal heart speed up and interrupts the respiratory movements that are the baby's rehearsal for breathing. In effect, the unborn baby coughs and splutters. Smoking also affects the efficiency of the placenta and is the most efficient way of pumping a powerful poison into an unborn baby's bloodstream. Nicotine makes the blood vessels in the placenta constrict so that less oxygen and fewer nutritional substances reach the baby. Mothers who smoke bear babies who weigh less than babies of nonsmokers—the baby's weight drops in relation to the number of cigarettes smoked.* This does not mean that some smokers do not have good-sized babies, but that, statistically, babies of smokers are deprived of

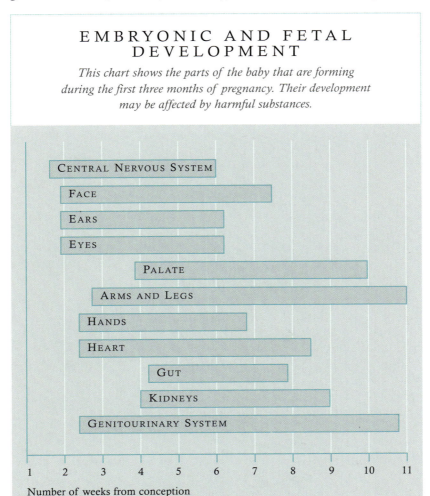

EMBRYONIC AND FETAL DEVELOPMENT

This chart shows the parts of the baby that are forming during the first three months of pregnancy. Their development may be affected by harmful substances.

Central Nervous System
Face
Ears
Eyes
Palate
Arms and Legs
Hands
Heart
Gut
Kidneys
Genitourinary System

1   2   3   4   5   6   7   8   9   10   11

Number of weeks from conception

the best possible nutrition. It is not just that a woman who smokes tends to eat less. Cigarettes have a direct effect on the baby's growth and development.*

Some women make the mistake of thinking that labor will be easier if their babies are lighter. Labor with a tiny, underweight baby is no easier or shorter than labor with a good-sized baby, and your baby is much more likely to be healthy and easy to care for if you have not smoked during your pregnancy. Underweight babies also cope less well with the stress of labor.

Smoking after the fourth month of pregnancy is a major cause of prematurity and the birth of underweight babies who are stunted in development and may have to be cared for in the intensive nursery. Smoking also increases the chances of bleeding, miscarriage (women who smoke are twice as likely to miscarry as those who do not), premature rupture of the membranes, premature separation of the placenta, hemorrhage before or early in labor, hemorrhage after delivery, congenital abnormality, stillbirth, and death of the baby in the week following delivery.* The more a woman smokes, the higher the risk.

If a woman does not smoke herself, but her partner does, she and the baby are exposed to secondhand smoke, and fetal growth may be affected.*

HOW TO GIVE IT UP If you are a heavy smoker and dependent on cigarettes to get through the day, it may be very difficult to give them up, even for the sake of your baby. Fortunately, the nausea of early pregnancy or just a sudden dislike of cigarettes prompts many women to cut them out.

"ACTUALLY, IT WAS VERY EASY TO GIVE UP SMOKING BECAUSE I COULDN'T STAND THE TASTE OR SMELL OF CIGARETTES IN THE FIRST COUPLE OF MONTHS. I CUT OUT COFFEE FOR THE SAME REASON."

If this does not happen spontaneously, you can use the techniques of aversion therapy to condition yourself to break the habit. Every time you feel queasy or vomit, make yourself think "cigarette" and use the association between vividly picturing the act of smoking and the overwhelming sensations of nausea to train yourself to develop a dislike of cigarettes.

HOW TO CUT DOWN If you are past the nauseous stage of pregnancy or feel perfectly fit throughout, as many women do, you can still try to reduce your cigarettes to at least half the usual number. Ask your partner to help by cutting down his consumption in the same way; if the two of you are making the same effort, your determination is strengthened. Also, cutting down on smoking is a concrete way in which your partner can contribute to your baby's health, by reducing the amount of passive smoking to which you are subjected. The more you can both cut down on your general consumption of cigarettes, the better.

You may be feeling guilty about smoking while still being unable to give it up, but the guiltier you become the more you want a cigarette in order to help you calm down. It is certain that guilt and emotional stress can also affect your metabolism adversely, including your heart rate, blood pressure, breathing, muscle tone, and the adrenaline in your bloodstream. So how much stress should you tolerate in trying to give up smoking? If you know how to release tension, you may be able to cope by smoking each cigarette only halfway down and still find that it helps you enough to be able to "unwind."

This is where your own judgment of the relative importance to you of smoking or not smoking in pregnancy is essential. Every pregnant woman has the right to be fully informed of the risks of smoking and to make her own decision on the subject during pregnancy. No one can *make* you stop smoking, however many warnings they give: you decide. On the other hand, your baby cannot choose whether or not to smoke. You choose for your child.

ALCOHOL

Alcohol may be socially acceptable, but you should limit your intake in pregnancy. Fortunately, many women develop an aversion to it. Alcohol crosses the placenta, and the baby's blood levels are about the same as the mother's. The risk the baby incurs from alcohol depends on how often you drink, how much you drink, and the baby's stage of growth. Alcohol in early pregnancy is more likely to have a bad effect, and even a single "binge" can cause damage to the baby.

"AT THE RESTAURANT, I ORDERED A GLASS OF WINE. THE WAITER SAID, 'HAVE APPLE JUICE!' I FELT SO ANGRY; I HAD NO RIGHTS, NO CHOICES."

It depends on your metabolism, too. Some women cannot break alcohol down into harmless substances, so it passes through the placenta in its poisonous form. Heavy, chronic alcohol use can cause fetal alcohol syndrome (FAS). The baby looks a bit like a pixie with big ears and may be mentally and developmentally retarded.

It is probably best to avoid alcohol altogether during your pregnancy, as some fetuses may be more susceptible to even small amounts.

BEING CAREFUL ABOUT DRUGS

Ask your doctor's advice about any drugs you may be taking when you intend to conceive. Do not wait until your first prenatal visit or even—if possible—until you are sure you are pregnant. If there is a chance that you might be pregnant, avoid taking any drugs that are not essential.

If a doctor other than your obstetrician is treating you, especially in the early months of pregnancy before it is obvious that you are having a baby, make sure that he or she realizes that you are pregnant before prescribing. This is particularly relevant if you are ill when away from home and have to consult a different doctor.

Go through your medicine cabinet and ask your doctor which drugs are likely to be unsafe during pregnancy. Any that your doctor advises you to get rid of, as well as those that were not prescribed for you or that are out of date, should be disposed of in the same way you would dispose of toxic waste.

MOOD-ALTERING DRUGS

Because so little is known about the effect of mood-altering drugs, it is wise to limit their use or cut them out altogether. You may feel that marijuana or Valium helps you to relax on occasion when you cannot "switch off." But explore other ways of releasing tension. The effects of relaxation (see pages 189–191) are likely to help your unborn baby much more than anything you take in through your mouth. There are some positive things you can do, ways of tuning in to your body rather than making an attempt to escape from it or deaden its sensations.

MARIJUANA Little is known of the effects of marijuana on the baby. Its strength varies widely, and its effects on the user vary. It has been claimed that marijuana can be teratogenic, but this is still being investigated.

COCAINE Whether inhaling a powder (snorting), smoking it (crack), or injecting it (shooting up), a woman using cocaine is very likely to have a baby who is small for dates or premature, and who is addicted to the drug. Cocaine can also cause placental abruption (separation prior to birth). These babies tend to be irritable and jumpy, and it is difficult to calm them down enough to take a satisfying feeding.* Heroin has similar effects.

TRANQUILIZERS Powerful tranquilizers such as chlorpromazine (Thorazine) and haloperidol (Haldol) should be avoided in pregnancy unless essential. If you think you might have conceived, talk it through with your psychiatrist and with a pediatrician. A milder tranquilizer may be sufficient to control your anxiety and reduce tension. Strong tranquilizers taken in labor may make the baby lethargic or stressed and trembling at birth.

SLEEPING PILLS

Try to avoid sleeping pills in pregnancy, even though your sleep may be disturbed. Avoid long-term use. Your baby will be affected and may suffer withdrawal problems after the birth. Treat insomnia with relaxation, exercise in the open air, an aromatherapy bath at bedtime, and lavender essential oil sprinkled on your pillow.

PAINKILLERS

It is best to avoid painkillers in pregnancy. Acetaminophen is the safest. Try relaxation, slow, full breathing, and fresh air (pages 189–191) to avoid headaches, and gentle exercise (pages 130–132) for muscle aches and pains.

ASPIRIN is best avoided at high, painkilling doses, though it is used in much smaller doses for women with recurrent miscarriages or a history of severe preeclampsia. In high doses it can affect labor or your baby's blood clotting and its heart. Codeine is safe to use occasionally. But taken for long periods, it can result in withdrawal problems for the baby after birth.

ACETAMINOPHEN is the best painkiller, since it seems to be safe for the baby. But don't exceed the dose stated on the package.

IBUPROFEN, mefenamic acid (Ponstan), Naproxen, and all other nonsteroidal anti-inflammatory drugs (NSAIDs) are best avoided. There are safer alternatives.

ERGOTAMINE, used in drugs to treat migraines, can cause your uterus to contract, possibly endangering your baby. Discuss alternative ways of treating migraine with your doctor.

ANTINAUSEA DRUGS

Drugs for nausea and vomiting are of three different kinds: anti-cholinergenic drugs, antihistamines, and phenothiazines.* All have side effects. The first category treats nausea by acting on your nervous system; it reduces secretions, including stomach acid, and relieves muscle spasm. No one can be sure whether these drugs are completely safe for the fetus. Antihistamines block the action of histamine (a substance produced in allergic reactions) and may cause drowsiness. The newer antihistamines are best avoided, but promethazine (phenergan) appears safe for occasional use. Phenothiazines are major tranquilizers and should be avoided.

Drugs to control nausea should not be used unless prescribed by a doctor who knows you are pregnant, and then only when you have weighed the advantages and disadvantages of taking the drug. Do not take any pills for motion sickness if you think you may be pregnant.

ANTIBIOTICS

Antibiotics may be prescribed in pregnancy. They are sometimes necessary, and any disadvantages to the baby are outweighed. Tell your doctor that you may be pregnant, or remind a doctor that you are pregnant when antibiotics are being prescribed for you. Never use leftover antibiotics that were prescribed for a previous infection, even if you know you have the same type of illness.

PENICILLIN (and derivatives such as ampicillin and amoxicillin), cephalosporins, and erythromycin can be taken without risk, but avoid co-amoxiclav. Do not take nalidixic acid, nitrofurantoin, or chloramphenicol in the last three months of pregnancy.

METRONIDAZOLE is generally safe during the second and third trimesters, but not in high doses.

AMINOGLYCOSIDES (gentamicin, tobramycin, and streptomycin) cause deafness in the baby (especially streptomycin).

TETRACYCLINES should not be used. They can affect the baby's bones and discolor the teeth.

DRUGS TO TREAT CONSTIPATION

Constipation is common in pregnancy, but extra fluids alone may be enough to cure it, especially if you adjust your diet to include a regular intake of bran. (See page 135 for more advice and information.)

STOOL BULK PRODUCERS, such as Metamucil, do no harm if taken with plenty of fluid and used in moderation.

STIMULANT AND SALINE LAXATIVES, which include senna-based laxatives such as Senokot, and milk of magnesia, seem to be safe, but they may cause premature contractions.

VARIOUS TYPES OF OIL will lubricate the bowels. However, avoid mineral oil, because it reduces the absorption of vitamins A, D, and K. Lack of vitamin K may lead to disorders of blood clotting in the baby.

DRUGS TO REDUCE FLUID RETENTION

Diuretics increase the excretion of salt and water from the body, and make your kidneys work very hard. They should not be used unless with the guidance of a hospital obstetrician or physician. Contrary to previous beliefs, diuretics are not the right treatment for preeclampsia.

STEROIDS AND DRUGS TO TREAT ASTHMA

Steroids are used for the treatment of asthma and hay fever, eczema and other skin disorders, and rheumatism and arthritis. Severe and prolonged asthma attacks are more likely to harm the baby than the drugs that are used to control asthma.*

ANTIDEPRESSANTS

There is very little known about the effects of antidepressants on a baby's development. But tricyclic antidepressants do not seem to be teratogenic. The risk of miscarriage or of congenital abnormalities does not appear to be greater than if a woman is not taking these drugs. Because drugs like Prozac—which are very long-acting—have been around for a shorter period of time, psychiatrists frequently err on the side of caution and do not prescribe these drugs during pregnancy, even though there are no reports of harm to the baby.

If you suffer from depression in pregnancy, you may need treatment with drugs, and the possible risks of medication must always be carefully weighed against the risks of not having it. Doctors sometimes decide to take women off antidepressants once they are known to be pregnant. If you do need antidepressants, talk to your doctor about tapering them off gradually so that you are no longer having them about four weeks before the baby is due. Then you can, if necessary, go back on them after the birth.

ANTIPSYCHOTIC DRUGS

Clozapine should not be taken during pregnancy, since it affects bone marrow. It makes sense to avoid using antipsychotic drugs that have been on the market for only a short time, and to stick to what has been tried and tested, and to those drugs the side effects of which are already known. Antipsychotic drugs affect the newborn baby's behavior, and side effects in the mother will also appear in the baby after birth—if she is sedated, the baby will be too, for example—but these are reversible. However, in such cases, a pediatrician should be standing by at the birth to ensure that the baby is stabilized. Babies who have received antipsychotic drugs are more likely to have convulsions, and diazepam causes babies to

"I DISCUSSED TAKING THE DRUG WITH MY PSYCHIATRIST AND SHE SWITCHED MY MEDICATION TO ONE LESS LIKELY TO AFFECT THE BABY."

get jittery as they come off it. So these drugs should be tapered off four weeks before the birth or reduced by half. To give the baby the best chance of dealing with the stress of being born, as little as possible of any drug should be taken.

DRUGS TO TREAT THYROID CONDITIONS

You may need to take drugs for an under- or overactive thyroid, but these can affect the baby's thyroid. You should be referred to an expert. Discuss the drugs you are taking with your doctor, if possible before pregnancy.

ANTICOAGULANTS

These drugs are prescribed for deep-vein thrombosis or for a pulmonary embolism—both serious conditions that are caused by blood clots. Taken early in pregnancy, they may cause miscarriage. Anticoagulants can also cause hemorrhage in the baby. Warfarin is teratogenic and should be avoided in the first three months of pregnancy and the last six to eight weeks. If an anticoagulant needs to be given toward the end of the pregnancy, heparin by injection is the safest. Any adverse effects can be reversed by small doses of vitamin K given to the baby after delivery.*

DRUGS TO TREAT DIABETES

Injections of insulin are quite safe. If you are diabetic and want to get pregnant, let your doctor know so that you can discuss in advance exactly how you can have a healthy pregnancy (see page 142).

ANTICONVULSANTS

If you normally take anticonvulsants or antiepileptic drugs, discuss with your doctor the possibility of modifying or even stopping them before you conceive. They may cause cleft palate and other disabilities. No anticonvulsant is free of risk. Ask to see a specialist before you start your pregnancy, and begin taking 5 mg of folic acid daily while you are trying to conceive.

GENERAL ANESTHETICS

There are times when a general anesthetic may be necessary during pregnancy; but, if possible, it should be avoided because the baby will be knocked out, too. Make sure that your doctor or dentist knows that you are pregnant if he or she recommends general anesthesia for anything.

OTHER RISKS

If you are paying close attention to your own general health, there are only a few other risks to your baby that you may want to consider in pregnancy. They range from environmental hazards, such as X-rays and food poisoning, to pregnancy problems such as an incompetent cervix.

X-RAYS

The American College of Radiology advises "no single diagnostic procedure results in a radiation dose significant enough to threaten the well-being of the developing embryo and fetus." However, the cumulative doses from multiple procedures may enter the harmful range. Radiation can partially destroy the genetic material that acts as the blueprint for the normal development of each cell of the body. A damaged cell is called a mutation. Radiation can have the strongest effects on an embryo in the initial stages of development. A badly affected embryo is then likely to be aborted spontaneously. But X-rays taken in pregnancy can also have an effect after birth:* they have been associated with a higher than usual chance of the baby developing diseases of the respiratory system, blood disorders, and infectious illnesses in childhood.

There are some cases in which diagnostic X-rays are particularly important and the only means of discovering certain disorders during pregnancy. If a doctor or a dentist advises X-rays, take professional advice, but check first to ensure that they really are essential. Your abdomen and thyroid should be protected, where possible, during the X-ray by a lead shield.

HIGH TEMPERATURE

If you are running a temperature, go to bed, drink plenty of fluids, and sponge yourself down with cold water, or take cool baths or showers to lower your body temperature. Do not just let your temperature rise, since there is a slight chance that a very high temperature—say, over 102°F (39°C)—in the first four months of pregnancy can damage a baby.* The most crucial time is during the third and fourth weeks after conception. This is a horrifying thing to learn in late pregnancy if you know you had the flu earlier on, but most babies are born whole and healthy even when the mother has run a high temperature. Include a high intake of vitamin C in your diet, and have some protein each day to reduce the risk of infection. As far as we know, there is no real risk of serious damage to the baby from a high temperature after the 16th week of pregnancy, but you could make the developing baby's heart race by getting overheated yourself.

"IT'S LIKE WALKING IN A MINEFIELD— THERE ARE SO MANY RISKS! IN A WAY I THINK I'D ACTUALLY BE HAPPIER NOT KNOWING ABOUT ANY OF THEM."

Saunas and long, very hot baths can also produce a temperature high enough to harm a developing baby, so be sure to keep temperatures down. Your own comfort usually acts as the best guide to your baby's safety.

FOOD POISONING

There are very few foods that you absolutely must avoid in pregnancy, although you may develop strong cravings for some foods and an aversion to others. However, there is a handful of foods that are more likely than others to cause food poisoning, so it is best to steer clear of these.

LISTERIOSIS Soft and blue-veined cheeses and chilled foods like precooked delicatessen meats are sometimes contaminated with listeria if they are not stored at sufficiently low temperatures. Goat's milk, cheese, and yogurt should be pasteurized. The symptoms of listeriosis are similar to those of the flu. If a pregnant woman suffers from this, she may have a miscarriage, or her baby may be stillborn or have birth defects.

SALMONELLA Raw as well as partly cooked eggs are sometimes contaminated with salmonella, which causes food poisoning. It is wise for a pregnant woman to eat only eggs that have been thoroughly cooked, and to avoid eating mayonnaise and other dishes with raw egg as an ingredient.

TOXOPLASMOSIS This disease can have serious effects on the fetus. You can catch it from handling cat litter or soil containing cat feces, so always wear rubber gloves when emptying a litter box and then wash your hands. Also wear gloves when gardening and wash your hands afterward.

Toxoplasmosis is also a food-borne infection. Eat only meat that has been completely cooked. Be careful at barbecues, especially with kebabs. Meat should never be pink or bleeding, as it is with a rare steak. Do not eat raw, cured meat such as Parma ham. Wash your hands after handling raw meat and wash kitchen surfaces and wooden utensils. Because toxoplasmosis may be present in soil, vegetables and fruits should also be well washed. For more information see page 428.

MERCURY POISONING Mercury can cause birth defects. Fish contains higher levels of mercury than other foods, since metal is washed into the sea from natural and industrial sources. Carnivorous fish store methylmercury that they absorb from the smaller fish they eat, so avoid eating swordfish and any other large predatory fish.

VACCINATION

Vaccinations are not recommended during the first four months of pregnancy, when there is a small risk of damage to the fetus. In the later months, most vaccinations (apart from rubella; see below) are considered harmless, but you should avoid smallpox vaccination throughout pregnancy, especially if you have never been vaccinated against it before. If you are traveling to a country that insists on smallpox vaccination, obtain exemption with a certificate of pregnancy from your doctor.

RUBELLA (German measles) is such a mild disease that many people have it in childhood without knowing it. If you contract rubella when you are pregnant, the virus may cross the placenta, and in the first 20 weeks it can have a serious effect on the baby. Even if you were vaccinated against rubella as a child, it is sensible to have a blood test before you become pregnant. If the test shows that you have never had rubella, you can be vaccinated against it. If you are already pregnant and discover that you are not immune, you can be vaccinated immediately after the birth.

The protection afforded by rubella vaccination lasts at least seven years, and probably much longer. After vaccination, it may take as long as three months to build up immunity to the virus. It used to be thought that rubella vaccine was dangerous in early pregnancy, but research now suggests that babies of women who were vaccinated without realizing that they were pregnant are not at increased risk.* However, it would be sensible to use contraception during these three months.

If you were not vaccinated against rubella before pregnancy and have never had the disease, avoid all contact with children who might have it. If you think you have been in contact with rubella, your doctor will offer an injection of gamma globulin. The risk of the baby being damaged in the first three months of pregnancy is high, especially in the first 8 weeks. If you contract rubella, you may want to consider a termination.

THE RH NEGATIVE WOMAN

All blood is either Rh positive or Rh negative. By far the most common type of blood group is Rh positive. Some 86 percent of people are Rh positive, which means that their blood contains something known as the Rh factor. This factor is tested for early in pregnancy as part of your routine blood test. Its presence or absence is noted on your records but is important only if you are Rh negative and the baby's father is Rh positive. There is no problem if the baby is Rh negative. However, a small number of Rh positive babies of Rh negative mothers become anemic, and if this goes untreated the baby may die before or after birth. If you are Rh negative with an Rh positive baby and some of the baby's red blood cells leak into your bloodstream, a risk arises with the next pregnancy. This can happen after an accidental hemorrhage in pregnancy or at delivery, or if you have miscarried or had a termination. Your body responds to the Rh factor in the baby's cells as it would to an invader, and manufactures antibodies against it. When these antibodies pass from your circulation into the baby's circulation they start to destroy the baby's own red blood cells.

The flow of red blood cells each way across the placenta is not usually substantial enough during a first pregnancy to cause your body to develop antibodies, but it can occasionally happen. When your first baby is born, some of its blood may flow from the placenta into your circulation. This triggers antibodies to the Rh factor in your blood. From then on you produce antibodies, and the next time you are pregnant with an Rh positive baby your antibodies may increase rapidly if further Rh positive cells enter your circulation, and they will attack the baby's blood vigorously. It may get jaundice, its brain may be damaged, severe anemia may develop, and, in the worst cases, the baby may not even survive.

There are several things that can be done. The first and simplest is an injection of anti-D immunoglobulin at 28 and 34 weeks of pregnancy and another immediately after the birth of an Rh positive baby. This serum stops the mother's biological defense mechanisms from acting against foreign Rh substances. A fresh injection of this serum is given during and after each subsequent pregnancy. The same routine is followed after a miscarriage or a termination, since the fetus may have been Rh positive and some of its blood may have entered the mother's bloodstream.

It is no good giving this serum *after* a woman's body has produced antibodies. If a high proportion of antibodies is detected in your blood during a second or subsequent pregnancy and your baby is known to be at risk, you can have amniocentesis (see page 232). The amniotic fluid is analyzed for the presence of bilirubin (bile pigment), because an anemic fetus excretes large amounts of bilirubin from destroyed red blood cells.

A woman who is Rh negative and whose partner is Rh positive is tested for Rh antibodies at intervals throughout the pregnancy. If there are antibodies present, a blood test can be done on the baby inside the uterus, ultrasound being used to guide the needle into the umbilical cord. If necessary, the baby can be given one or more blood transfusions before birth, again using ultrasound to guide the needle. If the baby is sufficiently mature, labor may be induced early. The baby can be treated immediately after delivery, too, and given a complete blood transfusion that will eradicate all the antibodies from its bloodstream.

Since the introduction of routine anti-D protection for Rh negative women, and the administration of anti-D after birth to those with Rh positive babies, this problem is now rare.

THE RH FACTOR

An Rh negative woman rarely has problems with her first baby, since little blood crosses from the fetus to the mother during the pregnancy. However, at delivery some of the baby's blood cells can enter the mother's bloodstream. If the baby is Rh positive, the mother's blood develops antibodies. In a later pregnancy, these antibodies will cross the placenta and attack another Rh positive baby's blood.

The first pregnancy

The Rh factor is important only when an Rh negative woman is carrying an Rh positive baby. At delivery, some of the baby's blood may leak into the maternal blood. As a result, the woman develops antibodies that destroy Rh positive blood cells.

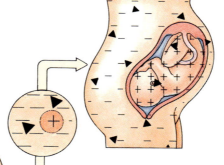

Each subsequent pregnancy

In a second pregnancy, these antibodies may cross the placenta. If the new baby is also Rh positive, its blood is damaged by the mother's antibodies.

The solution

Doctors inject a serum into Rh negative women at 28 and 34 weeks and within 48 hours of childbirth, or after a termination or miscarriage, to prevent creation of antibodies to Rh positive blood.

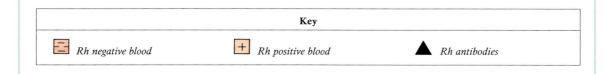

Key		
⊟ Rh negative blood	⊞ Rh positive blood	▲ Rh antibodies

AN "INCOMPETENT" CERVIX

Occasionally, a woman's cervix may be torn from a previous difficult labor or mid-pregnancy termination, or be damaged by a cone biopsy. She would not find this out until her next pregnancy, when she might lose her baby after the fourth month as a result of "cervical incompetence" (see page 388). The term "incompetent" is an unfortunate one and makes women feel as if they have failed to reach some standard of reproductive ability.

An obstetrician may recommend cervical cerclage—sewing the cervix closed for the duration of any subsequent pregnancy. This is a relatively simple procedure: once the pregnancy is established, a suture is inserted under anesthesia and is threaded through and around the cervix like the drawstring of a purse. It is removed at about the 36th week of pregnancy or later. Some obstetricians like to induce labor at this point because they say it is simpler, since contractions often start shortly after the removal of the suture anyway. You are not compelled to have labor induced, however, and should decide whether this is what you want. There is wide variation in the degree to which obstetricians in different countries use cervical cerclage. It is used a lot in some countries where there is a fee for performing the procedure. A random trial of cervical cerclage, conducted on women at high risk of giving birth prematurely, produced no evidence of its benefit.* Since twins and triplets are often born early, some obstetricians use cervical cerclage to try to prolong a multiple pregnancy. This does not work.*

PRETERM LABOR

If you pass blood (which could be coming from the cervix), feel a sudden rush of warm liquid from your vagina (which could be the membranes rupturing), or have regular contractions like menstrual pains that get longer, stronger, and closer together over several hours, chances are that you are going into labor. If this happens before you have reached the last month of your pregnancy, the baby may need special care at birth. So call your doctor or midwife, or go straight to the hospital. It is best for the baby to be born in a center that has intensive care facilities, with a neonatologist standing by in case the baby needs help with breathing.

If the baby is very premature, you will be given corticosteroids to mature the fetal lungs, which gives the baby a much better chance. Betasympathomimetics such as ritodrine and terbutaline are often used to stop contractions, but they don't work if your membranes have ruptured. These drugs may have side effects—a racing heart and high blood pressure, for example—so they are not always a good idea.

YOUR PHYSICAL WELL-BEING

To make the most of the experience of being pregnant,
you will want to get your body in good condition.
Healthy activity can be pleasurable in itself as well as
being an excellent preparation for labor.

Sometimes books on pregnancy and even childbirth educators give the impression that childbirth is an athletic event for which you have to train like a marathon runner, a kind of examination for which you must study assiduously, or even an ordeal with which you are unlikely to cope but which will be quickly forgotten afterward. No wonder expectant mothers become anxious! No mention is made of the excitement, joy, and sheer pleasure that many women experience in childbirth.

Most women look forward to childbirth with excited anticipation. They know that there is a slight chance of something going wrong but that the better they have prepared themselves with body-toning movements and exercises, the more likely they are to be able to handle any problems.

GETTING TO KNOW YOUR BODY

Before beginning exercises, it is useful to gain an awareness early in pregnancy of how your body works and what is taking place in your reproductive organs. One way of doing this is to have a closer look at your genitals. To get a clear view, you can kneel or squat over a mirror. A flashlight might help you to see the area better.

YOUR PERINEUM

The perineum is the tissue around your vagina and over the area between your vagina and anus. Just before delivery the perineum begins to bulge and its tissues fan out and open up as the ball of the baby's head begins to press through it.

YOUR VAGINA

The vagina is the soft, cushioned canal that is the passage through which the baby comes to birth. The outer part of the vagina is the vulva, consisting of layers of outer and inner lips (labia) constructed like the overlapping petals of a rose. During pregnancy, they change in color from red to violet as the blood supply to them is increased. Pregnancy hormones also darken your nipples, and you may notice dark patches on your face and on other parts of your skin.

Insert one or two fingers gently into your vagina and feel around the stretchy folds inside. Although the sides of the vagina normally touch each other and there is no space, notice how readily they spread apart. They open like an accordion when the baby is pressing down through them to be born, and the hormones that are released into your bloodstream make them even more flexible during the last few weeks of pregnancy.

YOUR CLITORIS

The clitoris is like a bud rising from the inner lips at the upper (front) end of your vagina. The base of the clitoris and the inner lips around it are very sensitive, and pressure on or stroking of these parts produces sexual excitement. As you touch its root, you may notice that it swells up. There is a hood or fold of skin surrounding the clitoris, and this connects up with the inner lips. So anything in your vagina that stretches the inner lips apart will also pull on this hood and stimulate the clitoris.

Women's genitals vary as much as men's. Just as penises are different sizes, the clitoris may be the size and shape of a small pea or more like the curved center of an orchid. Women's labia vary, too. Some are firm, some soft, some large and fleshy, others smaller. A woman may worry that masturbation might have changed their shape, but these organs are so flexible that pulling, pressing, or rubbing them does not produce permanent structural changes. Doctors and midwives cannot tell anything about your sexual habits by examining your vulva, although many women harbor a secret fear that they can, especially if they have suffered sexual abuse.

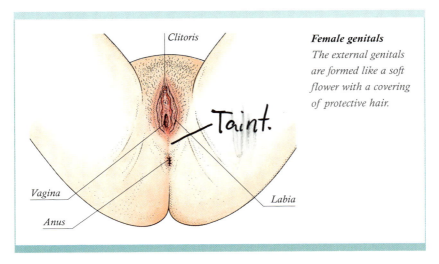

Clitoris

Taint.

Vagina

Anus

Labia

Female genitals
*The external genitals
are formed like a soft
flower with a covering
of protective hair.*

As it is born, the baby presses against this area, easing forward the tissues so that they open up like elastic, and then slides out with a rush of liquid. After the baby is born, these flexible tissues spring back again. At first they will not be as firm as they were before, but they will gradually gain in tone.

YOUR CERVIX

Now introduce your longest finger deep inside your vagina and you meet the rounded, firm cervix (the neck of the womb), the part of the uterus that will open (dilate) when you are in labor. Early in pregnancy it feels like the tip of your nose. You may notice a little dip in the middle, like the dimple in the center of a buttoned cushion. This is where the mucous plug is situated, and this plug, like the cork in a bottle, seals off the uterus from the outside. At the end of pregnancy, the cervix will have softened and, when you touch it, will feel more like your mouth when it is soft and relaxed than like your nose. This is a sign that you are ready to go into labor. The cervix is "ripe," and ready to open up.

YOUR PELVIC FLOOR

The muscles that support everything inside the pelvic cavity (including the uterus, the bladder, and the rectum) form the pelvic floor. They have special significance for your health, whatever age you are and whether or not you are pregnant. The upright position that humans have adopted in preference to the all-fours stance puts extra stress on these muscle layers in pregnancy.

Although these muscles form a coordinated working structure, they are not really a "floor" at all. They are slanted at different angles and levels and can be held with varying degrees of firmness. A woman may feel she is contracting her pelvic floor when she is contracting muscles in her buttocks or abdomen instead. The easiest way to feel these muscles is to

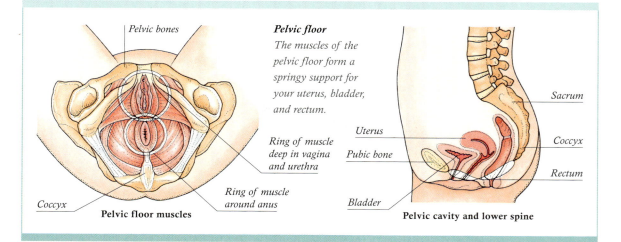

Pelvic bones

Pelvic floor
The muscles of the pelvic floor form a springy support for your uterus, bladder, and rectum.

Ring of muscle deep in vagina and urethra

Ring of muscle around anus

Coccyx

Pelvic floor muscles

Uterus

Pubic bone

Bladder

Sacrum

Coccyx

Rectum

Pelvic cavity and lower spine

interrupt a stream of urine, since you bring all of the pelvic floor muscles into play when you do this. Or you can think of them as forming a figure eight around the vagina and anus. In the middle of the eight is a horizontal bar, the transverse perineal muscle. When the muscles of the pelvic floor are contracted, the circular shapes of the figure eight change to almond shapes and the transverse perineal muscle is pulled toward the pubic bone (the firm ridge of bone just above the clitoris) like the opening lid of an old-fashioned rolltop desk. You can feel this from both inside and outside if you put one finger inside the vagina and a thumb over the pubis.

Your pelvic floor muscles contract spontaneously during lovemaking, increasing your sensations of pleasure and those of your partner. Awareness and control of these muscles is important in labor, too, when you need to release them as you press the baby down to be born.

Some people can hold their pelvic muscles contracted for much longer periods than others, and you may notice, when you first try to contract them, that they tire and tremble. To exercise your pelvic floor muscles gradually, pretend that this area is an elevator that you are taking up to the first floor. You hold it there, then move on to the second floor, and so on until the muscles are fully contracted. Then release them gradually to the ground floor. End with a toning movement by drawing the muscles up to the first floor again. If you do this 10 or 12 times a day, you will be able to hold them firm for longer periods, building up to a count of eight or nine without holding your breath or tightening your shoulders. But always remember to alternate tightening movements with resting spaces to allow the muscles to be reoxygenated in the intervals between activity.

CARING FOR YOUR SPINE

The spine is a flexible column of vertebrae that acts as the central scaffolding of the body and, because it is sinuous and lithe, enables all the parts that are attached to it to move freely. Your spine is not rigid like a lamppost. It is both strong and elastic. Caring for it properly depends on using it well. When it is used like a crane, you run the risk of backaches and back injury.

The section of the spine at the rear of the pelvis is the sacrum. It is the central pillar to which the pelvis is fixed. The large, flaring ilia, the bones that look rather like elephant's ears, are fixed to the sacrum by the sacroiliac joints.

The spinal vertebrae are cushioned by disks, rather like a dynamic hydroelastic pillow.* When you bend, these cushions soften the movement. When the vertebrae are pulled apart, the disks open up like segments of garden trellis. The disks contain fluid that is gradually lost during the day if you have been in an upright position, especially when you have been sitting a lot. For this reason, a person is nearly 1 in (2.5 cm) shorter at the end of the day than at breakfast time. Lying down enables the disks to fill up again, but they depend on *movement* to suck in fluid. In pregnancy, the sheer weight of your body, and the extra weight of the baby and its luggage, also sits heavily on disks in your lower spine. The result is that all this extra weight squashes them even more. The forward load produced by the increased size and weight of your uterus puts strain on the small of the back, and your upper spine may then be pushed into the wrong position in order to compensate. So to have a healthy back in pregnancy you need to use it wisely. This means knowing how to lift without strain and varying your position so that you do not sit still for long periods of time. It is a good idea to get your weight off your spine and on to all fours now and again and to have rest times when you lie on the bed. But rest is not enough. It is important to move around as well so that you plump up the disks. Dancing, pregnancy exercises, and swimming are effective ways of keeping the spine flexible and revitalizing the disks.

TONING YOUR ABDOMINAL MUSCLES

Four-legged mammals take the extra weight of pregnancy on their abdominal muscles, which are slung evenly between the front and back limbs. Despite their upright stance, human beings also need well-toned abdominal muscles because, if these are flabby, the back muscles are forced to compensate by taking on too much work to support the spine. When this happens, the vertebrae of the lower spine are forced into an unnatural position and the disks between them are subjected to a great deal of pressure. They may slide and become displaced. This leads to exhausting backaches. Girdles or "tummy control" panty hose and pants just take over some of the work that healthy muscles should be doing. The best girdle is composed of your own tummy and buttock muscles, and both sets need to be toned to provide mutual support.

The muscle running from top to bottom down the front of the abdomen, the rectus muscle, bears much of the load of late pregnancy. It is separated into two halves by a line down the center that is like a seam. When you are about halfway through pregnancy, this may show as a dark line in your skin from your navel down to your pubic hair line, although it does not occur in all women. You can see the same line as an indentation about the width of a pencil in photographs of Mr. Universe flexing his muscles and caving in his abdomen. The two sides of the rectus muscle can be pulled apart if it is subjected to great stress. Then it "unzips." Constipation and straining on the toilet can sometimes cause this muscle to separate as well.

You can test to find out if there is any separation of the rectus muscle. Lying on your back with a pillow under your head, rest your hands on your tummy and *very slowly* lift your head and shoulders with your chin tucked in.

If you feel a soft bulging area the width of a finger or more, the muscle has separated. You can rehabilitate it with exercises after the baby is born (see pages 416–419). Meanwhile, concentrate on leg sliding (see page 123). Some exercises intended to strengthen the abdominal muscles can cause the rectus muscle to separate. Do not try double-leg-raising exercises while you are pregnant, or even single-leg raising unless the muscles are already in very good condition. Nor should you do exercises that entail putting your feet under heavy furniture and then raising the upper body, or try sit-ups without using your hands. Not only can these exercises damage abdominal muscles, they can also strain the back.

EXPLORING PELVIC MOVEMENT

The bones that form the pelvis are like a cradle for the baby growing inside you, a cradle that can rock in all directions. Feel your pelvic bones with your fingers. Start with your hip bones. Press in over their upper ridges and then walk your fingers around and down into the small of your back where your hip girdle joins your spine. The point at which it does so is the sacrum, the bone that forms the back of the pelvis and the outlet through which the baby descends. Now walk the fingers around again to the big bones at the side, then down into the groin and around the front until they meet at your pubic bone. This forms the front of the pelvis, and the baby dips down under this bridge of bone just before birth. Notice that your pubis is much lower than your sacrum. The human pelvis is tilted. Once you have found exactly where these bones are and have a clear picture of them, get your partner to feel them, too. Guide his hands so that he is able to track your pelvis accurately.

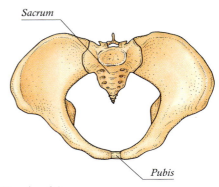

Sacrum

Pubis

Female pelvis
The female pelvis forms a kind of cradle for the developing baby.

PELVIC ROCKING

Lie on any flat surface (it can be a firm bed) with your head and shoulders supported by two pillows and your knees bent with the feet down flat. Explore the capacity for movement in your pelvis. Experiment with some gentle, rhythmic rocking. Then try rolling the cradle around as if you were doing a very slow hula-hoop movement. This is a kind of belly dancing while lying down, in which you tighten your tummy muscles while pressing your buttocks together. As you do so, notice how the different sets of muscles are alternately tightened and released and the way in which your tummy and buttock muscles work together in a coordinated fashion.

KEEPING IN SHAPE DURING PREGNANCY

When you are pregnant, it is easy to assume that sagging muscles are an inevitable accompaniment to weight gain and a changing figure. However, gentle toning exercises, aimed at firming up your abdominal muscles and avoiding back strain, do nothing but good. Stay aware of your breathing while you exercise, and never hold your breath.

PELVIC ROCKING

For this exercise, lie on a firm bed or on a mat on the floor with your head and shoulders supported by pillows, your knees bent and your feet flat. Experiment by pressing the small of your back against the floor or the bed and then releasing it so that you produce a gentle, rocking movement. Then roll your hips around in a slow, circular, hula-hoop movement.

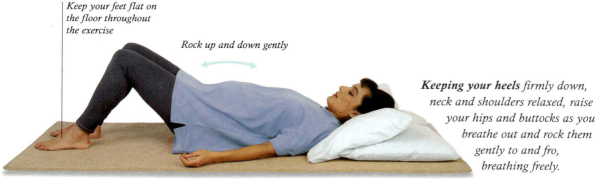

Keep your feet flat on the floor throughout the exercise

Rock up and down gently

Keeping your heels firmly down, neck and shoulders relaxed, raise your hips and buttocks as you breathe out and rock them gently to and fro, breathing freely.

Roll your pelvis in a circular motion

Relax and breathe easily as you roll your pelvis around, as if you were doing a slow, languorous belly dance while lying down.

EXERCISES TO AVOID

Double-leg raising and sit-ups are not recommended for pregnant
women. The abdominal muscles are not designed to cope with the effort
involved in raising the legs or trunk. If they are not strong to start with,
the result is back strain or torn abdominal muscles.

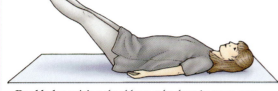

Double-leg raising *should never be done in pregnancy
or during the four weeks following birth.*

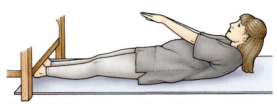

Sit-ups *should not be done with straight knees or back in
pregnancy or during the first six weeks after childbirth.*

LEG SLIDING

Leg sliding is a gentle exercise that allows
you to tone up your tummy muscles both pre-
and postnatally. Do it 5 or 6 times at first, and
gradually build up until you can do it comfortably
10 or 15 times. If you feel your back aching, stop.

Leg sliding is best done lying on your back on a firm
surface with a pillow under your head. Keep your
neck, shoulders, and arms relaxed. Follow your
breathing rhythm, moving on an out-breath, allowing
your breath to flow in between movements.

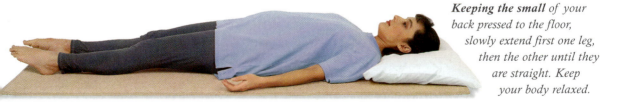

Keeping the small *of your
back pressed to the floor,
slowly extend first one leg,
then the other until they
are straight. Keep
your body relaxed.*

*Draw up each
knee alternately*

Draw one knee *back up,
then the other, without
lifting the small of the
back off the floor.
Breathe freely
between movements.*

A TEST FOR SEPARATION OF THE RECTUS MUSCLE

In the last months of pregnancy, you can check whether the rectus muscle, which runs down the front of your abdomen, has begun to separate.

If it has, be careful when doing exercises to tone your abdomen (see pages 122–123). You can repair the damage with exercises after the birth.

Lying on your back with your knees bent, tuck your chin down, and slowly raise your head and shoulders about 8 in (20 cm). Place your hands on your tummy. A small, soft bulge below your navel suggests the rectus muscle has probably separated.

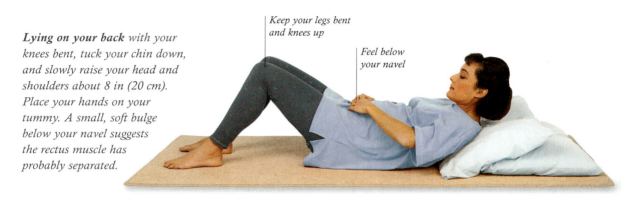

Keep your legs bent and knees up

Feel below your navel

PELVIC ROCKING AND BREATHING

Now combine pelvic rocking with controlled breathing. Each time you pull your tummy muscles *in* and press your buttocks together, give a long breath *out* through your mouth. Then, as you release the muscles and rock your pelvis gently forward (it is a very slight movement), allow your lungs to fill up with air, breathing in through your nose. Do it at your own pace, emphasizing the breath out and letting the breath in take care of itself. This movement done in early pregnancy is a good way of toning abdominal muscles in preparation for the work they must do later.

Now rest your fingers on the big bones at the front of the pelvis on either side. Continue the movement with the breathing and notice the swing up and down of these bones. This is the distance the bony cradle rocks as you walk and move around in pregnancy. The baby is thoroughly accustomed to these movements during its intrauterine existence, and it is therefore not surprising that rocking a newborn baby quiets and soothes it. Research shows that a baby who is being rocked is most likely to be comforted by a swinging movement of 3 in (7.5 cm) to either side of the central position.* This corresponds exactly with the arc of the pelvic rock.

A position with firm support for your spine is best for practicing pelvic rocking. Other positions may hollow your back, which can be harmful, especially in advanced pregnancy, because it puts stress on the sacroiliac joint at the top of your buttocks. In late pregnancy, your ligaments are softened by the hormones that make the vagina and cervix more flexible in preparation for the birth, and any form of pelvic rocking that involves back hollowing can cause more backaches.

THE WAY YOU MOVE

Exercises to help you cope with the stresses of pregnancy should be matched by others designed to help your adjustment after childbirth, since this is the time when the speediest and most dramatic physical changes are happening to you. Postnatal exercises are simply a modification of the ones you learn in pregnancy, so there is no need for you to learn completely new ones after the birth. These are described on pages 416–419.

POSTURE AND BALANCE

Good posture every day is more important than pregnancy gymnastics. Since the load you are carrying changes during pregnancy, give thought to balance and body mechanics, something usually taken for granted. It is not just a matter of "standing straight, head up" like a Victorian young lady walking with a book on her head, but of understanding how to economize on muscle work and use only those muscles that are needed for a particular task. This results in graceful and comfortable movement without strain and effort.

WALKING Whenever possible, walk rather than stand. The healthiest, most rhythmic and natural all-around exercise is walking. If you have to stand around, exercise your feet while you do so, even if only by scrunching up and extending your toes, going up onto the ball of the foot and down again, and shifting weight from one foot to the other. Muscles in the feet and legs pump blood back to the heart, so movement is important to maintain good circulation in the legs.

You can also increase the tone of your buttock muscles and help the circulation in your legs by bridging (see page 127).*

"I'VE ALWAYS BEEN VERY ACTIVE PHYSICALLY AND WAS DETERMINED I WASN'T GOING TO GIVE UP BECAUSE I WAS PREGNANT. SO I'VE CYCLED EVERYWHERE AND GONE ON WITH MY YOGA AND BEEN SWIMMING EVERY DAY."

STANDING For good posture, stand with your back to a wall, heels far enough away from it for your seat and shoulders just to touch it. Release your chest, press the small of your back toward the wall, and feel your seat tucking under and your tummy muscles working to straighten your spine. Make sure not to tighten your shoulders. Keep them dropped. Now imagine that a string is pulling your head up from the center at the top and notice the back of your neck lengthening. Relax your jaw. (Your jaw muscles cannot force your head up!) Walk a few paces away from the wall. You are standing in a stiff, exaggerated stance like a soldier on duty. Let the muscles settle into a more comfortable state. The rocking-chair exercise (see page 128) encourages good posture, too, and can be done with the help of your partner.

POSTURE AND BALANCE

Good posture is essential to your physical well-being during pregnancy. This means not only learning to stand and walk in the best way so that your baby is cradled in the pelvis in a position that is comfortable for both of you, but also performing other everyday movements, such as getting out of bed, in a way that avoids unnecessary strain.

STANDING WELL

Stand with your feet evenly planted, as wide apart as your hips, and parallel to each other. Keep your knees loose. Release any tension across your buttocks. Listen to your breathing. As you breathe out, feel the weight of your seat bones and sacrum pressing down through your heels, and imagine a thread attached to the crown of your head, drawing you upward through your spine and neck. Let your shoulder blades drop apart and relax, and your arms hang loosely by your sides. Visualize your baby nestling toward the inside of your spine. Be aware of your breathing.

*Relax
shoulders*

Keep knees loose

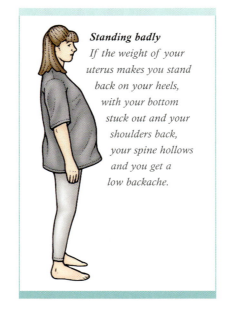

Standing badly
*If the weight of your
uterus makes you stand
back on your heels,
with your bottom
stuck out and your
shoulders back,
your spine hollows
and you get a
low backache.*

126

TAILOR SITTING

This is an ideal way to release tension in the lower back. It can be one of the most comfortable sitting positions during pregnancy, as long as you make sure you keep your spine lengthened upward and resist the temptation to slouch. Be conscious of your breathing while you are sitting.

Sit on your seat bones, *cross-legged, and let your knees drop naturally toward the floor. Allow your spine to lengthen upward as in the exercise "standing well." You could try sitting with your back against a wall for support.*

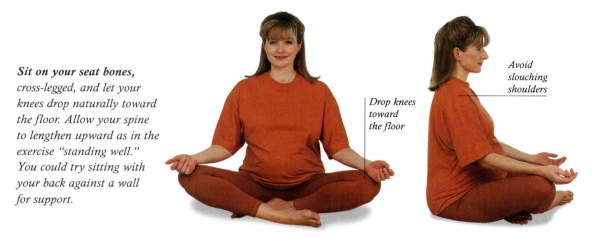

Drop knees toward the floor

Avoid slouching shoulders

BRIDGING

In late pregnancy, tummy muscles feel stretched, and it may be difficult to exercise them. It helps to exercise your buttock muscles in a relaxed position, since this means that you exercise tummy muscles, too. Bridging improves the muscle tone of your buttocks and helps the circulation in your legs. Do this exercise only if you feel comfortable on your back.

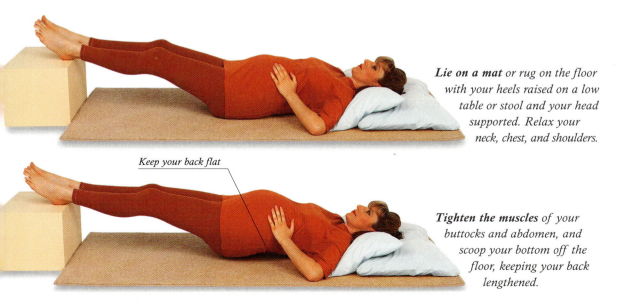

Lie on a mat or rug on the floor with your heels raised on a low table or stool and your head supported. Relax your neck, chest, and shoulders.

Keep your back flat

Tighten the muscles of your buttocks and abdomen, and scoop your bottom off the floor, keeping your back lengthened.

THE ROCKING-CHAIR EXERCISE

This encourages good posture during pregnancy by allowing you to press out the small of your back, while keeping the rest of your body aligned. For the exercise, you become like a rocking chair that rocks to and fro, and you need a partner to set you in motion. Avoid hollowing your back at any time as you do this. Stay relaxed and be aware of your breathing while you rock.

Stand well, as described on page 126. Your partner should face you, with her hands resting firmly on your hips.

Rest hands on hips

Bend your knees slightly and breathe easily as you rock your pelvis gently backward and forward between her hands.

Rock pelvis backward and forward

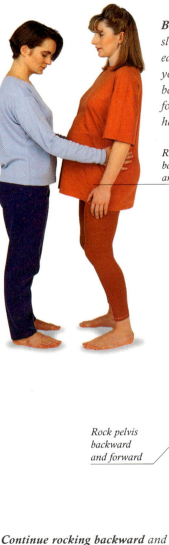

Rest hand under lower tummy

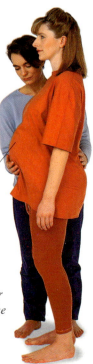

Rock pelvis backward and forward

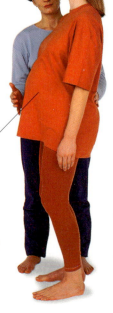

Your partner should stand at your side and put one hand firmly on the small of your back and the other under your lower tummy.

Continue rocking backward and forward, pressing against her hand with the small of your back, then releasing away from it.

GETTING UP FROM LYING DOWN

If you sit up suddenly after you have been lying on your back, you put great pressure on your tummy muscles, especially in advanced pregnancy. The method shown below helps you avoid strain on these muscles, and since it involves changing from a horizontal to an upright position in gentle stages, is also good for a healthy circulation. Aim for a smooth sequence of movements.

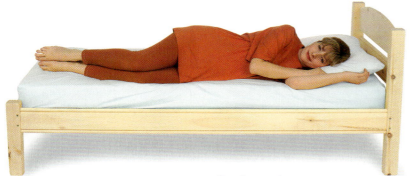

Roll over to one side, *swinging your shoulders around and drawing up your knees slightly. Use only those muscles you need to tighten to do this.*

Keep legs together as you swing them over onto the floor

Without tensing *your neck, draw your knees upward, and bring the top shoulder around, avoiding all strain on your neck. Push yourself up gently with your arms, in a smooth, coordinated movement.*

Swing your legs *forward from the hips over the edge of the bed and sit up. Drop your shoulders, press with your hands, and stand.*

ACHES AND PAINS

In late pregnancy, you are carrying extra weight that is centered in one area and so affects your balance. This alone can cause aches and pains by straining muscles and causing you to adopt an unnatural stance, leading to further strain. These exercises will help you ease your aches and pains.

FOOT EXERCISES

Foot exercises discourage varicose veins in the legs by stimulating the blood flow back to the heart. When you are sitting down or taking a rest, practice drawing the alphabet with your feet, one foot at a time, keeping your legs still. You will find that you can easily read or do some work at the same time.

THE SHOULDER ROLL

Upper backache that is caused by poor posture or heavy breasts can be relieved by doing the shoulder roll exercise.

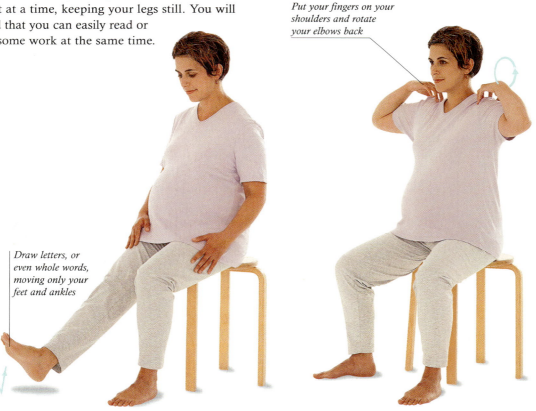

Put your fingers on your shoulders and rotate your elbows back

Draw letters, or even whole words, moving only your feet and ankles

THE ANGRY CAT

However many exercises you do with your back supported, it feels good to get the weight of the baby off your spine occasionally. You can do this by going onto all fours and rocking your pelvis, an exercise sometimes known as "the angry cat." This is a kind of pelvic rocking.

Spread your shoulders wide

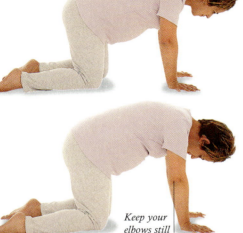

Keep your elbows still

***Get onto all fours**, keeping the small of your back flat, not hollowed, and your neck aligned with your spine. Your palms should be placed flat on the floor.*

***Without moving your** elbows or knees, keep breathing as you tighten your tummy muscles and hump up your lower back. Relax back to the flat position after holding for several seconds.*

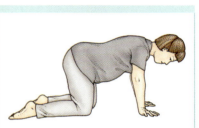

Incorrect posture
Never, under any circumstances, allow the lower back to cave in while doing this exercise.

THE WHEELBARROW

Toward the end of pregnancy, many women have pain in the groin. This usually occurs as a result of pressure from the baby on the joints of the pelvis. To relieve the discomfort, try this exercise, with your partner kneeling very close to you.

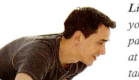

***Lie on your back** with your knees bent. Your partner holds your hips at either side. Let him take their weight.*

***Your partner slowly lifts** your hips, holds them up for a moment, then lowers them. Let him do all the work.*

WALL STRETCHING

A good way to lift your ribs off your expanding uterus is simply to stretch up your arms. Raise one arm up in the air and then the other, until you are comfortable. A similar result may be achieved if you do the exercise while sitting with your back pressed firmly against a wall to help alignment.

Sit with the base *of your spine pressed against a wall and lengthen. Keep your shoulders soft and wide and breathe easily. Keep your seat and legs grounded and your back flat against the wall as you swing your arms out to shoulder height. With your palms pressed against the wall, walk your fingers up the wall.*

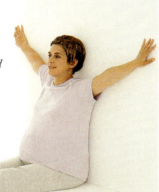

When you have *reached as high as you can, turn your palms outward and spread your shoulders wide. With each out-breath, let your seat bones drop and your spine lengthen up the surface of the wall.*

SITTING Sit back on your chair and make sure that your spine is well supported. If necessary, put a small cushion in the small of the back to provide support. In the last few weeks of your pregnancy, you may need more support than this; try sitting well back against a large beanbag or a firm floor cushion. If you have to write or use a computer at a desk for any length of time, rest your head down on it occasionally and gently stretch the back of your neck. Use a low footstool (so that your knees are level with or slightly higher than your hips) to rest your back when you sit for a long time.

BENDING AND LIFTING Use your legs, not your back, when you reach down for anything. This means that, whenever possible, you should bend your knees and get right down in order to grasp the load. Kneel or squat when you are working low down—cleaning the bathtub or making a low bed or lifting a heavy package, for example. Avoid misusing your spine as if it were a crane. For some household jobs, such as wiping or polishing a floor, get onto all fours. This takes the weight of the baby off your spine and is surprisingly comfortable, especially if you have backache.

LYING DOWN AND GETTING UP The front-lateral or "three-quarters-over" position is often most comfortable when you are lying in bed. It may help to put a pillow under your upper knee. Allow adequate space between your legs. Avoid hollowing your back when lying down, too. If necessary, put a small pillow under your hips so that your back does not cave in.

Whenever you get up from lying on your back, roll over onto one side first, swinging your shoulders around and drawing up your knees. Push yourself up gently with your arms. Swing your legs forward from the hips over the edge of the bed and sit up. Press with your hands and stand. It may sound complicated, but it can come to be a beautifully smooth, coordinated movement, like Cleopatra rising from her barge.

ACHES AND PAINS

Although bad posture is often responsible for aches and pains, you may have other aches and pains that are just the result of being pregnant. If this is the case, all you can do to relieve them is concentrate on relaxation and experiment with different positions in which you feel more comfortable.

If you have a backache, a chiropractor may be able to lessen it and show you how to use your muscles more effectively and avoid strain. Chiropractors use a table that can easily be adjusted to leave room for your tummy, and they can make spinal adjustments right through pregnancy without harming the baby.

LOW BACKACHE In late pregnancy, if the baby is facing your front and engages as a posterior (see page 270) with the back of its head pressing against your sacrum, you may develop a backache. Rest in positions in which the weight of the baby is tilted off the spine, and take every opportunity to get on all fours. Washing a kitchen floor can provide extraordinary relief from backaches. The angry cat (see page 131) is an exercise that combines this position with pelvic rocking to relieve your spine of the baby's weight.

UPPER BACKACHE This occurs when you try to compensate for the weight of your pregnancy dragging you forward by flinging your shoulders back and tightening muscles in the upper back. To relieve it, roll your shoulders backward when you have the opportunity and do the shoulder roll exercise (see page 130).

PUBIC PAIN The cartilage of the joint in the front of the bony pelvic girdle is softened and stretched by hormones in your bloodstream during pregnancy. This makes more room for the baby to come down during birth. Sometimes from around the middle of pregnancy this stretching starts to cause pain. Your pubic symphysis may be tender to touch and you may have low back pain as well as pain along your inside thighs. A pelvic support belt can help, so ask your doctor or midwife about this. A bag of frozen peas or corn wrapped in a cloth placed over the painful area may give some relief when you are resting. When you roll over or get out of bed, make sure that you keep your knees together.

TINGLING AND NUMBNESS You may feel tingling and numbness in your hands. This is known as carpal tunnel syndrome. It results from pressure on the nerves and tendons caused by swelling of the hand and wrist. You will be most aware of it in the morning, after your wrists have accumulated fluid during the night. To relieve the discomfort, hold your hands above your head for a few minutes and flex and gradually extend the fingers upward.

PAIN UNDER THE RIBS You may feel pain below the ribs when the top of the uterus (the fundus) is high after 30 weeks of pregnancy (see page 78). This pain tends to be on whichever side the baby is lying.

You will discover that you are only comfortable when sitting straight on a rather high chair and will not want to slump down onto your uterus. In spite of folklore about the dangers of an expectant mother lifting her arms above her head, it helps to stretch upward so that your whole ribcage is lifted off the uterus. You can also do stretching exercises while sitting with your back against a wall for support (see page 132).

PAIN IN THE GROIN In late pregnancy, this is the consequence of the stretching of the round ligaments that go from either side of the uterus into each groin. Avoid rapid movements such as standing up too quickly. Also avoid standing for long periods, and even when sitting, change position frequently. Symptoms can be relieved by doing the wheelbarrow exercise (see page 131). Some women get a stitch in the side because the broad ligament on either side of the uterus is stretched. If you are lying down on your side, place a small pillow beneath your uterus to prevent this from happening.

CRAMPS IN THE LEG Occasionally, pregnant women get recurring cramps, especially if they are trying to maintain a salt-free diet. Eating something salty before you go to bed may make the cramp disappear. A magnesium supplement can reduce cramps in the leg. Sometimes calcium tablets are prescribed for cramps on the grounds that your body must be short of calcium, but research shows that this is a useless treatment.* Avoid curling your toes. Use a light quilt or make up the bed loosely so that your toes are not pressed down by the weight of bedding at night.

"I ALWAYS WAKE HIM UP TO MASSAGE MY LEG CRAMPS. AT LEAST HE'LL BE WELL PREPARED FOR CARING FOR THE BABY DURING THE NIGHT!"

Lifting your feet above the level of your heart will also help circulation and relieve cramps. However, in advanced pregnancy this position may give you indigestion, so you are left with a choice between two discomforts. While you are lying with your feet up, roll them around in circles from the ankles to help stretch the calf muscles, or draw the letters of the alphabet, one foot at a time, keeping your legs still. If you do get a cramp, ask your partner to grip your heel and, using a forearm, push your foot up while holding your knee straight with the other hand. It may help to do this regularly, about ten times, before you settle for the night.

COMMON PROBLEMS

Although your baby can grow inside you without your having to think consciously or do anything about it, the baby's development affects your whole body and every system in it.

VARICOSE VEINS

The valves that help direct the blood through the veins back to the heart may soften in pregnancy and become unable to propel the increased amount of blood through the legs. This causes pooling of blood and swelling of your veins, especially when standing.

Avoid positions that allow pooling of blood in the legs: prolonged standing, or sitting with legs crossed or thighs pressing against the edge of your chair, for example. Foot exercises will help keep the blood moving. If you are advised to wear elastic stockings, choose semi- or full-support styles and put them on before you get up. Bend a knee, put one leg on, and wriggle it up; then do the same with the other.

VAGINAL VARICOSE VEINS Sometimes a woman develops varicose veins in her vagina and labia. The discomfort may be eased by wrapping some ice cubes in a handkerchief, knotting it, and packing it against the sore areas. Obviously you cannot walk around like this, but it is a good excuse to lie down for a while, in a position in which the whole weight of your uterus is not pressing down on the swollen veins. Some-times vitamin B_6 (pyridoxine) helps.

HEMORRHOIDS Also known as piles, hemorrhoids are varicose veins of the rectum and can be caused by constipation. If you have piles, avoid any straining on the toilet. This condition should be treated quickly because hemorrhoids can become prolapsed (protrude through the anus), causing extreme pain. Your doctor may give you a prescription for a relieving cream. A cotton pad soaked in witch hazel will help.

CONSTIPATION

You are more likely than usual to be constipated during pregnancy because the extra hormones that are produced while you are pregnant cause the intestine to relax and become less efficient. Eat plenty of fruit, vegetables, fiber, and whole grains, and drink as much water as you can. When you are on the toilet, allow your pelvic floor to be fully released and bulging down. Give yourself plenty of time to empty the bowels, and take a brisk walk every day if possible. If you are still constipated, ask your doctor to prescribe a stool softener.

BLADDER CONTROL AND INFECTIONS

In the first three months or so of your pregnancy, the developing baby and enlarging uterus are pressing against your bladder, and extra progesterone flowing through your bloodstream softens the tissues. So it is quite normal to urinate very often. This may be even more noticeable at the very end of pregnancy when the baby has gone down into your pelvis.

CYSTITIS Engorgement of blood vessels in the pelvic area means that there is a risk of urinary infection. A stinging, burning feeling when you urinate suggests cystitis. If left untreated, cystitis rapidly becomes very uncomfortable and can lead to pyelonephritis (see below).

If you suspect that you have cystitis, go to your doctor, who will prescribe antibiotics. It is sensible to seek help when you first notice the symptoms, since delay can allow the infection to take hold more firmly.

As a general treatment for cystitis, drink plenty of liquid. Drink a glass of water every time you have used the toilet. Cranberry juice or an alkaline drink, such as a mixture of sodium bicarbonate and sodium citrate, may help. One natural remedy is marshmallow root tea. Wear cotton underpants, and avoid any clothing that is tight on the crotch. Wear tights that have a cotton panel or air holes between the legs. Spend time on the toilet to empty your bladder as completely as possible. When the baby is pressing against your bladder in late pregnancy, you will be able to shift position so that the baby moves a little, allowing you to void some more.

PYELONEPHRITIS If you have a temperature and low back pain, and if it hurts when you apply pressure over your kidneys on one or both sides, you may have pyelonephritis (a kidney infection). Sometimes the infection also causes nausea and vomiting. Seek treatment immediately, since this is not only painful but can be dangerous for your kidneys. Antibiotics are effective, but all the measures suggested for coping with cystitis are also helpful, and you will probably appreciate a hot-water bottle against the painful area. Women with pyelonephritis are often admitted to the hospital for diagnosis and treatment. Antibiotics will clear the infection quickly, but you may have pain or discomfort for up to two weeks.

YEAST GROWTHS

It is normal to have an increased vaginal discharge in pregnancy, but if your vulva becomes itchy and your vagina is red, sore, and burning, you probably have thrush (candida or monilia). Suppositories or vaginal creams containing a group of drugs called imidazoles are the most effective treatment for thrush. If you get repeated infections, cut out sugar and white flour and base your diet on whole grains, fruit, vegetables, and protein. Thrush is very common in pregnancy, and frequently recurs, so it is often sensible to treat mild attacks simply by changing your diet.

BREAST TENDERNESS

The normal breast tenderness of the early weeks of pregnancy can be acutely painful for some women, and they walk with stiff arms to protect themselves in case anyone brushes against them. A good supporting bra is important, since if breasts are increasing in size, as they usually are at this stage, their weight can be uncomfortable. If your breasts get extra-sensitive like this, you will not enjoy your partner's most gentle touch until mid-pregnancy.

INVERTED NIPPLES

Some women have one or both nipples shaped like dimples. These are called "inverted" nipples. If you have a nipple like this but can press it out, or if it projects when you are sexually excited, the baby will be able to get hold of the nipple well and draw it out farther. Otherwise you may find it difficult to fix the baby onto the breast with a good mouthful. But if you do manage to start the baby off, he or she will soon suck the nipple into a good projecting shape. It is a fallacy to think that you need prominent nipples to nurse successfully, and there is no point in pulling and squeezing your nipples in pregnancy in an attempt to make them project.*

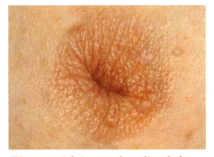

Women with inverted or dimpled nipples can still breast-feed. The baby soon sucks them into shape.

VOMITING

For some women, the nausea and vomiting common in the first three months of pregnancy (see page 27) go on much longer. This prolonged sickness is hyperemesis. A woman with hyperemesis is really ill because she cannot take any food by mouth. Surprisingly, the cure may simply be admission to the hospital, and often no further treatment is necessary. This is why some psychiatrists and obstetricians have suggested that hyperemesis is a symptom of disturbed relationships and that if you can get away from the relentless day-to-day contact with a partner, mother, mother-in-law, or anyone who is stressing you, the vomiting will ease. But part of the cure may simply be that you do not have to do any cooking or smell kitchen odors.

If you are vomiting at all hours of the day, cannot be sure of keeping any meal down, and are feeling wretched, it is worth trying to get away from your normal daily routine and surroundings. Spend time with people you know only slightly or not at all, who will not fuss over you. If this gives you the opportunity to do something that you have never done before (not hang-gliding!)—go off to a spa for a weekend or see something that you have never had the chance to see before—so much the better. There is a phrase that is sometimes used about a person who is run-down: "she needs to be taken out of herself." A woman who is vomiting almost without interruption may need to be taken "out" of herself and her usual relationships until she can cope emotionally. When her pregnancy has settled down, she can come back "into" herself with new strength.

NASAL CONGESTION

Some women seem to have permanent nasal congestion during pregnancy, particularly in the last few months. However, a blocked or runny nose is usually a by-product of the effects of pregnancy hormones rather than a viral infection such as a cold.

SINUSITIS Mucous membrane inside the nostrils and sinuses often swells during pregnancy because hormones liberated in your bloodstream are softening up your vagina and cervix. Try eucalyptus oil on a cotton ball or use an inhaler stick to relieve your stuffy nose. Sinusitis does not interfere with breathing during labor, so there is no need to worry about this, though you may be more comfortable breathing through your mouth. You will feel better if you take frequent sips of water or have a small spray bottle filled with ice water to spray into your mouth between contractions. A lip salve to smooth on your lips will help to prevent soreness. You will find that the symptoms of sinusitis disappear completely after you have given birth.

> "I SEEM TO HAVE HAD A STUFFED-UP NOSE FOR MONTHS—SOMETHING I DIDN'T EXPECT. IT'LL BE GOOD TO BE ABLE TO BREATHE EASILY AGAIN."

NOSEBLEEDS These are common in pregnancy and are also associated with higher hormone levels and congestion. A tiny blob of Vaseline in your nostril will usually stop a nosebleed. Avoid blowing your nose hard.

VAGINAL BLEEDING IN EARLY PREGNANCY

Bleeding from the vagina at any stage of pregnancy is always worrisome. In early pregnancy, it may be that the level of your pregnancy hormones is not sufficiently high to avoid breakthrough spotting. There is no way you can stop this without possibly affecting the developing baby. Cut out unnecessary exertion and, if the bleeding started at a time when your period would have been due, take life gently then and see if you can manage a few days in bed. Practice deep relaxation every day. There is further information about how to deal with a threatened miscarriage on page 386.

VAGINAL BLEEDING IN LATE PREGNANCY

If you notice any bleeding in late pregnancy, it may be a sign that labor is about to start. It is usually blood from around the cervix and, except where there is a polyp in the cervix that has started to bleed, shows that thinning out and some dilatation is taking place. If your baby is due within a month and the bleeding looks like the beginning of a period, a bloodstained mucous discharge (a "show," see page 250), do not worry. Accept it as a normal sign that your body is in good working order for labor and that you may start within a week or two.

Bright red bleeding, which flows as if you were at the height of a period, is another matter entirely. It is known as antepartum hemorrhage (APH) and, although quite rare, is serious. Call your doctor or go to the hospital immediately. Avoid both vaginal and rectal examinations because they can make things worse. An ultrasound scan is the best way of finding out exactly what is happening.

PLACENTA PREVIA Sometimes blood flows from the placental site when it is too low-lying and partly in front of the baby's head. Intermittent APH from 27 weeks onward is a typical symptom of this condition, known as placenta previa. Placenta previa occurs in about 1 in every 200 births, and it almost certainly means that the delivery will be by Cesarean section. During a vaginal birth, as the lower segment of the uterus thinned out, the placenta would be torn away from its roots, depriving the baby of both nourishment and oxygen. If you start to bleed, you are admitted to the hospital and, if bleeding continues, will be advised to continue to stay there until the baby is mature enough to be born.

Ultrasound at 18–20 weeks often reveals that the placenta is lying in the lower part of the uterus. This is not at all uncommon in early pregnancy and, by the end of pregnancy, when the wall of the uterus has stretched and enlarged, the placenta is usually in the right place in the upper part of the uterus. For this reason, it is not appropriate to plan a Cesarean section solely on the basis of this early scan. Only 6 percent of low-lying placentas that were detected by ultrasound in early pregnancy turn out to be lying over the cervix.*

PLACENTAL ABRUPTION APH can also mean that a part of the placenta, situated in the upper part of the uterus as it should be, has peeled away. This is called accidental hemorrhage (accidental in that the hemorrhage has occurred by chance) or placental abruption. Sometimes there is constant pain in the abdomen, and the uterus becomes and remains firm. The severity of placental abruption depends on how large a portion of the placenta has separated from the uterine lining, but it is a potentially serious problem, and the doctor should be told immediately. You will be advised to go to the hospital for bed rest and, if the bleeding stops and all is well with the baby, you will be discharged after four to five days. You should be able to resume your normal activities, but it is probably wise to avoid intercourse and orgasm until after the baby is born.

HIGH BLOOD PRESSURE

Every time you go for a prenatal visit, your blood pressure is checked (see pages 48–49). This is because, although slight fluctuations are normal, any significant rise may indicate preeclampsia. If the diastolic figure (the second number) in your blood pressure reading rises by more than 15, you are considered to have hypertension—high blood pressure.

Hypertension can be an early signal of preeclampsia. When a woman has preeclampsia, the placenta may not work as well as it should. But it is important that hypertension is not overdiagnosed. For every woman who has sustained high blood pressure, another is suspected of it because her blood pressure shot up at a prenatal visit. This may be because she rushed to get there, was sitting around for ages worrying about her older child, was made anxious by information she heard in the waiting room, or simply because having her blood pressure checked resulted in "white coat hypertension." If you can, refuse to be hassled, and stay relaxed about your blood pressure. The more checks that are made for hypertension in pregnancy, the more often it is found. They are often misleading.

Take some time to really relax each day, breathing deeply and concentrating on the new life within you.

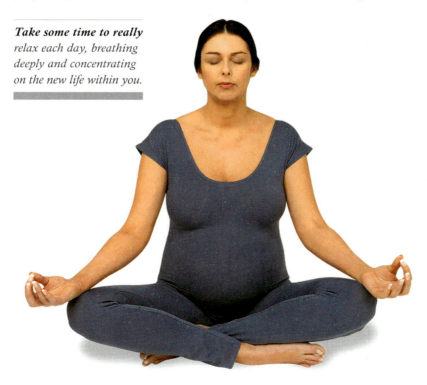

PREECLAMPSIA

The full name of this condition is "preeclamptic toxemia," but it is sometimes called simply "toxemia." In some countries it is "hypertensive disease of pregnancy" (HDP). It may also be called "pregnancy-induced hypertension" (PIH) or even "gestosis." All of these names reflect the fact that there is uncertainty as to its cause. A 19th-century doctor called it "the disease of theories," and this still remains true today. Preeclampsia affects between 5 and 10 percent of pregnant women but rarely occurs in early pregnancy, unless a woman has been malnourished for years.

SIGNS Preeclampsia causes symptoms only in its late and severe stages. The diagnosis is made if your blood pressure rises and you also have protein in your urine and fluid retention. On its own, a rise in blood pressure does not mean that you have preeclampsia. The risks to you are that, left untreated, it can lead to problems with your kidneys, liver, or blood-clotting system, as well as causing sustained high blood pressure. For your baby, the problem is that it can interfere with the way the placenta works, with the result that it is underfed in the uterus. With severe preeclampsia, you have headaches, visual disturbances, nausea and vomiting, and upper abdominal pain (particularly on the right side under the ribs) and feel very restless. If this happens, do not assume that it is a tummy bug. In extreme cases, a woman with preeclampsia may have convulsions. Then the diagnosis is eclampsia. This is rare, but dangerous. The baby is often delivered by Cesarean section.

CAUSES No one is certain what causes preeclampsia, but research indicates that it may be due to thinner-than-usual blood vessels in the placenta caused by an inappropriate reaction of the uterus to the presence of the placenta. The problem starts between the 6th and 18th week of pregnancy, when placental cells do not infiltrate arteries in the uterus deeply enough to make the blood vessels expand so that they can nourish the baby (see page 76). There is another element in preeclampsia, too; it seems to be a process similar to graft rejection. It is as if the baby is a transplant in the mother's body, and her immune system recognizes it and produces cells in order to expel the intruder.

The risk of preeclampsia is highest in the first pregnancy. But it also has something to do with the man; if a woman has a new partner for a subsequent pregnancy, the chances of her developing preeclampsia are about the same as if it were her first baby.

Poor nutrition may play an important part in preeclampsia. You may be able to avoid the disorder by eating well. If you had preeclampsia in a previous pregnancy, start on a program of good nutrition *before* you conceive again. Dietary restriction to prevent preeclampsia is harmful.*

You are more likely to get preeclampsia if any of the following apply: you have diabetes or kidney disease; you normally have high blood pressure

(140/90 or higher); you are having twins or more; family members have high blood pressure or have had preeclampsia; you are in your teens or are over 40; you are under 5 ft 3 in (1.6 m) tall; you have had preeclampsia before (there is a 1 in 10 chance of its recurring); you suffer from migraines.

TREATMENT Some doctors think that staying in bed at the first signs may avoid further developments. Certainly bed rest coupled with relaxation of body and mind will lower blood pressure and improve blood flow to the baby. Do not lie flat on your back in bed, but on your side or well propped up. Left-sided bed rest is best for blood supply to the placenta. It is fair to say that the current view is that no one really knows if bed rest is a good idea.

If you have high blood pressure with protein in your urine, or high blood pressure alone (above 170/110), your doctor will probably admit you to the hospital on the same day. Your blood pressure and urine will be checked every four hours or more frequently. You may have magnesium sulfate injections. This is an anticonvulsant that lowers your risk of developing eclampsia. If your blood pressure falls below 90 and stays there, and there is no longer any protein in your urine, you will probably go home after three or four days.

Many women feel trapped in the hospital when they have preeclampsia, because they may not feel ill. Knowing what is happening and why helps you to care for yourself rather than just put up with having things done to you. Ask questions: find out about your condition and understand the reasons for the treatment you are receiving. Nowadays you may not have to be admitted to the hospital, and high blood pressure is treated at home.

ECLAMPSIA

This is a very serious, but rare (1 in 2,000 births) condition, and skilled emergency treatment to control the seizures and lower the blood pressure is required. Once the immediate crisis is under control, your baby will be delivered, probably by Cesarean section, but in occasional cases vaginally.

DIABETES

For diabetic women with well-controlled blood sugar levels, childbearing is as safe as for others. It is important to control the condition carefully, particularly before conception and during the very early stages of pregnancy, since otherwise there is an increased risk of fetal abnormalities. The alphafetoprotein test, or the prenatal risk profile, which is the first screening procedure in a series that can reveal the risk of handicap, is more likely to yield an inaccurate result than in nondiabetic women, so this should be anticipated. It does not mean that anything is wrong. The accumulation of glucose in a diabetic woman who is pregnant is absorbed by the baby, who grows very fast. It is now common practice to monitor blood sugar levels at home using a glucose meter. When linked to a computer at the hospital, the meter provides details of the levels of blood sugar in the average day, so that you can adjust your sugar intake and insulin doses as necessary. A single ultrasound scan is an inaccurate way of trying to find out what the baby's size is likely to be at birth, so the obstetrician may recommend a series of scans during the later months of pregnancy. If it is thought that the baby is growing too big to pass easily through your pelvic outlet, induction may be recommended. If labor is induced, although the baby is large, it may not be mature, and so needs special care after birth (see page 380). Some babies of diabetic mothers are delivered by Cesarean section because induction is performed before the mother's cervix is soft and ready to open.

"THE DIABETES CAME AS A COMPLETE SURPRISE, BECAUSE I'D FELT SO WELL RIGHT THROUGH PREGNANCY UNTIL THEN."

There is no good reason why a diabetic woman should not breast-feed her baby, and many women do so very successfully. In fact, breast-feeding reduces the chances of the child's becoming diabetic later in life.

SUGAR IN THE URINE

Your urine is tested for sugar whenever you see the doctor or midwife (see pages 48–49). Nearly all women at some time during pregnancy produce sugar in their urine, indicating that they may have raised blood sugar levels, which contribute to a baby's growth. Very occasionally the presence of sugar in the urine can be a sign of diabetes, but most of these women are not diabetics. It is merely a biochemical variation, not an illness. When you are pregnant, you have more blood circulating in your system than normal, so there is more blood sugar that must be dealt with by your kidneys. You are more likely to have high blood sugar if you are an older mother, are overweight, have had repeated infections of the urinary tract, or if you smoke.

You can reduce the sugar level in your blood by modifying your diet: cut out sugary foods, bananas, and caffeinated drinks, and have small, frequent meals instead of a few large ones. If you go for a long time without food, body fat may be burned up and ketones appear in your urine. This is definitely not a good idea. It means that you are starving yourself. By all means restrict weight gain if it makes you feel better, but ensure that you have good nutrition. Sugar levels can also be reduced by making sure that you get some exercise each day.

GESTATIONAL DIABETES

Gestational diabetes is a condition in which excess sugar circulates in the mother's blood and causes a big baby. Some obstetricians recommend that all women take a glucose challenge test at some point in pregnancy. You drink a sugary solution, and a blood sample is taken one hour later. If this shows a high glucose level, a more rigorous test (a glucose tolerance test) can be done. Only 15 percent of women with a high glucose challenge test have an abnormal glucose tolerance test (and are diagnosed as having gestational diabetes). Other obstetricians perform a glucose tolerance test only on women in risk groups, such as those who show sugar in their urine, those who have had gestational diabetes before, others who have had unexplained late miscarriages or stillbirths or who have had very big babies in the past, and women who are very overweight.

If you have gestational diabetes, controlling the carbohydrate content of your diet and your calorie intake will lower blood sugar levels. Some obstetricians recommend insulin injections. This may reduce the size of the baby, but trials show no improvement in birth outcomes.*

ANEMIA

It is normal for your hemoglobin level to fall during pregnancy. Iron used to be prescribed automatically, but this can be harmful. When a woman's hemoglobin level does not fall, she is more likely to give birth preterm. Laboratory tests of hemoglobin concentration and ferritin levels (the normal range is 125–150) can be difficult to interpret, and there is a lot of disagreement about who needs iron supplements and who doesn't.*

If you are genuinely anemic, you feel very tired, get exhausted when you do anything vigorous, have dizzy spells, and are short of breath. Women with anemia are less able to cope with any heavy bleeding at birth and more likely to have an infection. Adjust your diet to include more iron-rich foods, protein, B vitamins (especially B_{12}) and vitamin C, and take the folic acid supplement that your doctor prescribes (see page 99). These are necessary to ensure that your blood can carry enough oxygen to all the tissues of your body. Your doctor will also prescribe iron tablets. If you find they make you constipated, ask for another kind. If you have a very low hemoglobin level (see page 42) after 30 weeks, injections of iron may be prescribed.*

HEADACHE

There is no reason why you should have more headaches when you are pregnant. In fact, some women who usually suffer from migraines find that they disappear throughout pregnancy. You can have tension headaches while pregnant just as at any other time. If your pregnancy is fraught with anxiety, or you are taking on more than you can handle, you may be prone to headaches. Decode your body messages, modify your lifestyle, and if you are worried about labor, find out how you can help yourself (see page 150). A sharp, blinding headache in late pregnancy that affects your eyesight should be reported to your doctor, since it could be associated with preeclampsia.

DIGESTIVE DISTURBANCES

Indigestion and heartburn are common problems in the last three or four months of pregnancy. There seems to be so little room in your abdomen, and it feels as if all your organs are being crushed.

It is better to have many small snacks than several larger meals a day, and sensible to avoid fried, rich, or spicy foods. Some people cannot digest bread or products containing yeast; cutting out these foods can eliminate heartburn. Many women discover that they cannot drink during a meal and that meals have to be taken dry. Experiment with different combinations of food and liquid to find the kind of diet that suits you personally. There is no perfect diet that is right for everyone. Since heartburn results from acid present in your stomach flowing back into the esophagus, find positions for sitting and sleeping in which the upper part of your uterus is not pressing against your stomach. You will probably prefer upright chairs and at night will feel better if you sleep well propped up with pillows. Make sure jeans, pants, and skirts are comfortably loose at the waist.

"WHEN I STOPPED TRYING TO FIGHT THE PREGNANCY AND ALLOWED MYSELF TO SLOW DOWN, I FOUND I WAS BEGINNING TO ENJOY IT."

SHORTNESS OF BREATH

When the baby is high, after about 34 weeks, and before it drops into your pelvis, you may find that you are short of breath whenever you exert yourself or even just climb the stairs. Your uterus is putting pressure on your lungs, and your diaphragm may be shifted out of place by as much as 1 in (2.5 cm). Again, sitting straight and sleeping propped up can help, and you will probably have to take life more slowly in order not to become breathless. There is a rhythm to everything in nature, and this is a phase of pregnancy when your body is telling you to slow down.

DAILY CARE AND COMFORT

When you are pregnant, you carry around your own central heating system. Your circulation is at peak efficiency and your metabolic rate has speeded up. You will find that you do not need to dress as warmly as usual, even on cold days when others say they are freezing. In hot weather, you will probably feel more comfortable in cotton dresses and skirts, and should avoid synthetic materials. Many pregnant women suffer from varicose veins in the legs, rectum, or vagina (see page 135). Boots should not grip so tightly that circulation is impeded. Make sure that jeans or pants do not interfere with circulation in the groin.

SHOES

Shoes should allow feet to keep their normal shape, and heels not be so high that your weight is thrown forward onto the balls of your feet. In late pregnancy, your feet may be wider than usual and so need a wider-fitting shoe or a half-size larger. Although lace-ups give good support to the arches, you may find that you cannot tie them so easily in late pregnancy.

BRAS

Breast changes and enlargement occur from the first days of pregnancy. You will need a bra that gives good support and, if you are heavy-breasted, one with straps that are sufficiently wide not to dig into your shoulders.

Heavy breasts, allowed to hang without support, may develop stretch marks (see below), which will leave you with silvery streaks after the pregnancy. If you have large breasts, you may prefer to wear a lightweight bra at night, too.

TEETH

Although the baby needs calcium in order to grow strong teeth, your own teeth are no more likely to fall out in pregnancy than at any other time. However, as your gums soften and become spongier along with other tissues in the body as the result of the action of pregnancy hormones in your bloodstream, you may get a gum infection. Good nutrition (see pages 96–100) is the first line of defense against this. Mouth hygiene is also important, with regular tooth brushing, especially after breakfast and before you go to bed at night. Arrange a dental examination and cleaning (but not X-rays) once you know you are pregnant. Have another dental checkup when the baby is about five months old.

SKIN PIGMENTATION

For many women, pregnancy is better than a beauty treatment: skin improves, eyes shine, and hair is in better condition. But some women develop patches of darkened (pigmented) skin on the face, which can be distressing. The technical term is "chloasma," but it is also called "the mask of pregnancy." It is a result of the high level of hormones, and also occurs in some women taking oral contraceptives. It is made worse by exposure to sunlight. The kind of cosmetic cream sold for minimizing birthmarks often disguises it effectively. The mask usually disappears once the baby is born.

You will notice that other parts of the body already pigmented become darker—for example, the circles around your nipples and the skin of your labia. You may also develop a dark line down the middle of your tummy from your navel, where the rectus muscle is stretched. It is particularly obvious in dark-haired women. All these colorations should disappear once the baby is born.

STRETCH MARKS

Stretch marks (striae) may appear over your tummy, buttocks, and breasts. They are dark streaks and are a sign that the skin has been stretched from underneath. They never disappear completely, but after the birth they change from brown or deep violet to a silvery shade, rather like the marks on some fine fabric that has not been properly ironed. Many women use a rich cream or oil to "feed" the skin, and there are some on the market especially for stretch marks. However, these are expensive, and any readily absorbed cream, or even vegetable oil, will do. If your skin is very stretched, and especially if you are having twins, it is marked like this because of pressure on the layers underneath the surface that cannot be reached by anything applied from outside. Still, it can be relaxing for you to stroke your tummy. Even though you may still have stretch marks, there is nothing to be lost and probably some pleasure to be gained from gentle massage with a rich, slippery cream.

ITCHING

You may get very itchy and uncomfortable in hot weather. Wear cotton rather than synthetic clothing and underwear that is as loose as possible. Calamine lotion, or an equal mixture of a few drops each of chamomile, lavender, and bergamot essential oils in 2 fl oz (50 ml) witch hazel or rosewater, is soothing when stroked into the skin.

If itching is really bothering you, consult your doctor or midwife. Rarely, it is a symptom of liver malfunction—a condition known as obstetric cholestasis—which puts the unborn baby at risk, and for which the only treatment is induction of labor.

SPORTS

Any sport you already do well is probably fine to continue with during your pregnancy: if you are really good at something, you do not waste muscular energy, and your movements are smoothly coordinated. As pregnancy advances, you will notice your balance changing as the center of gravity is becoming more concentrated in your tummy. Swimming is splendid, as are exercise and dancing, provided that you are not in a stuffy room. Strolling through a crowded shopping center does not provide you with good exercise and may make you feel stressed, but brisk walking in fresh air, wearing a comfortable pair of shoes, with arms swinging and breathing deeply, is excellent for you.

"I'VE CONTINUED WITH HORSEBACK RIDING BECAUSE IT'S WONDERFULLY RELAXING. BUT I TAKE THINGS EASY; I DON'T DO JUMPS ANYMORE."

Cycling is also beneficial, but be kind to yourself and your baby and avoid cycling trips in heavy traffic with its inevitable fumes. It is sensible in pregnancy to avoid all competitive sports because they may tempt you to overexert yourself.

TRAVEL

Travel is usually quite safe, but the exhaustion that may easily result from it is not. For this reason, divide up long journeys into short, manageable sections if you can possibly do so; rest in between. Do not sit immobilized in a car, train, or airplane for longer than two hours at the most without getting up and walking around for five minutes. Sitting for long periods reduces the circulation of blood in the pelvic area. Remember to empty your bladder regularly, since you are more likely to get a bladder infection during pregnancy (see page 136).

Travel in loose, comfortable clothing and shoes that allow for a little expansion. Soft slipper-socks are usually the most comfortable. Take any opportunity to drop off to sleep. Pack an eyeshade made of soft material to block out light.

FLYING On an airplane, drink water or fruit juice; avoid alcoholic drinks, since air travel is dehydrating, and alcohol will dehydrate you even further. If you are more than 36 weeks pregnant, some airlines will require a letter from your doctor saying that it is all right for you to travel. Your doctor will probably agree to write such a letter as long as the risk of your going into labor on board an aircraft is only slight. It would be quite reasonable to refuse consent if, for instance, your blood pressure is high, or if you suffered a threatened miscarriage in the early part of the pregnancy. In such cases, a change in altitude could bring on premature labor. Similarly, it is unwise to fly in a small, unpressurized aircraft, since the supply of oxygen to the fetus can sometimes be drastically diminished. Some airlines, however, place no special restrictions on travel for pregnant women. Bear in mind the strain of jet lag if you are thinking of flying a long distance, and wear compression stockings during the flight, since there is an increased risk of blood clots when sitting for a long time.

DRIVING This is perfectly safe if you do not find it exhausting, and if you are not subject to dizzy spells. Try to avoid driving in rush hour, and keep the windows closed and circulate the air inside the car if you are in a traffic jam with heavy exhaust fumes. If you have a heavy gearshift, the sheer hard work of changing gears can cause discomfort in the later months. Automatic transmission makes lighter work of driving. Make sure your seat belt strap is under your tummy.

WORKING

Only you can know when to give up work before the baby's birth. Do not let other people put pressure on you (easier said than done). Think through exactly what is best for you in the short and long term. Negotiate to avoid rush-hour travel if possible, work at home when you can, consider off-loading anything that is not important, and try to get to bed early. After the baby comes you will almost certainly be short of sleep. Stock up on energy by sleeping now.

If you decide to go on working until the last minute, build in spaces for relaxation, slow, full breathing, and just "being in the moment." Stay in touch with your body and with the baby. Make time to put your feet up, to sing (even if it is only in the shower), to do some slow, languorous belly dancing (not necessarily in the office), and to visualize your baby curled up in your uterus and ready to make the journey to birth.

You can be sure that there will be work crises, family crises, and people who need you. You can cope if you have harmony and balance in your life.

REST AND SLEEP

In the first and last three months, you will probably feel more tired than usual. Rest as much as possible, rather than trying to fight off the tiredness. It is much better to rest before you become completely exhausted and feel you cannot go on any longer. Toward the end of pregnancy there may be several reasons that you cannot sleep as much as you would like. Nearly every pregnant woman goes through a period when she either cannot drop off to sleep or she wakes in the night because the baby is kicking her, she needs to empty her bladder, or she has had a violent and disturbing dream and cannot get back to sleep. Sometimes the insomnia occurs because she is lying in bed worrying and in the darkness her fears gain the upper hand.

If you have just given up work, you may feel that your pregnancy has become a time of passive waiting and is stretching out longer and longer, so that you cannot see an end to it. You probably cannot sleep because you need action. Vigorous exercise during the day can be a remedy. You could also try the traditional remedies for sleeplessness, such as hot milk after a luxurious warm bath at bedtime. The problem with this, though, is that you are more likely to have to get up to empty your bladder.

The stillness of the middle of the night provides a marvelous opportunity for practicing your relaxation and breathing techniques and for getting in touch with your baby. Use the time to center down into your body and become more aware of the developing life inside you. Find a comfortable position to relax in, well supported by pillows wherever you need them, and let the pillows take the weight of your body, your limbs, and your head. Concentrate on your breathing and allow it to flow down through your body to where the baby nestles deep inside you. Cup your hands over the lower curve of your abdomen and breathe deeply so that the wave of the inhaled breath presses your hands up, and as you give a long breath out, your hands sink on the receding wave. Listen to the rhythmic sound of your breathing and think of it as being like waves breaking onto the shore.

Relax and enjoy lying there with your baby. Once you have begun to lose yourself in these feelings, you will find that your breathing has relaxed and you are drifting off to sleep. Talk and sing and have private conversations with your baby. In the later months of pregnancy, the baby can hear you, and this soothes you both.

EMOTIONAL CHALLENGES IN PREGNANCY

Many expectant mothers look and feel radiant. A healthy woman who is looking forward to a much-wanted baby, has a loving and secure relationship with a considerate partner, and has some knowledge about birth and what she can do to help herself, often revels in pregnancy.

Many women say, "I feel better than I have ever felt before" or "I'm really enjoying being pregnant" and are surprised at the vitality and sense of inner fulfillment that they experience. Yet probably all of us are assailed by darker thoughts at times when we are overtired or under some special stress. Some negative feelings that women experience in early pregnancy have been discussed on pages 28–30. But as your pregnancy advances, more specific anxieties may preoccupy you at times. Anxiety may grip you in the middle of the night when the baby has kicked you awake or when you have had to get up to empty your bladder and cannot get back to sleep again. Every fear is magnified in the darkness as you lie trying to sleep and unable to relax.

WORRIES ABOUT THE BIRTH

Labor can be an intensely pleasurable, all-absorbing, and deeply satisfying activity, which it is possible to enjoy. But just as some people do not like climbing a mountain, even though the view at the summit is magnificent, and just as some people feel that sex is overrated, whereas others think it is one of the best experiences that life can offer, different women have very different attitudes toward childbirth.

This attitude is not only a matter of what happens to you physiologically or how you are treated in the hospital, but also depends on what kind of person you are. Anxiety can cast a shadow over childbirth and produce the speeded-up heart rate, high blood pressure, muscle tension, and other physical results of stress that make birth more difficult.

Anxiety about labor is probably best dealt with first of all by finding out more about it—not just its mechanics, but the physical and emotional sensations each phase brings—and learning the relaxation, breathing, and focused concentration that can help you to work with your body instead of against it. The simple process of sharing fears also often results in feeling much more lighthearted, so that women begin to enjoy their pregnancies.

A good childbirth class where discussion is encouraged and you can talk freely about your apprehensions, as well as your hopes, is often effective in developing self-confidence and helping you to look forward to labor as a peak experience, not just an ordeal to be endured.

PAIN A woman having her first baby often thinks, "I have never had to experience anything really painful. How will I stand up to the pain of labor?" and since she has no idea what that pain is like or what contractions feel like, the thought can bring terror. Learning about labor, how contractions work, and how they may feel at different stages of labor is the most effective way of coming face-to-face with this anxiety and doing something about it. There is a whole section in this book about pain and pain relief (see pages 304–323). The important thing to understand is that for most women the pain of labor is different from the pain of injury. Some women describe it as "positive pain" or "pain with a purpose."

LOSS OF CONTROL For many women anxieties about labor are linked with a dread of losing control. For your whole life you have been taught to control physical processes and your behavior, and suddenly something is about to happen that clearly cannot be controlled and that will take over your body. You are told that you may cry out or groan, for example, that you may lose inhibitions, be impatient or irritable with your partner or whoever is helping you, and swear and say things you never meant to. You are horrified to hear that you may involuntarily empty your bowels or your bladder.

"I'VE ALWAYS BEEN A BIT INHIBITED ABOUT MY BODY. NOW I'M EXPECTED TO LIE DOWN, PART MY LEGS, AND LET COMPLETE STRANGERS GROPE ME."

You also learn that the waters may break suddenly. In any group of women discussing birth, first-time mothers nearly always ask those who have already had babies when their waters broke, whether it was sudden, and if so where it was; they express anxiety that the waters may break in the supermarket or on a bus or in another public place. What these women are saying is that they are fearful of letting their bodies function freely because of the embarrassment and social stigma attached. It is as if degrading physical processes—above all, dirty ones that involve getting rid of waste products from the body—are taking place in public.

Think through why you find the thought of your waters breaking in public so upsetting. You are having a baby, and it is perfectly obvious that you are going to give birth soon. If your waters do break in public, is it really so very terrible? You will attract interest and sympathy, but not disgust. You may see it as a kind of sexual act in front of other people. You are quite right, and understanding this can help you in labor. Birth, just like lovemaking, is a sexual process. If you can go with your labor instead of fighting it, the experience can be fulfilling in a strangely pleasurable way. Prepare the way to this through body awareness and relaxation. Touch relaxation (see pages 190–200) is a special kind of release that teaches you to flow toward sensations of pressure and heat. It will help a lot in labor.

FAILURE An anxiety closely connected with loss of control is the fear of making a fool of yourself. You may feel that you are on public display in labor and approach it as a test of endurance. You may also be anxious about "letting down" a partner who puts great faith in your ability to cope, or even of "failing" a childbirth teacher. Some men who participate in classes and the other preparations for the birth become so enthusiastic and obsessional that they are in effect "trainers," rather like athletic coaches. The woman then feels that she is expected to put on a performance and must excel in it. Childbirth classes that are geared exclusively to techniques, rather than focusing on wider aspects of the total experience, can reinforce this feeling.

"I WAS ALWAYS AWKWARD IN MY OVERWEIGHT BODY. BUT IN LABOR I SWAM THROUGH CONTRACTIONS LIKE A SEAL OR A DOLPHIN. I FELT TRIUMPHANT!"

In the same way that elaborate techniques performed to achieve sexual satisfaction can sometimes disturb the spontaneous rhythm of sex and interfere with the intense feeling and play of emotion between the couple, so breathing exercises and "distraction" techniques can sometimes intrude on the experience of labor. Exercises need to become "second nature" and to be made a part of yourself. It is like learning to play the piano: there is a vast difference between laborious scales and playing a sonata. The exercises are important because they prepare you for playing music. But the eventual aim is to let the music flow through you, rather than to superimpose tricks and techniques. Such a physical and emotional surrender is simple in labor because of its intensity. Birth involves mind and body working together in a completely absorbing, exciting, and passionate way. There is no success or failure in labor. You cannot make a fool of yourself, let anyone down, or fail an examination in birth.

FEAR OF MANAGING ALONE Some women approach labor as a medical incident like having an appendectomy, an unwelcome interruption of normal life rather than an experience that can be satisfying in itself. They feel totally dependent on the technology provided by the hospital and worry about whether they will get there on time, or whether the right people will be present to deliver the baby. Such dependence is reinforced by contemporary obstetrics and by every program on television that illustrates the latest marvel of science applied to childbearing. The impression is given that women must depend on lifesaving machines, and that without them it is not safe to have a baby. The fact is, however, that although these machines can be useful in diagnosing difficulties when a baby is at risk or when special problems arise in pregnancy or labor, the majority of women can give birth perfectly well without them. It is not advances in medicine but improved conditions, better food, and better general health that have made childbirth much safer for mothers and babies today than it was 100 years ago. The rate of stillbirths and deaths in the first week of life is directly related to a country's gross national product and to the mother's place in the social class structure.

Even in the West, it is twice as safe for a professional woman to bear a child than it is for a poor, unsupported mother. The challenge is to find out which mothers and babies are at risk and offer them everything that can make birth safer, and to enable all women to give birth naturally if they can.

LOSS OF AUTONOMY Another frequent anxiety is that of being denied the right to function as an adult. Many pregnant women resent the feeling that they cannot make their own decisions. Increasing numbers do not want to hand their bodies over to professional caregivers in pregnancy and childbirth, and seek maternity care in which they can take an active part, sharing the decision-making with their advisers.

If you are not sure whether your doctor is being open with you, or whether the hospital will really let you do the things in labor that you have asked to do, the uncertainty can produce a sick fear in the pit of the stomach. Too often, pregnant women are treated very much like children or as patients in categories, such as "high risk," "low risk," "primigravida," "multigravida," and so on, who have to be processed through the hospital system, passive receivers of care rather than active birthgivers.

FEAR OF HOSPITALS For many of us, hospitals are threatening places. People go to the hospital when they are ill. This may be the first time that you have been a patient in a hospital, and the sights, sounds, and even smells alarm you. Few maternity units are designed and decorated to be intimate, and to look more like home, or at least a good hotel. Some hospitals still have a forbidding atmosphere, with their long, green-painted corridors and white tiles and instrument carts. Delivery rooms in otherwise splendid modern hospitals can be windowless boxes, and prenatal clinics, your first introduction to the hospital, are often forbidding places without pictures and with backache-inducing chairs set in rows. Even more important than the surroundings are the attitudes of the staff and the ways in which they interact with patients. If you meet cool indifference, rigid authoritarianism, or patronizing behavior you may dread going for your prenatal appointments. This anxiety may color your whole approach to labor and childbirth.

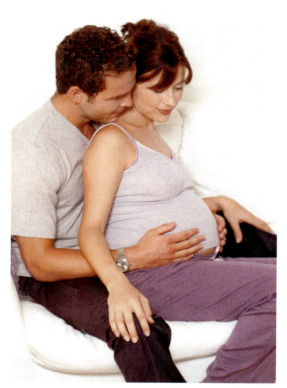

Being open to the changes in the shape of her body and ways in which their relationship unfolds helps to prepare couples for the day when they become parents.

There is a certain kind of emotional climate in which anxieties flourish, and unfortunately it is one that our society often provides for many pregnant women. If there is no one readily available of whom you can ask questions and who will answer in clear terms that you can understand, the seeds of anxiety are often sown. Then they are nourished over the months by the insecurity of seeing different members of the prenatal staff at each visit.

Women often feel apologetic about being anxious, about not being "sensible," as if they were revealing a shameful lack of emotional stamina. They are sometimes regarded as having something psychologically wrong with them if they show anxiety. But many fears are not the result of inadequacy but a response to stresses caused by an environment that is alien and unfriendly, and by care that is impersonal. In such a situation, anxiety is *realistic*.

Take a tour of the maternity unit. You can call the hospital to learn when tours are scheduled. Ask to see the birth rooms (see page 186), including the machinery that may be used. Although you might prefer childbirth classes that are run independently of the hospital, attend at least some of those at the hospital, too, so that you can get to know the staff, and talk with a nurse about the style of childbirth that you would like. Ask him or her to note down any particular requests on your chart. Read the section on talking to doctors (pages 53–56) before you go to see your doctor.

LOSS OF ATTRACTIVENESS Some pregnant women are deeply concerned that their sexual attractiveness may be completely destroyed by childbearing. They are frightened of losing their figures; they may also be anxious that the vagina will be slack and changed in shape and that they will never enjoy sex again. Fear of a tear or a cut (see page 331), often discussed in childbirth classes, is not so much about pain resulting from stitches. It is really anxiety about genital mutilation.

EPISIOTOMY Fortunately, only in a very few hospitals is episiotomy more or less routine for women having their first babies and for a large percentage of those having second and subsequent babies. Now this is changing fast. Women questioned the need for what amounts to surgical intervention in normal birth and the creation of an artificial and painful wound, and obstetricians and midwives responded by changing their practices. Obstetricians are asking why episiotomy became so widely used without proper evaluation. In fact, recent scientific trials have shown that this procedure, except in cases of fetal distress or other rare situations, has no advantage and causes unnecessary damage to the perineum. Women are often more anxious about episiotomy than any other invasive procedure. The thought of being cut or injured in such a sensitive place is horrifying. Many are concerned that giving birth will damage them, so they will never be the same again.

"I WAS READY TO GIVE UP. IT FELT AS IF I WAS SPLITTING IN TWO. BUT I PUT MY TRUST IN THE MIDWIFE, AND I DID NOT NEED A CUT."

There are various ways in which you can prepare the tissues of your perineum—the area between your vagina and your anus—to become soft and supple during pregnancy, so that you enter labor fully confident that you can give birth without injury. Pelvic floor movements (see pages 118–119) can contribute to the sensitive awareness, coordination, and control that help you in the second stage, allowing you to open your body for the baby to be born and reducing stress on the pelvic muscles and perineal tissues. Massaging the tissues with vegetable oil can also help. Getting in touch, literally, with this part of your body and feeling how flexible the tissues are will give you the confidence to know that your vagina and perineum are able to fan out and open wide like a great peony or a rose spreading thick, fleshy petals. Since in late pregnancy it can be quite difficult to reach your perineum and exert firm pressure, you may want to ask your partner to help you with this gentle massage. It feels especially good if the oil is warmed first and your partner's hands move slowly and rhythmically.

If you want to avoid an episiotomy, discuss the subject with your midwife or doctor in advance. Say that you would like them to assist the birth so that you can breathe the baby out rather than push it out, and ask for this to be noted on your chart.

All of this preparation is just as valuable even if you do end up with an episiotomy. You will be much better able to understand the healing process after a cut or tear if you already know where the soft tissues and muscles are: you will know precisely what has happened, and where. Exploring the vagina with your fingers during pregnancy (see page 117) and after giving birth, and looking at it in a mirror, helps you to feel that it belongs to you; you can gradually rehabilitate the muscles through practicing gentle pelvic floor movements (see pages 118–119).

WORRIES ABOUT THE BABY

Almost every woman wonders at some stage during her pregnancy whether her baby is normal. It may seem almost impossible that you could produce from the dark interior of your body anything that is completely perfect. This is probably the most persistent, gnawing fear of all, and the only way of coming to terms with it is to develop self-confidence, a process that, not surprisingly, takes time. This is where regular attendance at childbirth classes, which encourage you to trust your body and your ability to give birth, rather than depending on others, can help enormously.

WORRIES ABOUT THE FUTURE

After you have a baby, everything changes. How you see yourself, your priorities, and all your relationships, is affected in some way. To bring new life into the world is an enormous responsibility.

CHANGE When a woman is expressing anxiety about "things never being the same again," it helps to think through what exactly this means. One couple who had a deeply satisfying relationship saw the pregnancy and birth as an "interruption": "We don't want to change our lives for a child," the woman said, "to be swamped by it. How long will it take before we get back to normal again? Sometimes I'm frightened we'll *never* get back to normal." She said that she did not want to become the same kind of woman as her own mother. Most of all, she was afraid that her partner would not love her in the same way and that she would be desexed in his and her own eyes by maternity.

> "WE WERE HAPPY AND DIDN'T WANT THINGS TO CHANGE. BUT NOW WE'RE FALLING IN LOVE WITH THE IDEA OF EACH OTHER AS A MOTHER AND FATHER. WE'RE FALLING IN LOVE AGAIN."

LONELINESS Some women having their first babies move during pregnancy to a larger apartment or house, and find themselves in an area where they know nobody at all. They stop work in late pregnancy and no longer have daily contact with friends and colleagues. Home and alone for the first time, they are initially delighted, but quickly become bored and depressed.

If this is how it is for you, take up an activity that brings social contacts: learn something new; join a club of some kind; attend childbirth classes; track down interesting places in the locality; and invite people to your home. Your doctor or midwife may be able to tell you about other pregnant women or mothers with new babies who live near you and whom you can meet. Investigate the possibilities while you are pregnant. When you are busy with a baby, it may be difficult to make new friends, especially during the winter months, so take the opportunity to make them now.

SOCIAL EXPECTATIONS A woman once told me that her pregnancy made her feel that at last she was fulfilling a socially acceptable role, and her own mother was proud of her for the first time in her life. Doctors expected her to be a "good patient" and to be processed through the busy prenatal clinic like all the other women with their swelling tummies. She suddenly felt miles away from her former colleagues and others with whom she had shared a working relationship, separated by the fact of her pregnancy. But by the end she felt guilty that she had resented the baby at the beginning of her pregnancy. At night as the baby moved inside her, she lay wondering whether she would ever be a good mother. She said, "I sometimes feel so sorry for the little thing in there that I end up crying." In her prenatal discussion group, it emerged that several other women were also lying awake at night, preoccupied with similar worries. What each one had assumed to be a personal problem had turned out to be a shared experience.

If you realize that you are not alone with your fears, and are not being "odd" or neurotic, anxieties become much less disturbing. Thinking about inevitable change may worry you in different ways. You may be afraid that the relationship with your partner will deteriorate, or that you have no maternal instincts. If you are giving up your job and the money and freedom of earning your living, you may wonder if you will be able to tolerate being at home all day, and whether you will miss the order and routine of work and all the interesting people you meet there.

Although such anxiety is realistic in the sense that these changes are dramatic and demanding for many women, most expectant mothers worry more about labor and the baby than about how they will cope after the birth. Many take the unknown "afterward" more or less for granted. It is as if they can see only as far as the birth, which dominates the horizon. The postpartum experience may then come as something of a shock. So some anxiety about life after the baby arrives is a healthy sign, and it indicates that the emotional work is taking place that prepares you not only for birth but also for parenthood.

Many anxieties offer clues to the challenges confronting you during pregnancy. It is a waste of emotional energy to try to "forget" them or put them to the back of your mind. They are there to be worked with. It is often the man and woman who are determined to take it all in their stride and carry on as usual, and who do not acknowledge feelings of apprehension, who face the most shattering crises when they have the baby. The discomfort produced by anxiety can force you to think through the meaning for you of the coming of a child into your life. Without the stress and challenge of this kind, emotional preparation for birth and parenthood may be overlooked. Anxieties are a vital element in the emotional changes necessary to face up to the reality of birth and to the astonishing reality of the new baby.

BECOMING A FATHER

Becoming a father is a major step in a man's life.
It can also be a daunting one. Yet it is an experience
usually treated as insignificant in comparison with that
of becoming a mother. As a result, the stresses on the
future father are little understood, and men are not
prepared for the impact of pregnancy.

If people do notice that a man is finding the going difficult, they tend to laugh rather than sympathize. The nervousness and anxiety of the father-to-be are favorite subjects of jokes, ranging from the picture-postcard variety—a man wide-eyed and desperate in the hospital corridor as his wife produces triplets—to those amused tales about male ignorance and incompetence shared among women over coffee.

In classes for parents-to-be, a man is often discussed only in terms of how he can help his partner, and his own emotional needs are neglected. One result of this is to make him feel isolated, and it is difficult for him to reach out and give his partner the support she needs. She is the princess going to the ball—and he feels a bit like the back legs of a pantomime horse.

An expectant father may feel jealous of all the attention given to the future mother, absurdly envious of her reproductive powers, and sometimes even jealous of the coming baby. He feels guilty about these emotions and decides to concentrate on his work—because that at least is one thing he can do properly. And the more he immerses himself in his own preoccupations, the more left out of the pregnancy he feels.

Some men become depressed or experience violent mood swings similar to those that a pregnant woman may go through. A few even walk out of the relationship because the stress is too great for them to handle. Usually there are two people having a baby, and the man also goes through a transitional period of stress when deep emotions may be stirred and his behavior is difficult to understand.

REACTING TO FATHERHOOD

The sheer responsibility of having a baby can be frightening. The woman may be planning to give up work for a time, or even for good, and the man is expected to support the family. The financial burden may be too great for some men

A father discovers new depths of love and compassion, and life becomes more precious.

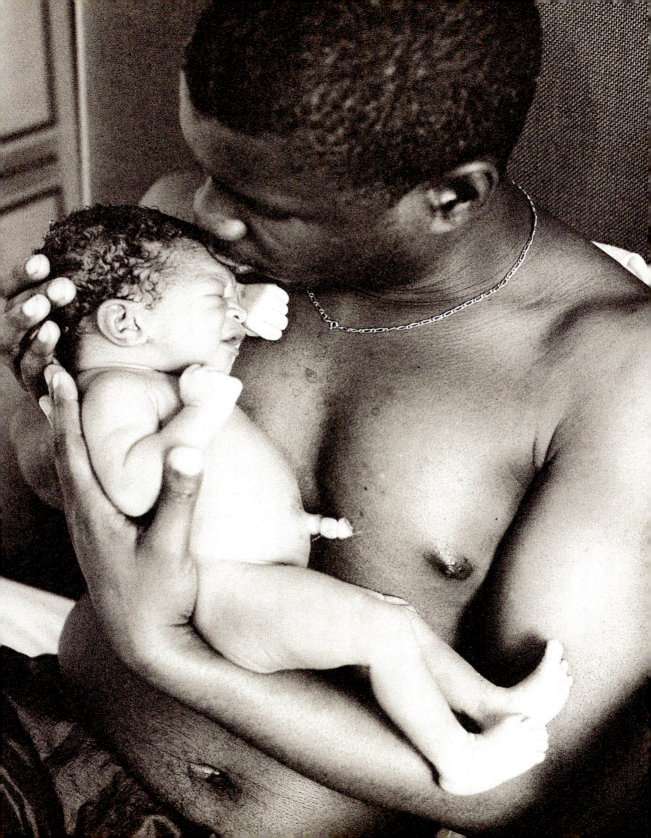

to shoulder without anxiety. For many men, money problems constitute a rationalization, a socially acceptable explanation for anxiety, without getting to the root of what they really find disturbing. In fact, some men find that the prospect of becoming a father brings with it a crisis of identity.

THE CHANGING RELATIONSHIP One element in this crisis involves grieving over a relationship that is bound to change. The easy ways, the lack of routine, the spontaneity of the early stage of the relationship, all have to give way to an existence centered around a baby. Some men see their partners as their mothers. When the woman becomes pregnant, it is as if the man is losing a mother and is being replaced in her affections by a new baby. As his partner becomes more involved in the pregnancy and the baby, he feels increasingly rejected and finds this shift of focus very threatening.

THE CHANGING WOMAN Some men acquire a woman as a kind of showpiece, proof of their success in hunting down and possessing a desirable sexual object, or evidence of their social success, a demonstration and a symbol of a lifestyle that embodies achievement. Delighted as such a man may be to be fathering a child, he may find it quite difficult to cope with his partner's new concentration on the pregnancy rather than on him. He feels that the physical changes in his partner's body are upsetting, as conventional attractiveness is replaced by a very different body—a melon-shaped abdomen and heavy, swelling breasts covered with a network of tiny blue veins. A man who has valued a woman as a status or sex symbol may feel cheated by her pregnancy.

THE DEVELOPING BABY It is sometimes difficult for a man, who does not have the baby growing inside his body, to acknowledge its reality. He often begins to become more aware of the child at about the time he feels it bump and kick at night. Some men find this sensation not only astonishing and exciting but rather eerie, and they take a while to adjust to the idea of another being living and growing inside the body of the woman they know so well.

THE FUTURE GRANDPARENTS When a couple has a first baby, they may have to work through a painful transitional period in which they must forge a new adult relationship with their own parents, one that allows for the responsibility and commitment they have to the child they are bearing. This may produce stresses with the future grandparents, and a man may get caught up in a difficult relationship with his own mother, just as a woman may with hers. When a man's mother is fearful that she is losing her son, she becomes demanding. He may feel the pull of her possessive love drawing attention away from the needs of his partner and baby. Sometimes a woman sees this, whereas the man is completely unaware of it. It is important to understand that the older women, the ex-mothers, are in the process of being replaced, and they may feel hurt and unwanted. If there is a problem of this kind, the couple should talk about it together and be honest about their feelings.

THE FATHER'S NEW ROLE

Having a baby used to be solely the concern of the woman, usually with her mother standing in the background giving advice. Today, it is much more something for a woman and a man to share.

There are still some men who say they do not want to get involved in "women's things" and who feel that their manliness is being threatened. They have the uneasy suspicion that learning about childbirth means that they will no longer be potent, virile males. Some hope to hand the woman over to experts and retire from the scene.

Forty years ago, some midwives and obstetricians looked askance at men who became involved in childbirth, as if they were slightly odd. Turn the clock back a hundred years or so, and men were kept at a distance from anything to do with birth: pregnancy was a "certain condition" in women that a man pretended he knew nothing about.

My mother told me that my father felt embarrassed to go out with her in advanced pregnancy, so that walks they took had to be after dark, with her enveloped in a wraparound coat. And as for a father wheeling a stroller, or changing a diaper—it was unheard of. Even a man who might have liked to try his hand at such things rarely got the chance. This was partly because in those days there used to be what one perceptive psychoanalyst called a male "taboo on tenderness." Men were frightened that to be seen to be involved with women's activities would humiliate them in the eyes of other men. And childbirth was the epitome of all feminine mysteries. Both women and men were prevented by these rules from discovering their full potential.

"HE FOUND IT REALLY HARD TO BELIEVE THERE WAS A BABY THERE UNTIL IT KICKED HIM ONE NIGHT. HE GOT VERY EXCITED."

Many modern men are determined to share as much as they can in pregnancy and birth. They enjoy the woman's changing shape and the reality of the baby's kicking against their hand. But often a man still feels he will be a novice at fatherhood. He wonders just how much he can do, since the baby is growing in his partner's body, not his. In a way, the partnership between the mother and her unborn child is already complete, and a man can sometimes feel like an intruder.

But a woman depends on her partner's support and needs the special relationship with him, which is quite different from any others that she has. She may not realize just how much he is sharing in the pregnancy emotionally, and the heights and depths of his own feelings about it. There is no longer any need for a man to square his shoulders and pretend he is not stirred by what is about to happen in his life. Take every opportunity to make plans and discuss your feelings about the changes to come.

FEELINGS ABOUT BEING AT THE BIRTH

Most expectant fathers today approach childbirth with curiosity and in a very different spirit from that of their fathers and grandfathers. Although they may wonder whether they are going to make fools of themselves while playing an unfamiliar part, and may be nervous about unpleasant procedures involved in labor, they want to understand what is going on and to support their partners. Hospital staff are usually extremely busy and working with more than one patient at a time. It is impossible for them to give the constant companionship and loving care that a woman craves as she is swept through the intensely powerful physical and emotional experience of labor, and the very unfamiliarity of the surroundings can make the most courageous woman apprehensive. She needs her partner or someone else who loves her. She needs someone there who is not simply an onlooker, but a companion who understands what happens, who knows what her prenatal preparation has been, and how to help her. (For more about the father's role at the birth, see page 287.)

> "I WOULDN'T HAVE MISSED IT FOR THE WORLD. I WASN'T SURE THAT I WANTED TO BE THERE, BUT IT TURNED OUT TO BE AN INCREDIBLE EXPERIENCE."

The man who fully involves himself shares in an experience that is exciting, challenging, intensely moving, and deeply satisfying. It is a question not only of helping his partner have their baby, but of an often surprising encounter with his own emotions. There may be an astonishing, incredible joy and wonder at being so close to the beating center of life. In a very direct way, love is made flesh.

BEING SUPPORTIVE ABOUT PRENATAL CARE

Pregnancy can be a time of great emotional upheaval as a woman adapts to the extraordinary things happening inside her body. She has to go through all sorts of physical examinations that are not always conducted in a warm, sympathetic way. Many women are made anxious by the kind of prenatal care they receive.

THE MEDICAL OR DOCTOR'S OFFICE

Some men find a woman's anxiety difficult to understand. They find the sophisticated technology used today reassuring and fascinating. But if a man imagines something happening inside his testicles or penis, it may be easier to comprehend. How would he feel if his testicles started to swell up and change shape dramatically, forcing him to visit a doctor regularly and be prodded, poked, and examined by strangers who seemed concerned only with the lower end of his body? It might be impossible to get information about what was happening to him, knowing only that he faced an ordeal at the end of nine months when whatever was occurring must be terminated and the thing inside him somehow gotten out. How would he like to be lying flat on a high table, sometimes with his legs up high and wide apart in metal stirrups, while various women in white coats peered at him with little lights and probed his body with special machines? Out of the corner of his eye he could see them writing up case notes full of technical terms and abbreviations that, for all he knows, could be suggesting some form of disease.

A man has to go to a medical office only once to discover how intimidating it can be. In the atmosphere of a medical office, women often feel that they have become part of a factory process. Questions go out of their heads, or seem to interrupt the smooth running of the institution and mean that other women waiting their turn have still longer to wait. Often a woman returns depressed and anxious. A partner who can attend occasionally can give her moral support and build the foundation for a good working relationship with those who will be present during labor.

CHILDBIRTH CLASSES

By attending classes in preparation for the birth with his partner, a man can learn a good deal about the physiological processes and emotional changes of labor. He can also begin to understand his own part in it, and often has the chance to see films of birth where men are giving support to their partners using skills learned in class.

EVERYDAY HELP

In the last three months, a man can help by seeing that his partner gets more rest and lies down every afternoon or evening. Extra labor-saving equipment or help in the home can ensure that she does not get worn out. She should not be doing heavy shopping, so he may take over supermarket duty, or go with her to load the car. If there are jobs in the house like moving furniture, these are his now. And if she cannot get down to bathe the toddler or strip the bed, the man can make these his responsibility now. On the other hand, the woman does not need to be treated like an invalid, and the couple can enjoy going out together, especially at the end of pregnancy, when time may seem to pass very slowly and she feels she has been pregnant forever. A man can also protect his partner from the well-meaning and often confusing advice that comes from other people both before and after the birth. He can support her in doing things the way that they have both decided is right for them.

YOU AND YOUR PARTNER

Pregnant women are not only obstetric patients or just future mothers. They are also usually in an intimate loving relationship. Pregnancy can be a time of great opportunity for both partners to discover things about themselves and each other. If they do not communicate easily, it can be a time when small irritants turn into major crises.

THE COUPLE UNDER STRESS

Some couples find the transition period of pregnancy an especially difficult time. It can put stress on the couple that has an informal relationship and marries when a baby is on the way. It can put equal stress on a couple when both partners enjoy their careers and have never seen themselves as parents, but decide to continue with the pregnancy when the woman conceives by mistake. It can bristle with challenges, too, when a woman has been on the pill, stops taking it because the couple thinks it might be a good idea to have a baby, and then immediately becomes pregnant before she has had time to switch her mind to the reality of motherhood. In these situations, rapid adjustment is necessary, and either or both parents may feel trapped at the same time as they are feeling delighted.

As soon as they tell other people about the pregnancy, they may feel that a social machine has swung into action. Some couples say that they felt strong disapproval from relatives, especially their parents, when they put off having a baby because they were both busy with their careers. Then when the woman became pregnant they were overwhelmed by the relief and pleasure expressed, as if at last they were doing the socially acceptable thing. Even positive reactions may feel like a public intrusion on their intimate personal relationship.

SHARING PROBLEMS

When a pregnancy starts, a man and a woman may begin inhabiting different worlds. He may think that she has become psychologically unpredictable and vulnerable. She may see him as unsympathetic, unloving, and crude. He may feel he can no longer talk to her about "rational" matters, and that she has lost interest in everything except the baby. He may feel pushed out into the cold, as if he were living with a different woman. Because they are often isolated from other couples facing similar difficulties, they may believe that such problems are unique to them. Talking to others expecting babies can help them to detect the social pressures on prospective parents that often create emotional stress. Attending classes together can provide a bridge between the socially assigned gender roles of man and woman, and can help draw them closer.

TALKING IN A GROUP

In a prenatal group where couples discussed the effect of pregnancy on their relationship, one woman who was feeling that she had lost her individuality in becoming an expectant mother remarked that she was frightened of what this was doing to her relationship with her partner. Would they, she worried, become just "Mom and Dad" and cease being lovers? Her concern about this was making her resent the baby at times.

The members of the group found that other couples, too, were experiencing the same anxiety. Some felt strongly that they wanted to be different kinds of parents from their own parents and to have happier marriages than them. It was agreed that it was important for a couple to share these thoughts with each other and to discuss not just the practical arrangements to be made for the baby, but their ideas about the kind of parents they hoped to be. Becoming a mother involves emotional "growing pains" that can be as disturbing as those of adolescence. A similar psychological process often occurs in a man, too, but he usually feels he has even less justification to talk about it because *he* is not physically pregnant. Yet to be able to nurture their young, both the man and the woman have to change.

Another couple who had been through this in an earlier pregnancy said that talking about it helped them to understand each other better and that they came to like their changed roles. At first they were merely playing the parts of "Mommy" and "Daddy," but then they found they were good at them, and became aware of qualities each had never imagined the other possessed.

"IT'S A WHOLE NEW WORLD FOR HIM BECAUSE HE DIDN'T GET INVOLVED IN HIS FIRST WIFE'S PREGNANCY, AND SHE DIDN'T EXPECT IT. IT'S INCREDIBLY EXCITING FOR US BOTH AND WE HAVE GOTTEN MUCH CLOSER— AND MORE IN LOVE EVEN THAN BEFORE."

DEVELOPING CONFIDENCE

Many couples have a private name for the unborn child. As a woman passes through the prodding and procedures of each prenatal visit, she and her partner may begin to feel as if their baby has become "the" baby, or even "the hospital's" baby.

Some couples have problems in family relationships (especially with parents), which they do not realize are shared by others. Each partner may resent the other for his or her insensitivity and ineptitude at handling these situations, or for being overdependent on their parents. At a childbirth class, there may be an opportunity to talk through these problems with others and to discuss the future grandparents' feelings and any other situations that might cause stress. The very fact of finding that they are not alone with these difficulties can help a couple overcome them.

GROWING THROUGH THE EXPERIENCE

Many of us have babies before we are emotionally ready for them. As a result, some babies come into the world in spite of, rather than because of, what their parents feel about each other. When a woman decides to continue with an unplanned pregnancy, she needs emotional support. If a man has nothing else to offer, he can at least give her this.

It is bound to be painful for them both if they decide to part with the baby, but the experience can help them to grow in understanding. When a couple is unhappy together, there is an even more compelling reason to use the months of pregnancy for joint preparation for the birth, if only because the task can bring a new perceptiveness and sensitivity to the other's needs. Preparation for birth is not simply a set of instructions and exercises, but a process in which two people start out together on a shared enterprise. It creates many opportunities for increased understanding of each other's needs and enrichment of the relationship. When a man and woman are able to fully understand what the pregnancy means to the other partner, they are well on the way to growing up together.

"THE FATHERS' EVENINGS WERE A BRAVE EFFORT BUT THEY PRESENTED THE MEDICAL VIEW OF CHILDBIRTH. OVERALL, I FELT EXCLUDED FROM THE PREGNANCY BUSINESS."

The emotional changes of pregnancy occur for all couples who are expecting a baby, and it helps to realize that others share these experiences and find them challenging, too.

SEX IN PREGNANCY

It is important to know that you are loved in pregnancy, whether or not this involves sexual intercourse. Stroking, massage, loving touch, and sexual pleasuring are all part of this physical expression of the relationship.

ATTITUDES TOWARD SEX

Many couples make love right through pregnancy. At the beginning, nausea and vomiting can mean that the last thing you want to do is to make love, but usually by the middle months lovemaking is enjoyable and satisfying. Pregnancy is a good time to learn more about how your body works. A woman who learns about her uterus, vagina, and pelvic floor muscles may become more sensitively responsive to this part of her body.

Many women do not realize the function of the pelvic floor muscles in lovemaking and some have never explored the way in which the vagina, labia, and clitoris are constructed. In fact, some women have their first orgasm when they are pregnant.

This is not a matter of intellectual information and diagrams of the genitals. Some women dislike and distrust their bodies. For the first time in pregnancy they come to know and be comfortable with themselves. If you have never before allowed feelings to sweep through you, preparation for the intensely emotional experience of labor, with its storms and currents, and the extraordinarily powerful drama of delivery, unlock a capacity for "letting go" that can apply to lovemaking also. But some couples (especially in the later months) feel that they do not have medical approval for lovemaking. You may have guilty feelings and be anxious that you are harming your unborn baby. Expectant parents often want to talk about this in childbirth education classes. Many couples say that sex is a difficult subject to discuss with their doctor.

BREASTS

Changes in your breasts in preparation for feeding the baby later are one of the first things you may notice in pregnancy. The little bumps around your nipples get bigger and the breasts themselves grow larger. If you had small breasts before pregnancy, you may enjoy your new figure. Your bra may feel uncomfortably tight, and some women say that their breasts are so sensitive that they feel bruised.

If this happens, it is difficult to think of your breasts as erotic. If you enjoyed a bit of sexual grappling before you became pregnant, you are most unlikely to now. In a state of sexual arousal, breasts swell by as much as 25 percent, as blood rushes into the veins and tissues become engorged. This is why you may not want your breasts touched at all. Any nipple stimulation should start with touch as light as thistledown, and only get firmer if it feels good.

At the very end of pregnancy, you may notice that if your partner plays with your nipples you get contractions. There is a neurological link between breasts and uterus, and nipple stimulation is sometimes used as a way of starting labor. If the baby is not yet ready to be born and you get contractions with nipple stimulation, it may be best to avoid it and have a lovely, slow back massage instead!

ANXIETY ABOUT MISCARRIAGE

If you have had a previous miscarriage—especially if there has been more than one—fear that you might have another may put you off sex. You may feel that you have to "hold on," both physically and emotionally, to your new pregnancy, and see sex as a threat to the baby. In this case, you are likely to be far too tense to relax and enjoy lovemaking.

Your partner, too, may be nervous and think that he is a danger to the pregnancy. When two people feel like this, they trigger further anxiety in each other and may even avoid cuddling and caressing because they fear sexual arousal. This is a pity, because they both need to relax. The stress of worrying about miscarriage, and the physiological changes that occur under acute stress, may actually increase the chance of its happening.

Doctors usually advise against intercourse if a woman has any spotting of blood in the first 12 weeks or has miscarried in a previous pregnancy, and most women probably feel safer avoiding intercourse if they have any bleeding. However, slight bleeding around the time when a first and second period is due is actually quite common. Up to a third of women in any childbirth class say that they had a slight bloodstained discharge at this time, and yet go on to have a normal pregnancy and a healthy baby. They often do not tell the doctor about this, so doctors may not realize just how frequently this happens.

A doctor who has advised against intercourse early in the pregnancy sometimes forgets to say later on, "It should be OK, now. You are past the time when you are most likely to miscarry," and the couple continue not only to avoid intercourse, but any lovemaking, right through pregnancy, or feel guilty about it if they do make love. This is another way in which pregnancy becomes hijacked by medical dogma, making it stressful for a woman and her partner. It might have been better for the advice not to have been given in the first place.

Couples who have enjoyed very active "angry" sex in the past will find that this type of "fighting" lovemaking is painful and does not work for most women when they are pregnant. You and your partner can explore new ways of making love or, if you prefer, avoid it altogether. The only thing we know for sure is that sex in pregnancy should always be gentle.

TIREDNESS

You may feel incredibly tired in the first weeks and worry that you will be like this until you have the baby. This physical exhaustion is linked with the major adjustments your whole body is making in those first few weeks, things you cannot see, but which are of far-reaching importance. The baby is fully formed in miniature by three months, and every cell in your body is directly or indirectly involved in adapting to meet the challenge of pregnancy. No wonder you are tired!

All of this is happening when you may have told very few people that you are pregnant, so no concessions are made when you are under pressure at work, for example. Or if you are busy at home with older children, you may want to prove to yourself that you are going to be able to handle a toddler and a baby, too. The result is that you drop into bed with relief and fall asleep as soon as you can. Sex is the last thing you want. However, if you feel confident about your sexuality and are in a strong, caring relationship, you are more likely to be able to take all this in your stride.

LIBIDO

A woman having her first baby tends to be less interested in sex at the beginning of pregnancy, though women having second or later babies often notice very little change in libido.

Some women actually enjoy sex more once they know they are pregnant. It may sound odd, but they find it easier to give themselves to their feelings when they are pregnant because there is no longer the risk of getting pregnant. For these women, contraception may be associated with holding back, being careful, remembering to take the pill, inserting a diaphragm correctly, making sure that a condom hasn't slipped off, recording the menstrual cycle, or having intercourse only when it is "safe," or even gambling with the withdrawal method. A woman who has worried constantly about getting pregnant or not getting pregnant discovers that she can now forget all these things and relax and enjoy it.

Even so, this is more likely to happen after about 10–12 weeks. Once the period of nausea, vomiting, tiredness, and anxiety about possible miscarriage is over, many women say they enjoy sex more than ever before.

"AFTER THE FIRST THREE MONTHS, WHEN I STOPPED FEELING EXHAUSTED AND THROWING UP, I GOT TURNED ON. THE TROUBLE WAS, MY PARTNER DIDN'T!"

The middle months of pregnancy are a time when they feel happy with their bodies: their skin has a healthy bloom, their hair is thick and glossy, and they glow with pregnancy radiance. However, this sense of well-being is less likely if you are under great pressure at work or if you are constantly worrying about money. Then the fatigue felt in the early weeks tends to continue and you never get "turned on" in mid-pregnancy. Nor is it likely to happen if you feel angry about being pregnant, unhappy about your relationship, or trapped by obligations at work or in the family.

POSITIONS FOR LOVEMAKING

Most couples want to adapt lovemaking techniques as pregnancy advances. The conventional "missionary" position (with the man lying on top of the woman) is rarely comfortable, unless he gets on all fours and puts no weight on you. Any weight on your breasts is extremely uncomfortable. It is worth experimenting with other positions in which the woman is uppermost or in which entry is from the side or from behind. A side-lying position in which you have your back to your partner and nestle into his lap is often comfortable. You may enjoy being on all fours or kneeling with your partner behind. No harm will come to the baby: the bag of waters cushions it and a seal is provided by the mucous plug, like a stopper in a bottle. Even when your abdomen is bumped in lovemaking, the baby bobs like a cork in a glass of water. In many ways, sex in advanced pregnancy is funny, and it helps to approach it in a lighthearted way.

THE MIDDLE MONTHS

By the start of the fourth month, the tissues around and inside your vagina have "ripened" and remain like this through pregnancy. They are thicker and swollen, rather like ripe soft fruit, similar to the way they are engorged during sexual arousal. Even the color has changed from shades of pale pink and red to purple, violet, and blue as a result of the increased blood supply. This means that a woman may be in a permanent state of gentle sexual arousal. She also feels very moist. Vaginal lubrication, which seeps through the convoluted walls of the vagina, may make her much more conscious of her vagina.

The pressure on the genital organs is so great for some women that they say they feel "lusty," like one woman, who says, "I can't wait for my husband to get home, poor man!" or another, who says, "I couldn't get through the day without masturbating—I felt so sexy. I thought I must be very peculiar until I talked to my sister-in-law who had a baby last year, and she said she felt just the same."

"MY BODY FEELS INCREDIBLY ALIVE. MY PARTNER LOVES MY BIGGER BREASTS AND MY NEW CURVES. WE BOTH FEEL SEXUALLY RECHARGED."

When a woman is feeling supercharged like this, she is sometimes aghast to discover that her partner does not want to have intercourse, or that he cannot get or maintain an erection. Yet many men are anxious that they can hurt the baby. This concern isn't a bad thing, because they become more thoughtful and considerate about lovemaking. But a man who is really frightened may believe erroneously that lovemaking can break the bag of waters, bruise the baby, or start labor immediately, and may refuse to touch the woman at all. It is as if he feels that self-control will guard the pregnancy. These beliefs are remarkably similar to those held in societies where taboos are imposed on a father to ensure the well-being of a baby.

CAN ORGASM START LABOR?

Although the female orgasm involves contractions of the uterus, it will not trigger labor unless everything is ready to start anyway. It is quite natural to feel contractions, which usually die down after a few minutes. The uterus is an active organ and contracts from the time of your first period right through to menopause. It is especially active in pregnancy, and the contractions (Braxton Hicks contractions) that you feel in the last months are rehearsals for labor. If you have had a preterm labor before, notice spotting of blood, or if the mucous plug is already gone, it is wise not to have intercourse. Once the cervical mucus has been disturbed by contractions (and this can happen in the last four to five weeks), ascending infection is a possibility.

THE LAST THREE MONTHS

By about seven months, indigestion or heartburn can be a problem when you lie flat, so you need to have your head and shoulders well raised with pillows. You may prefer making love in a sitting position, using a big floor cushion, chair, or the side of the bed.

Your fantasies about your body—your body image—are bound to affect your sexual feelings. Your body is going through such vast changes that you may get a very distorted idea of it. Some women think they are far bigger than they really are, or believe that their partners find them ugly, when, in fact, men often delight in pregnant women and think the physical changes exciting and beautiful. One woman told me she felt like a "hippopotamus wallowing in the mud" and felt completely sexless right through her pregnancy. Another said she saw herself as a "goddess, queen of all dark, growing things stirring deep in the earth," and she kept that feeling right through childbirth.

USING SEX TO INDUCE LABOR

If you are "due," especially if induction of labor has been suggested, lovemaking is one way in which you might be able to start things off naturally. Some women are believed to be particularly sensitive to prostaglandins in semen. (Prostaglandins cause the uterus to contract, and semen has a higher proportion of them than any other body substance.) It is best to choose a position in which the woman lies on her back with her legs raised on the man's hips or even his shoulders, so that the semen gets deposited right by your cervix. But since this is uncomfortable at this late stage of pregnancy, it should be done gently. Lie still with just one pillow under your head for half an hour afterward. Your partner then plays with your nipples to stimulate uterine contractions. You can go to sleep, but he may have to keep this up on and off for a few hours.

Breast stimulation in late pregnancy sometimes produces a strongly contracting uterus. This is worrying to some people, but unless you have reason to think that the baby may come too early, it is harmless. It may actually be a good thing, because the contractions that result can help to prepare the way for labor, softening and drawing up the cervix and dilating it a little before the actual labor begins.

NIPPLE STIMULATION DURING LABOR

Stimulation of the nipples can restart a labor that has come to a halt. Some doctors have tried it in place of the oxytocin drip. But it does not always work. It may depend on how the stimulation is provided: perhaps someone you love may be more effective than a breast pump. The nurse, doctor, or midwife may agree to go out and leave you. It makes sense to try the natural way of stimulating the uterus first. The emotions you have as lovers are not in conflict with the feelings of compassion and tenderness you have about a baby.

PREGNANT AGAIN

Pregnancy the second, third, or more time around is a new experience. It is never exactly like the first time. It holds different challenges. Coping with these changes involves flexibility and resourcefulness on the part of both parents.

In some ways things are much easier: you know what to expect and have probably developed self-confidence. You may sail through the pregnancy with style. But there may be difficulties that come as a surprise because you thought it would be simple this time.

REACTIONS TO ANOTHER PREGNANCY

You may have been longing to get pregnant again and it has taken a long time. Or this pregnancy may have come as a shock. However it is, a second pregnancy is often very different from the first.

OTHER PEOPLE'S REACTIONS The first problem you may encounter is the reaction of other people to a new pregnancy. Whereas your first was greeted with delight, friends and relatives are usually far less interested in the next pregnancy and may even raise their eyebrows and criticize you if you already have several children, or if you are pregnant again after a very short interval. They can make you feel that what you are doing is careless or irresponsible, or not very public-spirited and even socially harmful. Some women say they were asked "Do you want it?" or "Don't you think you've had enough?" Others cite sympathy offered by well-meaning friends: "How ever will you manage?"

YOUR PARTNER'S REACTION You may find that your partner is not so excited about the next pregnancy. He may be busy and preoccupied and even seem totally uninvolved. Even if you are still working, your partner may feel an extra burden of responsibility and financial anxiety when a second or subsequent baby is on the way—even more so if this is the point when the family will now rely on his salary alone. One baby was fun, but now he feels "trapped" into having to provide for a growing family for years to come. Some women are desperately disappointed at their partners' reactions to later pregnancies and feel that they are missing out on all the joy of the first baby, and the companionship that drew them close together the first time. Talk about your feelings so that you can come to appreciate what the experience means to each of you.

FINDING TIME TO RELAX

When you already have a lively two- or three-year-old or a group of energetic youngsters to look after, and perhaps a job as well, pregnancy can be very tiring. The first time around you were able to look after yourself, with time for thinking, planning, and dreaming. Caught up in the hustle and bustle of work and family life, doing the school run, coping with meals children can consume, and facing an everyday battle with chaos, you may have to relegate pregnancy to the back of your mind. You simply do not have time to think about it. This may result in your neglecting yourself, your nutrition, and your relaxation, and also missing out on time when you can focus your thoughts on your baby and yourself. When you realize this, in the short and infrequent intervals

"I FEEL THAT I'M CHEATING ON THIS SECOND BABY. I REVELED IN THE FIRST PREGNANCY, BUT THIS ONE OFTEN SEEMS TO BE JUST A DRAG."

between your commitments as employee, wife, mother, nurse, teacher, psychotherapist, hostess, chauffeur, house cleaner, chief cook, and bottle washer, the chances are that you will feel guilty. If you have no time now, you wonder what it will be like after the birth. You begin to feel apologetic to the little baby who is growing inside you, and perhaps also fearful that you cannot give him or her the love that you have devoted to the others.

This feeling may be intensified after the birth, when to some extent the new baby has to be fitted into family life rather than your own activities being modified to the baby's needs. If you are sitting a two-year-old on the potty, or trying to calm down three children in the bathtub playing a very splashy game that threatens to submerge the toddler, it is difficult at the same moment to fix the new baby comfortably on the breast, give him loving attention, and enjoy the release of milk.

Talk about these feelings of inadequacy with other women who are facing the same problems. If you do feel guilty, the only solution is to try to organize your life so that every day you have at least some time to think about and plan for the coming baby, and once the new baby is born, to give him or her your whole concentration.

TAKING CARE OF YOURSELF

A new pregnancy may produce aches and discomforts that you have not experienced before. Lifting bigger children and the inevitable clearing and cleaning may contribute to backaches and bad posture. This is accentuated by fatigue and doing things in a rush. If your child still wakes in the night, does not *ever* like the idea of an afternoon nap, or wakes very early in the morning and comes jumping into your bed during the hours after dawn, a restless bundle, you may be running short of sleep and longing for a solid uninterrupted 10 or 12 hours. Perhaps it is possible to arrange this when your partner is at home on the weekend.

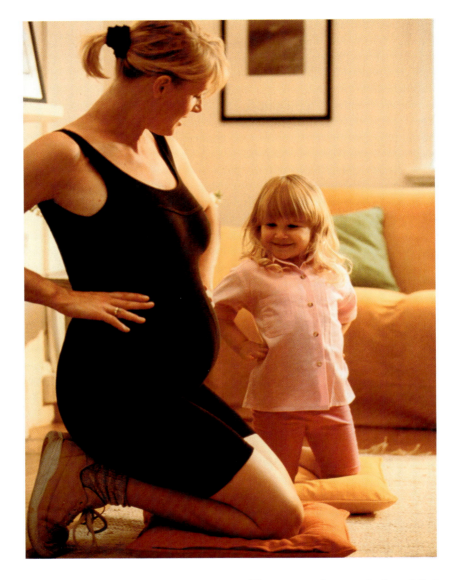

During a second pregnancy *you may be anxious that you will not have enough love to share between two children. Don't worry—you will.*

Chances are that you look and feel more pregnant with this baby, too, partly as a result of poor posture and tiredness, but also because of the stretching your uterus has already withstood during the previous pregnancy or pregnancies. This may mean that you do not feel happy about your body. A lack of pleasure in yourself is then expressed automatically in the way you stand, walk, and sit. It is a vicious circle only too easy to get into, so focus on things that make you feel better about yourself. Ask your childbirth educator to help you firm up your abdominal muscles. Use your buttock and leg muscles to help support your spine and tummy, and do a few rhythmic exercises daily (see pages 122–124). Your older child may enjoy doing them with you. Then make an opportunity to cherish yourself a bit. Ask your partner for a massage or try some other feel-good activities that would help to cheer you up.

DO I HAVE ENOUGH LOVE?

When you look at your first child you may wonder whether you can ever give as much love to another baby. And you may worry that you will somehow take love away from your older child when you share your affection with the new baby. Love isn't like that. The more we love, the more we are capable of love. When we spontaneously give ourselves in joy, love flourishes—and enriches us and everyone else in the family.

PREPARING AN OLDER CHILD

Some parents worry about how to prepare an older child for the new baby. This problem can seem almost insurmountable if the older one is clinging and very dependent. Childbirth educators* have come up with the idea of making a book for such a child, with photographs of himself, and starting with a simple description of how a baby grows inside its mother, complete with line drawings and a photograph of the mother when she was pregnant. You could show preparations being made for the birth, and then your child as a newborn baby, being nursed or bathed. These pictures could be followed by a series of photographs of the older child eating, drinking, playing, helping in the house and garden. Perhaps the last page could be left blank for a photograph of the new baby. All this helps an older child to prepare for the new baby and to realize that he was once just as small and incapable as this baby will be. If possible, borrow a baby for a few hours or have a mother and her small baby in the house for half a day or so. This will help your child to confront the reality of a baby and also observe how a mother cares for it. Many older children expect a new baby to be either a passive bundle that can be handled like a doll or a playmate who can join in their games immediately.

If you are moving an older child from a crib to a bed, do so several months before the birth, so that it does not seem a consequence of the baby's arrival. And if you are going to have extra help after the birth, encourage the helper to become friends with the older child well before the advent of the new baby.

When another baby is on the way, the relationship between the father and the older child is of great importance. It is a time when the two can draw closer together and enjoy each other's company for longer periods, something that will help you a great deal after the birth when you are busy with the new baby.

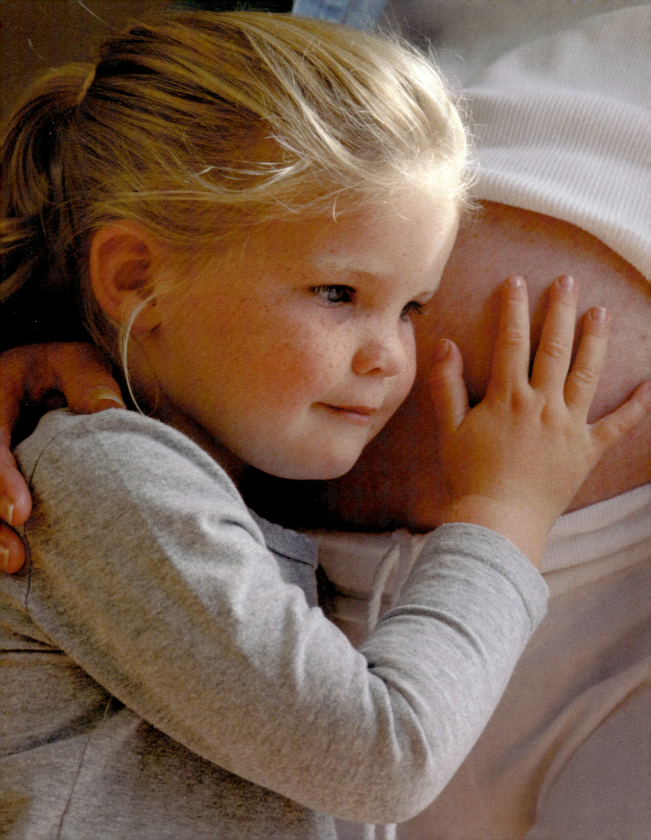

SIBLINGS AT THE BIRTH

If you are thinking about having your older child or children present at the birth of this baby, involve them in your prenatal care, and prepare them for the experience of birth by giving simple but vivid descriptions of how the baby is born, what happens in labor, and how you may behave. Children are fascinated by how the baby grows in the uterus. They need not only to see pictures of giving birth but also to get familiar with the breathing and other sounds you may make.

At the birth, children should have an adult companion whom they like who is responsible solely for that child. Labor is often long and children get bored. They want to play, to run around outside, to eat, drink, and sleep. They also need explanations of what they see and hear at the time: "She is grunting because she wants to push"; "That creamy white stuff kept the baby's skin soft, smooth, and watertight so it did not get all wrinkly inside." The child's companion should be well informed as well as comfortable with being at the birth. An anxious adult conveys this to a child. Whenever a child expresses the wish to leave the room or do something else, the companion should respond instantly. Your midwife or doctor should be involved in planning ahead for a child's presence at birth, and have a chance to get to know the child and build a friendly relationship. By the time a child is around four years old, you can help him or her to construct and write a birth plan: "I would like to cut the cord . . . hold the baby after mommy has cuddled it . . . cut the cake at the birthday party after the baby has come out." It may be a good idea for your other children to be present if you are having a home birth, and for some women this is a reason for choosing not to have a hospital birth.

"ONE OF THE NURSES CAME IN AND SAID, 'YOUR BABY'S BEING BORN.' I WENT IN AND SAW SAM'S HEAD COMING OUT. I STAYED HOME FROM SCHOOL THAT DAY TO SEE SAM."

Birth provides an opportunity for an older child to share in a major life transition, and to develop new social skills and awareness.

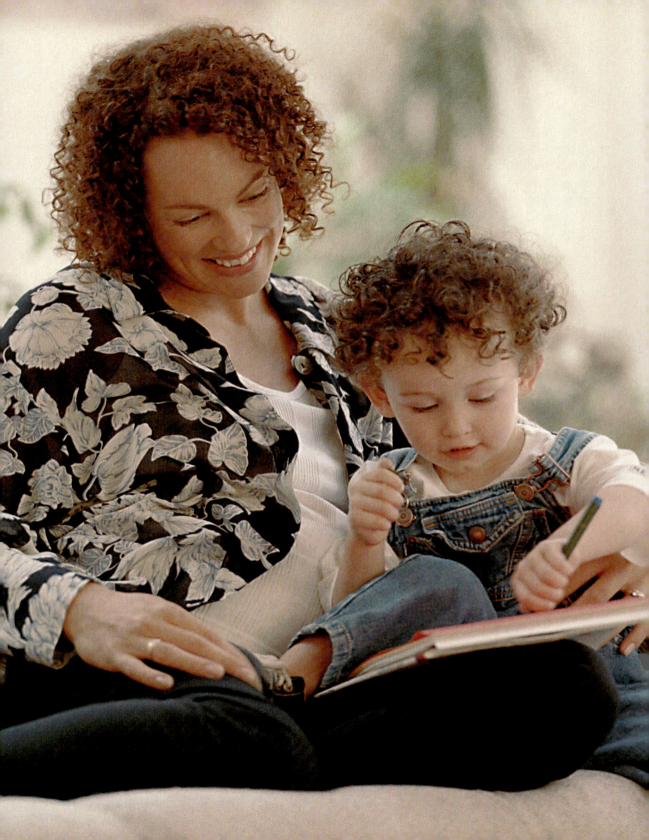

PREGNANCY

THINKING AHEAD *to* BIRTH

180 | IN TUNE WITH YOUR BODY FOR LABOR

226 | WINDOWS INTO THE UTERUS

238 | THE LAST FEW WEEKS

IN TUNE WITH YOUR BODY FOR LABOR

Part of preparation for birth consists of exercises, but it is even more important to *think* about labor in a constructive way. Give yourself time to imagine what is going to happen in your body and what you may feel.

Imagine the birth of your baby. Think of different kinds of labor (see pages 270–285) and how to cope with them. Don't restrict your fantasies to only one kind of labor, because life is not completely predictable and it may turn out that the labor you have is very different.

CHILDBIRTH EDUCATION

Education for birth helps you know more about your body and feel happy with it during pregnancy. You learn how to prepare yourself so that when you are in labor you can work with your body instead of fighting it, so that you understand the activity of the uterus, and through relaxation, breathing, and focused concentration, achieve harmony with the birth process. This is important not only for the hours that you are actually in labor, but also for how you feel about the whole experience, yourself, and the baby afterward. Birth is not "just another day in a woman's life." Women remember their births and the intense emotions that were stimulated with extraordinary clarity years later, often into old age. They remember vividly how they felt when labor started, when the bag of waters popped, how it was when they got to the hospital, what doctors, nurses, midwives, and their partners did, interventions that occurred in the birth and, of course, their first meeting with the baby. Positive experiences remain as good memories. Negative experiences, far from being forgotten, intensify over time.*

CHOOSING A CLASS

Once you have begun your prenatal care, it is time to think about arranging childbirth classes, so that you and your partner can learn about the physiological changes of pregnancy and labor and the possible emotional impact of the stresses involved. It pays to shop around for classes and discover different ones available in your area. You would not dream of walking into a hairdresser's and asking them to cut and style your hair without finding out what sort of work they did. Learning about childbirth is even more important, so approach childbirth classes with the same discrimination. For the quality of teaching to improve, critical, informed consumers are needed. Any prenatal teacher worth her salt learns from her students, and continues to modify her teaching on the basis of the feedback she receives from them and ideas they share with her.

FINDING OUT ABOUT CLASSES

When you inquire about classes, do not assume that they are successful only if those who have attended them have had easy labors and births. If you have to have a forceps delivery or a Cesarean section it does not mean that you have "failed" in applying what you have learned. Having a baby is not like passing an exam or winning a race. You are not expected to come out "on top" with a two-hour labor, or to take no pain-relieving drugs. It is much more a question of learning how to adapt your responses to the particular challenges of your own labor. So it can be useful to talk also to women who have experienced labors that were not straightforward, and to find out from them if attending classes helped them at all.

"I WAS WORKING HARD IN THE OFFICE THROUGH MOST OF MY PREGNANCY, AND THE CLASSES GAVE ME SPECIAL TIME THAT WAS JUST FOR MYSELF."

Even though women all over the world have babies in much the same way, birth can be a vastly different experience for different women. Just as sexual intercourse involves certain mechanical and physiological processes that are the same everywhere, what people feel about birth, exactly what they do, and the meaning of the total experience varies with the individual and the occasion. Childbirth is not primarily a medical process but a psychosexual experience. It is not surprising that adapting your responses to the stimuli it presents should involve a subtle and delicate working together of mind and body.

When looking into classes, ask a woman who has attended them whether she found the skills that she learned helpful when she was in labor, and whether she felt confident and understood what was going on. If she says, "Nothing helped," it implies that the classes did not relate in any way to the reality of labor; if she says that she was absolutely terrified from beginning to end, it sounds as if the classes did not help her, either, although she may have enjoyed getting to know the other expectant mothers.

Your local hospital may offer classes, although frequently they focus on the routines and procedures you may expect to have done in that hospital rather than on the choices, and on baby care rather than on what you can do to help yourself during labor. Your doctor or midwife may know of other classes. Contact the International Childbirth Education Association or Lamaze International (see page 427) to find out where classes are being held in your area.

WHAT MAKES A GOOD CHILDBIRTH CLASS?

Good classes are progressive in the sense that you learn a little more each time. You should not feel at the third or fourth lesson that you have sat through it all before. There should be opportunities for you to ask questions and discuss topics freely rather than listen to a formal lecture. Breathing and relaxation exercises that can be of practical use in labor should be included. Their relevance to labor should be specifically described, together with why and how they are used.

Relaxation is not as simple as it might sound. It is not just a question of flopping in front of the television or lying down with a bar of chocolate and a good book, but of learning complete awareness and control of muscle groups all over the body so that they can be contracted or relaxed at will, including muscles you may not even know you possess. Relaxation also means learning how to relax under stress, not just lying in a deck chair on a sunny day or in a classroom while a cool voice tells you that a contraction is beginning, continuing, and then fading away.

It helps to learn different patterns and rhythms of breathing for the different phases of labor (see pages 205–213). So when you are asking about classes, try to find out from any woman who has been to them whether she learned things like this.

"I DIDN'T JUST WANT REASSURANCE AND TO TALK ABOUT 'DISCOMFORT.' I WANTED COMPLETE HONESTY SO THAT I COULD MAKE RATIONAL CHOICES FOR MYSELF."

An effective teacher helps her students realize something of what labor feels like, and the reality and power of its challenge. She also explains things fully, without fear that she is burdening their minds, and does so honestly and clearly.

Unfortunately, in some classes there is far too much talking down to pregnant women. You have a right to understand what is happening to your body and what people are proposing to do to you. A good teacher does not answer your questions with "Oh, you don't have to worry about that," or imply that everyone will do what is best for you and your baby, and that all you need do is to have complete trust in your birth attendants. Discussion should always be a real exchange of ideas among you, your teacher, and the group, not simply a few questions to which answers are fired back without any recognition of the apprehension and the sometimes nightmarish fears that lie behind them.

You can see from this that a good deal depends on the personality of the teacher. It is not so much "the method" that is good or inadequate as the quality of the teaching itself, and perhaps most of all the relationship that the teacher has with her students. I have seen teaching that seemed woefully inadequate or mechanized, or that involved learning a number of rather irrelevant physical exercises, and, yet, because of the personality and attitude of the teacher, women enjoyed their births.

THE READ METHOD

There are different approaches to childbirth education, and the names associated with them can be confusing for expectant mothers. The Read method is named after Dr. Grantly Dick-Read;* it is the oldest method and is usually associated with "relaxation classes." The philosophy behind this approach is that ignorance produces fear, which leads to tension, which in turn quickly produces pain. So teachers concentrate on overcoming fear by teaching deep relaxation and the breathing that accompanies it, along with providing full and accurate information about the childbearing process, exercises to keep you supple and poised, and discussion of breast-feeding. Today, there are few Read method teachers, but most childbirth educators incorporate his concepts into their classes.

LAMAZE OR PSYCHOPROPHYLAXIS

Psychoprophylaxis is a highly systematized training centered on techniques of breathing rather than relaxation. It originated in the former Soviet Union, was developed in Paris, and was then introduced to the United States.* Psychoprophylaxis classes begin by deconditioning the women from their fear and doubts about childbirth, and then reconditioning them to respond to labor contractions as helpful stimuli and not as pains. Exercises are taught both for limbering up before the birth and for use during labor. Full information is given about the anatomy and physiology of pregnancy and labor. In the 1970s, many childbirth educators taught psychoprophylaxis with a lot of "huffing and puffing," distraction techniques, and strenuous exercises for pushing the baby out. They now have a much more broad-ranging and flexible approach.

In the United States, women know psychoprophylaxis by the name of its French originator, Lamaze, whereas in France itself it was often called *accouchement sans douleur* (birth without pain) or *asd*. This name is thoroughly misleading and might make any woman having pain in labor feel that something is going wrong. For most women who have been to classes, the pain of labor is not the most salient thing about the experience but is a side effect with which many of them, helped by techniques of adjustment and by emotional support and guidance at the time, can cope well without any pharmacological aids. Other women want some additional pain relief in labor, and should certainly have it.

In North America and Britain, psychoprophylaxis methods have changed radically since they were first introduced. Dogma has disappeared, breathing is no longer regimented, and the whole approach has become more relaxed.

THE BRADLEY METHOD

In the United States, an obstetrician, Robert Bradley, has created "husband-coached" childbirth, in which the man acts as the woman's teacher and supporter in pregnancy and labor. Breathing is slow and full, obstetric intervention is kept to the minimum, and pain-relieving drugs are not used. Many Bradley enthusiasts opt for home birth. The Bradley organization is known as The American Academy of Husband-Coached Childbirth.

THE AUTOGENIC METHOD

On the continent of Europe, a system of training for labor that is based on the Schulz methods of relaxation and breathing is taught in many hospital prenatal classes. Here women are taught to relax fully by conceptualizing warmth and weight in different parts of their bodies; their breathing should be slow and relaxed throughout.

ACTIVE BIRTH

Janet Balaskas has developed an active method of preparing for birth based on hatha yoga, with the focus on moving around and changing position throughout labor, and giving birth squatting, kneeling, or on all fours. To be able to do this freely and with comfort, it is very important to practice "stretching" exercises beforehand, and a woman learns how to adopt "open" positions with help from her partner.* Some methods of preparation for active birth are now often incorporated into other classes, and Janet Balaskas's great achievement is that in many hospitals all over the world she has succeeded in getting women off the labor bed and the delivery table and onto the floor.

THE ODENT APPROACH

For Dr. Michel Odent, it is important to provide an environment that facilitates a spontaneous psychophysiological process in which the woman is left undisturbed and feels as if she is "on another planet."

Instead of holding childbirth classes, Odent organized singing get-togethers for new parents, pregnant women, and their partners, midwives, doctors, and small children. He has rediscovered the use of water in birth, offering the woman a deep tub of warm water in which she can float in a peaceful, darkened room. For birth, he favors the standing squat, with the woman supported from behind by her partner or another helper.

THE KITZINGER PSYCHOSEXUAL APPROACH

My own "psychosexual approach" originally grew out of both the Read and psychoprophylaxis systems and incorporates many active birth positions and movements. It is based on my conviction that the woman can be an active birthgiver rather than a passive patient. It focuses on birth as experience rather than a series of exercises in breathing and relaxation.

Social anthropology has contributed much to my own approach, and especially my observations of how women behave in and feel about labor in different cultures. I have learned most from women themselves. Birth often involves barely glimpsed feelings about ourselves that have developed through the formative years of childhood: attitudes to and fantasies about our bodies, feelings about the relative size and positions of organs and orifices, and concepts of cleanliness and pollution, beauty and ugliness. All of these are partly social in origin, products of our upbringing and family relationships.

Labor is a social situation, not just a physiological or a private emotional experience. Since it involves human relationships at a sometimes tense and demanding time, it helps to know how to talk with the people assisting at the birth and how to understand what may be in their minds.

"THE ROLE PLAY HELPED A LOT, EXPLORING WAYS OF ENGAGING WITH DOCTORS AND NURSES, AND HOW TO HANDLE RESISTANCE."

All childbirth teachers agree that students need plenty of information about how their bodies work and what goes on in hospitals. Most classes make a visit to the hospital and take a tour of the delivery room. However, preparation for labor is not just a matter of knowing what will happen to you, but of learning how to negotiate to get the kind of birth you want, and acknowledging that birth is a matter of politics, too.

THE AIMS OF CHILDBIRTH CLASSES

As you will see, there is wide variation in exactly what is taught and how, although there is general agreement that six sessions of one and a half or two hours each are the minimum required. The aim is not to retreat from contractions but to adjust to them and respond actively. There is more and more emphasis on a woman's being in the kind of setting and having the loving emotional support that enables her to be confident in her own powers and to behave spontaneously, without having to do "exercises" or wondering whether her performance is good enough.

In classes, partners can learn how to help in pregnancy and labor and understand something about the feelings involved in becoming a parent. It is important that a woman be allowed to bring a female partner if she wishes, and classes should not be restricted to heterosexual couples. Your partner in childbirth classes may be male or female, a lover, husband, friend, or relative. If you are offered less than these options in the classes you attend, you may feel the need to supplement them with other classes, reading, or private tuition.

WHEN TO START CLASSES

Whatever method you opt for, do not leave booking classes or your reading until the last moment. Start finding out what is available in your area and begin your course of reading four or five months before the baby is due, even though classes may not be offered until the last nine weeks or so. You may find that classes are organized only for women in the last two or three months of pregnancy, but there is usually an opportunity for you to meet the teacher earlier.

A TYPICAL HOSPITAL BIRTH ROOM

If you plan to have your baby in a hospital it is a good idea to look at a birth room. Some equipment seems daunting until it is explained to you. Hospitals usually arrange tours of their maternity departments for expectant mothers.

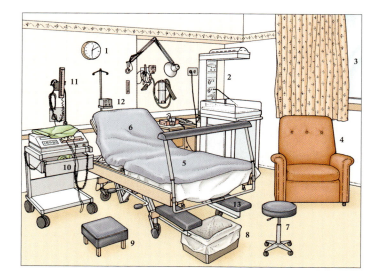

1 **The clock** *is used to record the length of each stage of labor and for noting the time of the baby's birth.*

2 **The resuscitation table** *for the baby is equipped with oxygen and suction apparatus to extract any mucus from the baby's lungs.*

3 **Curtains screen** *harsh daylight so that it does not disturb you. They are intended to provide a reassuring element in the birth room, and you can ask to darken the room for your first meeting with the baby.*

4 **Some hospitals have a chair bed,** *a comfortable seat for the birth partner that can be folded out as a bed.*

5 **A squatting bar** *gives firm support to hold on to if you want to adopt a squatting position.*

6 **The birth bed** *has three sections, head, middle, and foot, which are adjustable. The head can be raised or lowered. The entire bed can also be raised or lowered. The foot can be lowered or removed as shown here.*

7 **The adjustable stool** *is for the doctor or midwife.*

8 **A plastic container** *catches fluids and waste products.*

9 **A low stool** *is usually provided and is useful for helping you get onto the bed.*

10 **An electronic fetal monitor** *with sensing devices that are attached to your abdomen can be used intermittently or continuously during labor, or not at all. It detects and records the fetal heart rate and your uterine contractions.*

11 **Behind the bed is the apparatus for measuring blood pressure.** *There is also a supply of oxygen available and spare electric sockets for other purposes.*

12 **A pole** *will hold a bag of fluid if a doctor sets up an intravenous drip.*

13 **Adjustable footrests** *are on either side of the bed. When the mattress at the foot of the bed is removed, you can place your feet here.*

It is beneficial to learn good posture in early pregnancy, and something about how the baby develops inside you and how to cope with any minor discomforts of pregnancy. It is also an advantage at any time, whether or not you are pregnant (and for men as well as women), to know how deep relaxation can help you get to sleep.

Whatever approach you select, provided you are happy with your teacher and develop confidence in yourself, the teaching will be right for you, and you will have a variety of tools that you can use to help you cope with contractions in labor. Labor need not be a fearful ordeal but a positive, rewarding experience and a really *happy birthday*.

MAKING YOUR OWN SPACE

Some women want to be absolutely alone during labor. Most women, however, welcome understanding, support, and encouragement from someone in whom they have confidence and with whom they can "be themselves" and do what comes spontaneously.

Labor should not have to be a public performance. Unless there are especially urgent and demanding reasons for total strangers—nurses, doctors, students, medical auxiliaries, hospital porters and cleaners—to be there, you have the right to ask for privacy in the birth room and have only those people with you whom *you* have chosen to be there. You could make this absolutely clear in the birth plan that you hand over to be inserted in your chart (see page 52).

When women describe their birth experiences in hospitals, especially large ones, they often talk about all the people who wandered in and out, anonymous faces looking through the porthole window in the door, and conversations about them, not with them, conducted over their supine bodies. Can you imagine the effect of having strangers and other observers around you when you took a bath, sat on the toilet, tried to sleep, or were making love? Birth is a psychosexual activity that involves revealing that which is usually physically and emotionally private. It is patterned by rhythms similar to those in other physiological functions that entail letting your body open up. It involves strong emotions like those of intense sexual arousal. The tides and waves of labor culminate in the birth passion. To be watched by someone with whom you have no intimate and trusting closeness, to be inspected, criticized, applauded, and urged to do better, can interrupt and prove an obstacle to psychophysical coordination. This is why it is important to create your own space for birth, and to arrange to have one or more companions with you with whom you feel not just comfortable but completely at ease. If you are going to be giving birth in a large hospital with people whom you have never met before, this is all the more vital. You need to choose a birth companion who will be like an anchor for you in a stormy sea.

CHOOSING A WOMAN BIRTH COMPANION

Research shows that if a woman has another woman with her during labor and birth she has less need for pain-relieving drugs and her labor is shorter. There are fewer operative deliveries (forceps, vacuum extractor, and Cesarean sections) and episiotomies. Babies are in better condition at birth, and mothers are much more likely to look back on the birth as a positive experience. Studies have also revealed that these women have fewer perineal lacerations, are more likely to be breast-feeding at six weeks, and are less likely to be depressed.* Ten randomized controlled trials that involved 3,000 women in childbirth who did not even know their companions before they went into labor have confirmed the benefits of having a support person.*

"MY SISTER WAS MARVELOUS DURING MY LABOR—REALLY SUPPORTIVE—AND IT WAS LOVELY HAVING HER THERE AND SHARING THE MIRACLE OF THE BIRTH WITH HER."

The constant presence of a birth companion who is focused on your needs has turned out to be one of the most effective forms of childbirth care introduced in the last 25 years. It is the rediscovery of a practice that was elemental to birth in many different cultures all over the world, including Europe and North America, until professionals took over. Women have always had other women with them. In medieval Europe women birth companions were known as "God sibs"—literally, "sisters in God."*

Today, and increasingly in the U.S., the term "doula," which is a Greek word meaning "a female birth companion," is used to describe a supportive woman helper. A doula can be present at the birth either instead of the baby's father or to support the couple who want to be together.*

Doulas are women who are especially interested in birth and in helping women through birth. They know how to provide emotional and physical support. If you are thinking of who this person should be, consider your childbirth teacher, a student teacher, a close friend, or anyone in your family who has the right personality and experience and who will give you loving emotional support. Or you can contact a doula organization and arrange to meet with a registered doula who offers her services for a fee (see page 427). A doula is often described as someone who will "mother the mother." In fact, this may not be exactly what you want. Many women do not look for mothering but welcome understanding and practical help from someone more like a sister.

Hospitals used to lay down strict rules stating that only one other person could be with a woman in childbirth. This has now changed. More and more hospitals recognize that having not only your partner but also a friend or family member whom you know and trust, and whom you have selected, helps you relax and increases self-confidence, with the result that labor is more likely to go well.

QUESTIONS TO ASK A DOULA

Doulas come from a variety of backgrounds. Many are childbirth teachers; some have been midwives; others are mothers who have had good experiences of birth themselves. It is important that a doula does not intrude on birth in a way that disturbs you or makes relations with your other helpers difficult. This entails great sensitivity and skill on her part.

Before you make the decision to hire a doula, you will need to know more about her. Some of the personal questions you might want answers to include whether she has had a baby herself, what was her experience of birth, why she has chosen to do this work, and whether she has any particular or strong beliefs about it. Make a contract with her, which you both sign, including an agreement as to how often you will meet, what happens if she is with someone else or cannot come for any reason when you call her, and the financial arrangements.

RELAXATION AND MASSAGE

Relaxation is the art of letting go and allowing peace to flow through you. The skill is in being able to release your muscles at will and not only when you are in a special mood to relax. It is not just an exercise. Relaxation is as necessary as a partner to—and interlude in—strenuous activity as breathing out is to breathing in.

THE IMPORTANCE OF RELAXATION

Relaxation is vital for labor. If you cannot relax you are likely to become exhausted as muscles tighten up all over your body in reaction to the challenging stress of contractions. By tensing muscles unnecessarily you are wasting energy, and if you are exhausted, pain will be felt more sharply and your ability to control it is bound to be diminished.

Generalized tension and anxiety can sometimes affect the way the uterus contracts, producing incoordinate uterine action. This causes painful contractions that are not very effective in pulling open the cervix. Because it alters your whole body chemistry, marked tension lasting a long time can also reduce the oxygen supply to the baby. Just as the smooth coordination of your digestive system, the beating of your heart, and your breathing are all affected by acute tension, so stress and anxiety can slow down the unfolding process of childbirth and make it more difficult.

Relaxation helps keep your mind clear so that you are able to understand what is happening and can respond to it purposefully and creatively.

CENTERING DOWN

To explore and enjoy the skills of relaxation, you need to be able to "center down," to use an old Quaker term, and enjoy peace of body and mind. Lie down on your side, well supported with plenty of pillows, back rounded, head and shoulders forward, legs and arms bent. Or sit in a comfortable chair with cushions supporting all of your back, including the back of your neck. You may also like a cushion under each arm or underneath your thighs. Think of the journey the baby makes to be born. Focus on feeling your muscles and flesh heavy, all tension released.

TOUCH RELAXATION

With Touch Relaxation, a partner gives you a message of touch to say, in effect, "release here." You respond to the pressure and warmth of the hands with immediate relaxation. If you learn to respond to your partner's touch in this way during pregnancy, it will be a spontaneous reaction when you are in labor. In effect, your partner will be able to draw tension out of you.

To practice this, contract different sets of muscles one set at a time. Your partner then rests his or her hands over the area that feels tight, and as soon as you feel the touch, you release, as if you are flowing toward it. Sometimes it helps if the touch develops into a gentle massage over the part of the body that is tense. This should always be very slow. A partner who is worried or excited may massage in fast, jerky movements, and this has the effect of communicating tension rather than relieving it. Whenever massage is performed on bare skin, it is a good idea to use a little powder or warm oil, so that the hands glide smoothly and you do not feel itchy.

Between each exercise, it is important to discuss whether it feels right for you—whether you want the touch firmer, lighter, or in a slightly different place. During labor, too, you can talk together between contractions so that your helper understands exactly what you want. Some examples of Touch Relaxation for different parts of the body are shown on pages 192–200. In childbirth, touch helps you to release all the muscles you do not need to use in order to have the baby. It relieves psychological stress, too, because you feel secure and nurtured.

On the other hand, some women find that the experience of giving birth is so total, so overwhelming, that touch would be superfluous. While Touch Relaxation can be an important part of preparing for the birth, when you are in labor you may come to a phase when you do not want to be touched at all. If so, simply tell your partner this. It is vital that you have the kind of support *you* want and that your partner be willing to stand back and let you do things your way.

RELEASE OF TENSION By practicing relaxation techniques like this with you, your partner becomes aware of any tensions you are feeling and, when you are in labor, can notice if there is a buildup of tension in your body long before anyone who does not know you well realizes what is happening. Then, all that is needed is to reach out a hand with the message: relax! If your shoulders are getting tense, a firm hand rests on your shoulder. If your legs are knotting up, loving hands stroke your legs firmly.

One great advantage of this is that it does not involve giving directions and "coaching" in labor. There may be times—especially at the very end of the first stage—when positive guidance is invaluable, but there is no place at all for bullying a woman in childbirth. Through learning Touch Relaxation, your partner will have the self-assurance to give you the kind of help you need at exactly the right time.

RESPONDING TO THE DOCTOR OR MIDWIFE Experiencing Touch Relaxation together also prepares you to respond to the touch you receive when the doctor or midwife examines you. Instead of feeling threatened, tensing up, and pulling away like a snail drawing in its horns, you will be able to relax. This makes having your tummy palpated and pelvic examination much easier and more comfortable.

PRESSURE FROM THE UTERUS During childbirth, the stimulus coming from the uterus feels remarkably like a strong, intense kind of touch radiating from inside. As the uterus contracts it squeezes tightly. A powerful pressure builds up and there is a sensation of heat. When the cervix is being opened and pulled wider, still more pressure is exerted. Then, as the baby moves down through the cervix, pressure is produced by the ball of its head. It feels as if a grapefruit

"I HADN'T REALIZED THAT I CLENCHED MY JAW WHEN I TENSED UP AROUND MY EYES OR HOW OFTEN I CURLED MY TOES WHEN I CONCENTRATED."

were being pressed down first against the anus and then through the vagina. To all these stimuli a woman may respond either by tightening up or by releasing her muscles.

LEARNING TO FLOW WITH A CONTRACTION Imagine that you are in labor and that the pressure of the uterus is increasing with each contraction. Visualize the pressure of the baby's head, too. Then release and flow toward these sensations. Some women experience each contraction as warmth building up to heat and then dying down again. One woman told me that for her every contraction was like an oven door swinging wide open. At its peak she received the full blast of the heat and then the oven door swung closed again.

When the baby's head is on your perineum and coming through the vagina, all the tissues fan out like the petals of a flower. As they open, you feel a warm, tingling sensation, as if the whole area is being flooded with heat. If you have learned always to relax in response to the pressure and warmth from your partner's hands, you can respond to these physical messages from *inside* your body, too, not by pulling back but by releasing and *flowing toward* them. In this way you can use the sensations you get from within your body to guide you through labor.

TOUCH RELAXATION

Tension makes birth painful. If you learn how to relax in
response to your partner's touch, it becomes spontaneous in
labor. To practice, sit on the floor, propped with cushions.
Contract different muscles and notice how you feel when
they are tight. Your partner rests one or both hands over the
area and you relax as if flowing out toward the touch.

ABDOMEN

Under stress, your abdominal muscles tense up,
which can cause shallow breathing and may
make labor more painful. Practice relaxing your
abdominal muscles in response to your partner's
touch so that it becomes a spontaneous reaction
during labor. The pull of the dilating cervix often
feels painful. Light massage just above your pubic
bone can help to ease pain and tension.

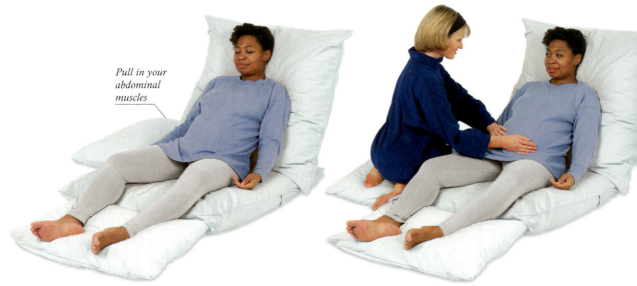

*Pull in your
abdominal
muscles*

Give a long breath out through a relaxed mouth. Tense
up by tightening your abdominal muscles and pulling
them in toward your spine. Notice how the tension feels.
You will find that you have also tightened the muscles
at the bottom of your back and that your breathing is
affected, too.

Sitting or kneeling by your side, your partner massages
your abdomen with both hands in a continuous,
flowing movement, one hand following the other slowly
and evenly over the lower curve of your tummy in a
half circle. Release your muscles to her touch. Light
massage just above your pubic bone usually helps, too.

SHOULDERS

Most of us tighten our shoulders under stress. This results in strained breathing and sometimes a headache because of tension in the back of the neck. In labor, tension in the shoulders results in heavy, panicky breathing, which in turn leads you to hyperventilate. A side effect is less oxygen reaching the baby. If you know how to release your shoulders, you will not hyperventilate. Try pressing your head and shoulders back into the pillows. A woman may tense her shoulders like this during strong contractions in the first stage. See how it affects your breathing.

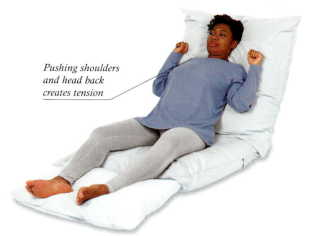

Pushing shoulders and head back creates tension

To feel what happens *when your shoulder muscles become very tense, concentrate on pressing your shoulder blades back toward each other as if they were angel's wings and you could make them meet at the back.*

Your partner rests *one hand firmly over each shoulder, applying pressure with the heels of the palms at the front of your shoulders. You release immediately, flowing out to the touch. The hands should be slowly removed.*

Focus on your partner's touch

When tension is *building up in labor, firm pressure on your shoulders, or the shoulder on the side nearest your partner, enables you to release it.*

Keep legs relaxed and spread a little

HEAD AND FACE

These exercises help to release tension in the head and face. You may not be very aware of your scalp muscles, but tension here causes a strained facial expression as well as head and neck aches. If a woman in labor is concentrating hard, or feels anxious, the muscles around her eyes become tense and her brow furrows. Her jaw stiffens, her mouth gets tight, and it is difficult for her to release her vagina and perineum.

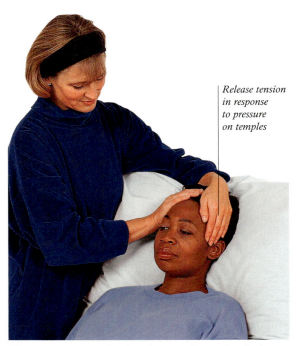

Release tension in response to pressure on temples

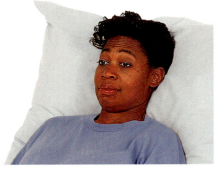

Push your eyebrows *up toward the top of your head. Notice how you feel when you do this. The scalp muscles can become this tense during labor, and over time you begin to develop a headache or neck ache.*

Your partner cups *her hands around your head. As you feel the pressure, release and slowly close your eyes. As she feels your tension easing, she reduces the pressure. Visualize any residual tension flowing out of your head.*

FACE TENSING

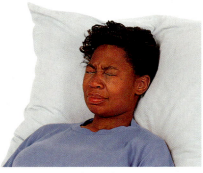

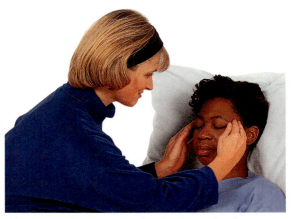

Frown as if you *have a headache and are in a very bright light. Notice how you feel when you screw up your eyes and forehead. This is what you might do while concentrating hard in labor.*

Placing two fingers *on each side of your head, your partner presses gently on the temple bones. Release tension as you feel this touch. As your partner reduces the pressure, visualize residual tension flowing out and away.*

ARMS

When you have a very strong contraction, it is tempting to grip someone or something and to contract muscles in your arms. This makes pain worse and, along with tension in the shoulders, interferes with breathing, so that you start to gasp.

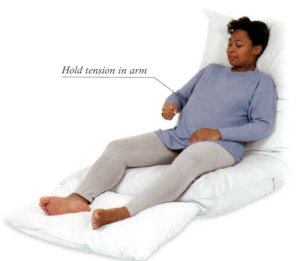

Hold tension in arm

Tighten the muscles in the arm that is nearest to your partner. Notice how your arm feels. Your partner watches to judge when the muscles look tight and then applies gentle pressure on the arm.

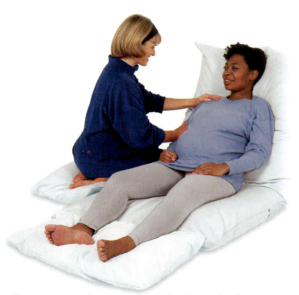

Your partner places one hand firmly on the front of your shoulder, with the other hand over the inside of your upper arm, cradled around the big muscle there, the biceps. The hands are held as if molded to your body. As soon as you feel the warmth and pressure of the touch, release your arm muscles completely.

The hand on the inside arm moves slowly and firmly, stroking down to your wrist. The other hand stays on your shoulder. As the hand moves, focus on residual tension flowing down your arm, out and away. This slow, firm stroking can feel very good at the start of each contraction.

LEGS

When a woman feels her baby pressing down to be born, she often tightens the muscles of her inner thighs. A vital part of opening up to allow your baby to be born is the complete release of tension in your inner thighs. Sometimes these muscles get so tight that your leg becomes stiff and your foot is drawn up in a painful cramp. This can be released with massage.

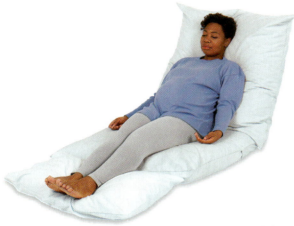

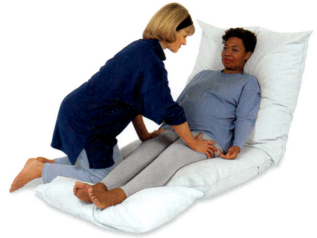

Press your knees very firmly together and hold the position. While you are doing this, notice how tense the muscles of your inner thighs feel.

Your partner rests one hand lightly on the outside of each leg and you relax toward the touch, letting your knees roll outward naturally.

EASING CRAMPS

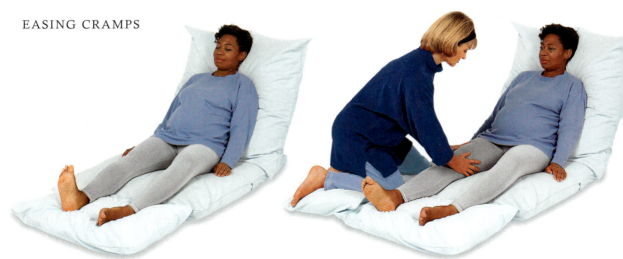

To practice easing cramps, stretch one leg out straight, so it feels stiff and taut, then flex your foot. Hold this position for a short time and concentrate on feeling the muscular tension that results.

To help release the tension in the muscles, your partner places one hand on the inside of your thigh, molding the hand to the leg, then strokes slowly and firmly down to your ankle. Release to the warmth of the touch.

RELEASING TENSION

This massage is useful toward the end of the first stage of labor, when contractions are close together and last a minute or more. At this time your legs may feel cold and tense, and your whole body may begin to shiver and shake. Firm massage to your inner thigh muscles releases tension and warms your legs so that you feel they belong to you again.

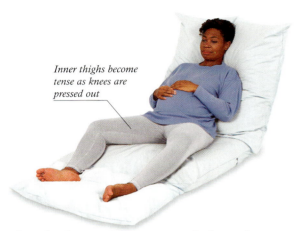

Inner thighs become tense as knees are pressed out

See what happens when you press *both your knees outward so that your inner legs are uppermost. Hold the position briefly and concentrate on feeling the tension in your inner thighs as you do so.*

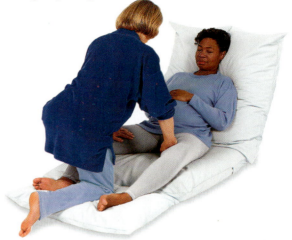

Your partner rests both hands *inside your upper thighs, and you relax toward the touch. She strokes slowly and firmly down to your knees, then gently as her hands come up over the outside of the legs in a continuous movement.*

RELEASING PELVIC FLOOR MUSCLES

This massage reminds you to release your pelvic floor so that you can help the baby's head bulge forward in your vagina. Each downward movement of the hands has the effect of releasing the muscles through which the baby is coming to birth.

To focus on this feeling, *first contract your pelvic floor muscles as if they were an elevator going up to the second, third, and then fourth floor of a building. Pull them up and hold them. Then your partner rests both hands on your inside thighs, and you release the pelvic floor muscles down to them, as if the elevator were going down. As your partner slides her hands toward your knees, release still more, letting your perineum bulge.*

BACK AND SHOULDERS

Lie on your side, making yourself comfortable with pillows. Your back is rounded, your head and shoulders well forward, and your underneath arm behind your back. If a woman is lying on her side and becomes tense in labor, she often adopts a fetal position. Having someone hold your shoulders is helpful if you overbreathe during contractions. A thumb massage over your upper back and shoulders or each side of the spine may help, too.

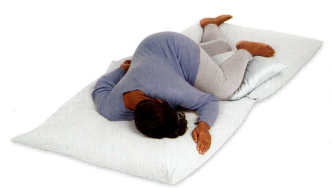

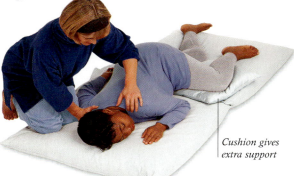

Cushion gives extra support

Curl up and hunch your shoulders. Notice how your shoulders tighten up so they are now near the level of your ears. Your breathing will probably be affected, too.

Your partner rests her fingers on your shoulders and applies firm pressure with the palms. You release, flowing out toward the touch.

SMALL OF THE BACK

Many women have backaches in labor, usually around the sacrum—the bone in the small of the back where the pelvis joins the spine.

Tension is created when the small of the back is pulled in

To find out where your sacrum is, your partner places her fingers over the large bones at the side of the pelvic cradle and traces the shape of the pelvis around to where it dips down at the back to meet your spine.

Still on your side, pull in the small of your back to tense up muscles all down your back. You will find you stick your bottom out and throw your shoulders back. This is what happens if you have back pain in labor.

RELIEVING BACKACHES

The tension that results from a backache can be greatly relieved by your partner's applying firm pressure over this area. Relax your muscles and let go of tension while your partner presses along each part of your lower back or massages your back with firm strokes. A partner doing back massage may get a backache too, so make sure your partner relaxes and rests from time to time.

To help you release, your partner presses firmly and steadily over the sacrum, using the heel of the palm (not the fingers). As soon as you feel the warmth and pressure, relax, letting go and flowing out toward the hands. Muscles down your back soften and loosen immediately.

In childbirth, firm counterpressure can feel good, or you may prefer this type of massage. It is best done by moving the flesh—both skin and muscle—on the bone, rather than by merely creating friction. Your partner can use a firm, circular motion with hands more or less stationary, or slide the hands across the top of one buttock to the top of the other and back again.

Partners using counterpressure or doing back massage often get a backache, too, because they are relying on muscle strength in the arms rather than allowing their body weight to flow down through their arms. Your partner may want to rest one hand on your hip but should be careful not to exert pressure there or lean on you, since that will cause you discomfort.

BUTTOCKS AND TAIL MUSCLES

A woman may tense her buttocks in labor because the baby is pressing against her rectum and anus as it comes around the curve of the birth canal, and she feels as if it is coming out of the wrong hole. She is often convinced that she needs to go to the toilet. She tries to resist the sensation by tightening up her muscles, but when she tightens her buttocks she also tightens her pelvic floor muscles against the baby's head. It is as if she is shutting the door on it. Contracting these muscles can delay the descent of the head and cause unnecessary pain.

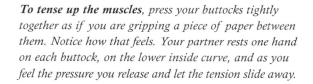

To tense up the muscles, press your buttocks tightly together as if you are gripping a piece of paper between them. Notice how that feels. Your partner rests one hand on each buttock, on the lower inside curve, and as you feel the pressure you release and let the tension slide away.

Your partner can help you relax by firmly massaging your buttocks as if kneading bread dough. It is important to get down into the fat and muscle, very slowly kneading both buttocks at once. As soon as you feel this firm, reassuring touch, you relax.

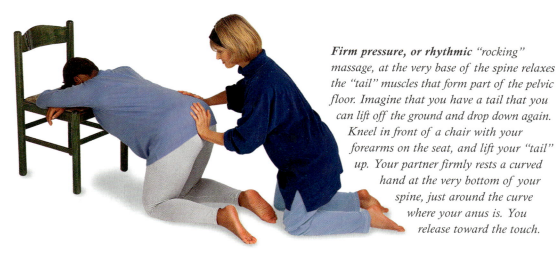

Firm pressure, or rhythmic "rocking" massage, at the very base of the spine relaxes the "tail" muscles that form part of the pelvic floor. Imagine that you have a tail that you can lift off the ground and drop down again. Kneel in front of a chair with your forearms on the seat, and lift your "tail" up. Your partner firmly rests a curved hand at the very bottom of your spine, just around the curve where your anus is. You release toward the touch.

PUPPET-STRINGS RELAXATION

Of course, you do not always have someone to help you with relaxation. You can practice relaxation by yourself, using a method that I call the "puppet-strings" method.

Lie in whatever position you usually sleep. Make yourself really comfortable, well supported by pillows, and give a long, sighing breath out and relax. Imagine that strings are attached to all your joints. Think of one fixed to your elbow, being tightened gradually so that your elbow is pulled up with the string. Depending on the position in which you are lying, your elbow may be moved a lot or a little. Then let it go. Notice the different feelings. Now the angle of the string is different, so feel the pull in a different direction. It lifts your elbow higher and higher. Now the string is released. It may take a little practice, but try not to allow any parts other than those operated by the string to move. The hand hangs limp at the wrist. The shoulder is not lifted. Only the elbow is activated.

Now do the same thing with an imaginary string attached to the other elbow. Let it be pulled in various directions. Continue as if a string were fixed to one big toe, then the other one, the back of one ankle, then the other, the left knee, the right knee, the left wrist, the right wrist, the index finger, the middle joint of a finger, one shoulder, the other shoulder, your left hip, your right hip.

Then imagine two strings, attached to your right elbow and right wrist, for example, tightening one after the other until both are drawn taut; first the wrist string is released, then the elbow string. Experiment with the strings working in a different order. Keep your mind focused on the tightening string rather than on the muscle you are contracting. Only when the invisible string is taut should you turn your mind to analyzing which muscles are tightened.

Imagine one string fixed to the top of your head, another to the base of your skull. First one is pulled, then the other. One goes slack, then the other. You will find that you can make the strings pull in different directions and at varying angles. This saves it from being a repetitive exercise that you do from habit, not focusing on what your body is doing. It is important that any body movements you do bring awareness, an increased sense of working *with* your body. Mechanical exercises have no place in learning to relax.

STANISLAVSKY RELAXATION

There are acting techniques for increasing body awareness and learning which muscles contract and work together. The precise combination of muscles working together varies with each individual and with the nature of the task, the angle at which you tackle it, the weight, dimensions, and even the texture of tools used. You will find that tasks you perform, even ordinary, everyday tasks, often cause you to change your breathing, and sometimes you hold your breath altogether. You may also discover that you tense up muscles that you do not need to use because you tackle a job in the wrong way or overwork at it, or because you are emotionally keyed up about what you are doing. All this is a valuable process of self-discovery as you gradually learn more and more about yourself.

The method of relaxation that is based on Stanislavsky's acting techniques explores different sets of muscles in the body that naturally function together and the ways they work in response to imagined activities and tasks and even thoughts and feelings. You think of certain situations—things you might be doing with your body—and mentally involve yourself in these as if you were actually performing them. Notice which muscles have become tense. Once the observation is made, switch off the picture in your mind and deliberately release those muscles. Start by sitting or lying against a firm support and let the pillows take the whole weight of your body. Listen to the sound of your own breathing. Breathe so that you can just hear yourself—in through your nose, and then out through your mouth. Allow the breathing to flow through your mouth, letting the breath out be long and slow. The sound is like a little sigh as you breathe out. You may notice that there is a slight pause after you breathe in, as if you have reached the crest of a wave. Enjoy that slight pause. Then give a long breath out. And with each breath out, relax a little more.

SUGGESTED EXERCISES FOR STANISLAVSKY RELAXATION

You need a vivid imagination to act out these scenes! Nothing should distract you. Find a quiet place where you can be alone, because it is best if no one is watching to make you feel self-conscious. You need to focus entirely on what you are doing.

THE JAW Imagine that you have some very sticky toffee in your mouth, and chew it well. It is sticking to your teeth. Work this great hunk of toffee out of your teeth. Notice what is happening. Then rest and drop your jaw. Let it relax, quite soft and loose. Notice the different feeling of complete release of the jaw muscles.

THE EYES We do not usually notice when our eye muscles become tense. Imagine that there is a firefighter climbing a ladder to rescue a little dog stranded at the top of a house. Focus on the firefighter as he climbs all the way up. Observe the feeling in the muscles behind and around your eyes. Follow him with your eyes—up and up—until he is at the top. He has the little dog under his arm and is bringing it down and down. Now he is at the bottom. Relax your eyes, and if you want to, let them close. Notice how different they feel.

THE FEET Imagine that you are at the seashore standing on a very pebbly beach with no shoes on. Making very slight movements, imagine that you are walking on the beach with the sharp pebbles underfoot, and really feel them under your bare feet. Pick your way carefully over them. Oh! That was a sharp one! Observe the tension in your feet. Now go on to the soft sand. Really feel the difference. Then imagine lying down and letting your feet relax completely.

THE HANDS Can you recollect the feeling of making a snowball? Imagine that you are picking up snow and are patting the hard, cold mass into a firm snowball. You are hurrying so that you can throw it at someone. As you quickly make your snowball, notice the tension in your hands. Then drop them and let them relax beside your body on the bed or floor and notice how warm, soft, and loose they feel. Now scoop up some more snow, repeat the actions, and then relax.

TASTE Imagine that you are sipping some water. Place the imaginary glass to your lips. It is sharp, straight lemon juice! Really taste it. Notice what is happening in your mouth and the tension that is spontaneously produced. Now it is gone. Let the muscles of the mouth soften. Now you have a large, ripe peach. Take a good bite of it. It is very juicy and the juice is dribbling down. You need to suck it and draw in the juice. Smell it, too. Chew it, swallow it. Now it is gone. Notice the very different feeling this creates in your mouth. Relax completely and think through what happened to the muscles inside your mouth and nose and to the other facial muscles as you imagined yourself eating the peach. You may want to try this one a second time.

SMELL Muscles around the nostrils and in the cheeks and the mouth work together as we smell and taste things. Imagine that you have in your hand a bottle of liquid. Take out the stopper and take a good sniff—it is ammonia! Notice your reaction—how you have become stiff down the back of your neck. Then deliberately relax. Breathe in fresh, pure, clean air. Let yourself breathe easily.

Here is another bottle. Do the same with this one. It is perfume this time: lily of the valley. You will find yourself drawing in the scent of lily of the valley in long, slow breaths, holding the fragrance as if it were suffused behind the surface of your face. Now the fragrance is gone and you are just breathing air. Relax.

Go on from this to recreate in your imagination actions that you usually do without thinking, simple things like writing a shopping list, tying shoelaces, or unlocking a door. Try to imagine the sequence of actions and sensations to discover exactly how you use your body while doing them. After each acted scene, take some time to relax completely.

VISUAL IMAGERY IN CHILDBIRTH

Preparation for birth is not merely learning techniques for handling pain. It is much more positive than that, and at best enables you to draw on your own inner power. Ninety percent of birth, like 90 percent of sex, has to do with what is going on in your head. One woman experiences a long or physically difficult birth with elation. Another finds a straightforward birth distressing. It is in large part a result of the quality of the relationships between her and her caregivers. It is difficult for a woman to have a positive experience in an unsympathetic or hostile environment.

The mental images a woman has of labor and birth are vitally important, too: how she imagines all the intense physical sensations as they well up in her, and the meaning that these have as contractions sweep through her body and the baby's head descends. Pain may be seen as destructive and produce pictures of internal organs tearing and the baby being damaged, or be seen as purposeful, an effect of strong muscles working and the body opening. It helps to focus on creative images, and to rehearse them ahead of time. Imagine being in labor, welcoming each contraction with relaxation, rhythmic breathing, and a vivid mental picture that enables you to go *with* the work of your birthing body, instead of resisting it. These pictures inside your head may be enough for you to get in tune with your labor.

"I ENJOY WINDSURFING, SO THAT'S HOW I PICTURED MYSELF WHILE I WAS GIVING BIRTH—AN ACTIVE IMAGE THAT FITTED MY STRONG, RAPID LABOR EXACTLY."

You may want an entirely internal focus and feel that anything else would be distracting, or you may prefer to concentrate on something that you can see during contractions: a photograph, painting, the pattern on your partner's shirt or a piece of pottery, sculpture, or some intricate tiles—something that represents for you the energy and flow of birth. Sky and seascapes, a range of mountains capped with snow, a path through the forest, great trees with their branches spread wide, a waterfall cascading into a lake, a field of wheat with the wind sweeping across it, a flower opening from bud to full bloom—perhaps a waterlily or a rose—are images that may be right for you.

In some Mediterranean cultures, women have a flower beside them when they are in labor. It is the rose of Jericho, which looks dried up and lifeless but in the heat of the birth room opens and spreads its petals wide. In southern Italy they call it "the hand of the Mother of God." It is both a symbol of the help that Mary gives them in childbirth and of the cervix that is opening wider and wider so that the baby can be born. In Mediterranean cultures, too, there is a tradition of ritual actions that provide a powerful sense for the woman in labor of everything being opened and released, so that she can feel her body opening in a similar way. In Greece, grain or water may be poured, windows and doors flung wide, and clothing unbuttoned.

As labor progresses and contractions get stronger and longer, you may want active images that express the extraordinary power unleashed in your body. It often helps to focus on imagined actions, and to feel that you are swimming over waves, windsurfing, climbing a hill and skiing down a slope, swinging and flying, or roller-coasting over contractions. You can use music in a similar way, selecting tapes that echo your images of birth and represent for you the elemental forces of earth, air, fire, and water.

In many cultures, women are drawn to images of water. Contractions are like great waves bringing the baby to birth as if on the swell of the incoming tide. Women poets writing about birth use water imagery, too. For the poet Kathleen Raine, contractions are "waves that break on the shore of the world" and she calls to her baby, "Child in the little boat, come to the land." An ancient Armenian poem expresses the overwhelming feelings of giving birth: "The skies were in labor and the muscles of the earth and the ripe red seas were in labor."* Some women have a poem, a chant, a prayer, or a song that has special significance for them and helps them to keep on top of contractions.

"A PAINTING OF MARY GIVING BIRTH TO HER BABY, HIS HEAD CROWNING IN A HALO OF LIGHT, WAS MY VISUAL FOCUS. I HELD THE IMAGE IN MY MIND."

If when you are in labor an image turns out to be unsuitable or irritating, simply discard it and choose others, or focus on your uterus squeezing in and hugging the baby, your cervix opening in increasingly wider circles, the tissues of your vagina fanning out, your baby pressing deeper and deeper to be born, and reaching down to lift your baby into your arms. The essential element in the use of images like these is to achieve focused concentration, rather than letting your thoughts be dispersed by pain, and interpreting physical sensations in a positive, creative way, instead of feeling under attack. A woman uses the power of her mind, in harmony with the power released by her uterus, to help her body work freely.

BREATHING FOR LABOR

Relaxation and breathing are so closely associated that it is important to explore them as parts of a unity. You will not be able to breathe easily in labor unless you are relaxed.

As labor progresses, you may spontaneously breathe more rapidly. If you breathe more quickly and at the same time heavily, you will hyperventilate and flush carbon dioxide out of your bloodstream. This can make you feel uncomfortable, and, if it is severe enough, you may even pass out. Ironically, when you hyperventilate, you feel that you cannot get enough air in, and you tend to gulp air that makes the hyperventilation worse. In fact, it is possible to correct the effects of hyperventilation by

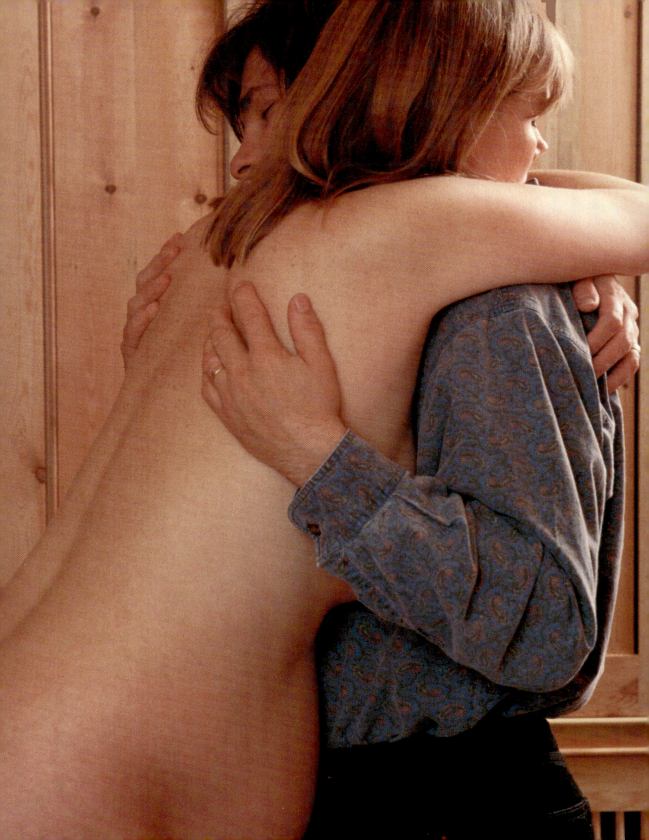

holding your breath for short periods, or by rebreathing carbon dioxide (breathing in and out of a paper bag). This restores carbon dioxide levels and the symptoms disappear.

The opposite—underbreathing or even not breathing at all—results in lack of oxygen and is more likely to happen if you have Pethidine or other opiates to relieve pain. Although you can cope with this, your baby needs you to breathe normally. Overbreathing, "forgetting" to breathe, and holding your breath are all harmful to the baby during childbirth.

"AS MASSIVE CONTRACTIONS SWEPT OVER ME, I COULDN'T HELP HOLDING MY BREATH. MY MIDWIFE SAID, 'SHOUT, MOAN, SING! THAT'LL HELP!'"

In many cultures, breathing in labor is deliberately "tuned" to help a woman work with the forces bringing her baby to birth. Among the Zulu, for example, breathing exercises are taught in pregnancy. A woman goes to the door of her hut each morning as the sun rises and takes careful, controlled, full breaths through each nostril alternately.* She uses the same breathing in labor. In other cultures, breathing is patterned by background sounds, including prayers, music, the beating of hands, repeated phrases of encouragement, or the swaying of women holding the mother.

BREATHING TO GO WITH THE FLOW

Smooth, easy breathing rhythms can help release tension and create a sense of pleasurable relaxation. Contractions come like the waves of the sea; there is a strong natural rhythm. You can either resist this, trying to "switch off," escape from, or dominate it, or go with it and adjust your breathing to the compelling sweep of uterine power. You can only go with the rhythm if you accept what is happening in your body.

So the breathing I suggest for labor is not to do with "distraction techniques" and is no magic method of eradicating sensation or guaranteeing that you do not feel pain. It is simply another way of getting in tune with your body, and especially with your uterus.

Rest your hands over the lower curve of your abdomen. In late pregnancy you have a lovely melon shape there. Breathe as slowly as you comfortably can. As the breath enters your nostrils, allow them to dilate, notice the slight pause between the breath in and the breath out, and then breathe out through a soft, relaxed mouth as if you had on a new and glossy lipstick. Enjoy that breath out. Notice what is happening to your abdomen.

Having someone you love with you makes for the best atmosphere in which to relax.

Feel it rising under your hands as you breathe in—a gentle swelling, like a wave building up. Then as you breathe out, the abdomen sinks back and the wave recedes. Be aware of the slight pressure under your hands as you breathe in, and the pressure withdrawing as you breathe out.

BREATHING DOWN YOUR BACK

You need someone to help you rehearse this. Try kneeling in front of a chair with your forearms and head resting on the seat and your knees well apart. Ask your helper to rest one hand firmly on each side of the base of your spine. Then breathe slowly right down your back, noticing the pressure against your helper's hands as you inhale and how it gradually falls away as you exhale.

THE GREETING BREATH

When you are in labor, meet each contraction with your breathing, giving first of all a complete greeting breath. This is a deliberate, slow breath *out*. Imagine an early first-stage contraction lasting 45 to 60 seconds. Breathe slowly through the contraction, with the lower back spreading out and pressing slightly against the bed or floor as you breathe in, and the pressure being lifted as you breathe out.

THE RESTING BREATH

As a contraction fades away, you give a long, slow, complete breath out through your mouth—a resting breath. This is important partly because it offers complete relaxation at the end of a contraction so that you rest and get refreshed before the next one, and partly because it signals to everyone in the room that your contraction has finished. If the midwife or obstetrician has something to say to you, now is the time, between contractions—never during them.

"I WAS UNDER STRESS AT WORK, CLEARING THE DECKS BEFORE GOING ON MATERNITY LEAVE. I DID THE FULL BREATHING DOWN MY BACK. IT HELPED ME FOCUS AND GAVE ME ENERGY."

In strong labor you may want to give several of these complete resting breaths once a contraction finishes. Do whatever feels good. If you always respond to the end of a powerful contraction by one or more resting breaths, you can be sure that, however difficult contractions are, you are giving your baby oxygen by breathing fully.

FULL CHEST BREATHING

You need a partner to help you practice full chest breathing. Begin by lying on your side with your back well rounded, your head and shoulders curved forward, your legs well apart, and the upper leg drawn up and bent at the knee. Now lift your head as if stretching your spine all the way up the back so that you feel taller. Stretch your neck at the back and stretch all the way up your spine. Let your head drop back into place and settle comfortably on your shoulders. Make sure that you leave a good space between your legs. Then give a long breath out and relax completely. Allow your eyes to close if they feel heavy.

Think of your back. Your spine is not stiff like a lamppost. It is constructed of small vertebrae in a curving shape like a string of beads. We often act as if our spinal columns were very stiff. Yet think of the way a cat moves and how the movement ripples up and down the back.

Now your partner rests one hand on each of your shoulders and massages with the flat of both hands from the top of your back right down to the bottom. The hands should be relaxed. Say if you would like the massage to be heavier or lighter, slower or quicker. Is it in the right place? It should feel good. Concentrate on relaxing toward the hands.

Then your partner rests the palms of both hands firmly above your waist on either side of the spine over the rib cage. They should be in a position that is comfortable for you and should not be pressing in on your waist (or where it once was!). Notice their warmth and strength. Breathe in through the nose and out through the mouth again so that the main level of breathing awareness is where you feel the pressure and warmth of the hands, and listen to your breathing. Breathe right down to where you feel the hands, expanding your rib cage so that it is swelling out under the hands as you breathe in, and then falls away from the pressure of the hands as you breathe out. Listen to it for a moment. Can your partner feel the pressure, building up as you breathe in and falling away as you breathe out? This is full chest breathing.

This kind of breathing can help you cope effectively with early first stage contractions. You may be happy to breathe like this all the way through the first stage, concentrating on breathing into the area against which your partner is pressing. When you are actually in labor you will not need the hands there because you will do it automatically, and the contracting uterus itself will provide sufficient stimulus.

UPPER CHEST BREATHING

As contractions strengthen, you may want to lift your breathing above them, as if over the crest of a wave. Contractions like huge waves come every four or five minutes and last about a minute. You may find that you can cope with them more easily if you breathe more lightly and more quickly.

To practice breathing with these contractions, your partner rests the palms of both hands on your upper back just below your shoulder blades. Breathe so that your main level of breathing activity and awareness is where you feel the pressure of the hands. You may want to breathe more rapidly, perhaps through parted lips. You should be able to hear a crisp little sigh or "huff" with each breath out. Now if you rest your hand over your upper chest you will feel it rising and falling at the same time, rather like a seagull floating on a wave. In labor, the wave of a contraction will be underneath and you will be breathing over the top of it. Relax your shoulders; they are not doing any of the work. If you find that you can still breathe with your full chest, do so. Only "lift" your breathing if you really need to.

REHEARSING BREATHING AND CONTRACTIONS

Prepare yourself to ride the waves of contractions during labor with the type of breathing that feels right for you. Breathe easily and without strain as contractions sweep through you. There are no rules about breathing. When you are in labor your body will tell you what to do.

SIMULATING CONTRACTIONS

It is best to practice this technique with your partner, who acts as your "uterus" by pinching a little flesh on your inside thigh between her fingers.

To simulate a contraction your partner simply lifts a fingerful of flesh off the leg and gradually increases the pressure for 30 seconds or so, and then reduces it. If you need to, allow your breathing rhythm to get lighter and quicker as the pressure builds to the maximum. Then breathe slowly and fully as the contraction fades.

Be careful that the pinching is not over a varicose vein or so strong that it causes a bruise. There is no need to press down on blood vessels.

BREATHING

You learn to respond to painful stimuli with breathing, so that you can work with your body in a positive way instead of fighting pain, which only increases tension and makes labor more difficult.

Full chest breathing can be helpful if you no longer find it easy to breathe all down your back. Your partner rests her hands at waist level and you concentrate on breathing down to where you feel the pressure.

Upper chest breathing is useful if you feel the need to soar over the top of stronger contractions. Your partner rests her hands at the base of your shoulder blades and you focus on breathing where you feel the pressure.

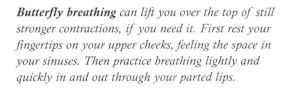

Butterfly breathing can lift you over the top of still stronger contractions, if you need it. First rest your fingertips on your upper cheeks, feeling the space in your sinuses. Then practice breathing lightly and quickly in and out through your parted lips.

BUTTERFLY BREATHING

This is a kind of breathing that you may never need to use, but which feels lifesaving in a speedy labor when contractions seem to hit you like enormous waves in rapid succession.

When the going is hard, women tend to raise their chins in the air, tense the muscles of the neck and jaw, and start to gasp and overbreathe. Instead, let your head drop forward onto your chest like a heavy flower on its stalk. Remembering to keep your shoulders loose, the back of your neck long, and your jaw released will help you to keep a steady rhythm.

Butterfly breathing is the lightest, most rapid breathing you may want in labor. With most breathing techniques you are consciously using your diaphragm and lungs, but butterfly breathing is easier if you think of it as being centered in your mouth and behind your cheeks and not in the throat. If you center your breathing in the throat, you will probably tense up your neck. Think of the space in your mouth, the space behind your warm, plumped-up cheeks. Either sit up in a chair or lie well propped up on the bed. If you are lying flat, you can find yourself panting heavily. So pile three or four pillows behind you, or try a squatting, kneeling, all-fours, or standing position.

"IT WAS AGONY TO LIE ON MY BACK DURING MY LABOR, SO ALTHOUGH THE MIDWIFE SAID IT WAS INTERFERING WITH THE PRINTOUT FROM THE MONITOR, I KNELT AND HELD ON TO THE BED. THAT WAY, I COULD COPE MUCH BETTER."

Resting the plump pads of the tips of your fingers against your cheeks will help you to concentrate on this area. Part your lips in a slight smile like the Mona Lisa. Relax your mouth. You will probably salivate a little. Breathe lightly in and out through your parted lips. Start gently, then allow your breathing to speed up till it is like little dancing waves.

Butterfly breathing may be quite difficult at first. You may feel that you are taking in or letting out too much air. Most people do to begin with. They think that they will never be able to manage it in labor, but then it comes quite naturally and they do not know how they could have coped without it.

It may help to think in terms of a definite rhythm in which one beat is slightly accentuated: *one*, two, three, four; *one*, two, three, four; or one, two, three, four, five, *six*. If you do this, be careful not to expel a great deal of air on the accentuated breath or you will gasp in the following breath and start to hyperventilate. If it is difficult to keep the rhythm, or your throat is getting tight, give a quick blow out through pursed lips and carry on with the light breathing immediately after.

After you have experimented with this breathing, try it once again, and this time notice especially if your shoulders or the back of your neck becomes tense. Drop your shoulders and relax. Under stress, it is tempting to breathe too heavily and sound as if you are a chugging piece of machinery. Try to keep your breathing as light as a whisper. When you rehearse, think of the sound of leaves in the forest floating to the ground. Bear in mind that in childbirth you will naturally make more noise than that. You will want to use this sort of breathing only when you are coping with the strongest contractions, at the end of the first stage. You may discover that full chest, upper chest, or even breathing all down your back works well for you at this time. Do whatever feels right for you.

When you reach this point, you may feel like a little ship in a storm at sea in the midst of huge waves and confusing crosscurrents. For most women this is the most difficult time of labor. Grantly Dick-Read used to call it "the pain period of labor." This does not mean that you may not feel pain at other times, but this is when you will need all your concentration and control.

SHEEP'S BREATHING

If we watch any mammal giving birth, a cat, for example, or a sheep, we notice that it does not take great breaths in and then "block" the birth canal by holding its breath. A sheep gives birth with rather light, quick breathing. Its breath is involuntarily held as it bears down and then it continues the light, accelerated breathing again.

During the second stage of labor when the baby is traveling down the vagina or birth canal (see pages 260–263), most women feel the urge to push during contractions. As a contraction builds most women move from full to lighter, quicker breathing. Then the surge of desire to bear down comes and you hold your breath. As soon as you can breathe again you do so, then feel you have to bear down again—and so on until the desire fades, breathing slows down, and the contraction ends. Practice this with only a very slight push, with a hand resting over your perineum so that you can feel its gentle bulge forward.

THE BIRTH DANCE

Once you are fairly confident about your ability to relax and breathe rhythmically, explore some different positions that you may want to use in labor. There is no reason that you should have to be tucked up in bed. There are definite disadvantages to the supine position (lying flat on your back) for your baby, since the blood flow in the large veins in the lower part of your body may be obstructed by the heavy weight of your uterus, and this can reduce the blood flow through the placenta to and from the baby.

Through the first stage of labor you will almost certainly feel happiest walking around or standing up. During contractions you will probably want to lean against a wall or your partner. If you have a low backache, you can lean forward onto a heavy piece of furniture. Once labor is advanced, it will be easier if you already know the positions in which you are likely to feel most comfortable. Avoid getting stuck in one position.

THE BIRTH DANCE IN LABOR

There is no reason to spend labor in bed. In fact, lying flat on your back diminishes the oxygen supply to your baby and prevents the uterus from contracting efficiently. While you are pregnant, try different movements to find those that are most comfortable for you.

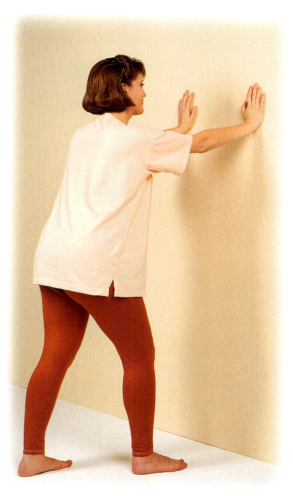

STANDING

In early labor, you may feel happiest walking, standing, or even dancing. During contractions you may need something to lean against.

Stand with your feet well grounded and wide apart. Place the flat of your hands against a solid surface, such as a wall. Try rocking and rolling your hips in this position.

ON ALL FOURS

The essence of labor is movement, so explore different ways to rock, circle, and tilt your pelvis, changing position as and when you feel like it.

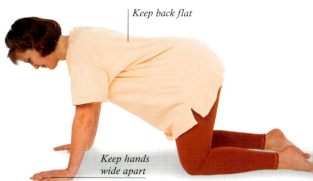

Keep back flat

Keep hands wide apart

On all fours *To relieve a low backache in labor, get down on all fours and place your hands flat on the floor, as wide apart as your shoulders. Remember not to arch your back.*

KNEELING

Try not to get stuck in one position. From kneeling you can explore a range of movements that will help you to keep your pelvis flexible and open. Your shoulders should stay soft and loose, too.

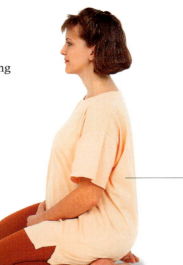

Keep your back straight

Kneeling up *Kneel on the floor with your back straight, legs apart, ankles turned out, and toes turned in toward each other. This position opens the pelvis and releases any tension in the back.*

Kneeling forward *In the same position as before, lean forward with your forearms flat on the floor. This is good to open the pelvis, too, taking the baby's weight off your back and relieving backaches.*

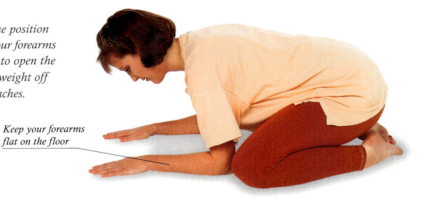

Keep your forearms flat on the floor

Hanging abdomen *Try kneeling on all fours, with your forearms on the floor, your knees spread wide, and your abdomen hanging between them. In this position you may like to rock backward and forward. Keep your lower back flat.*

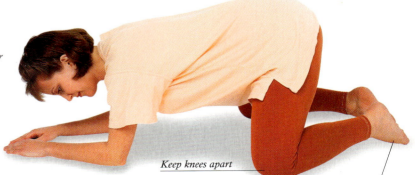

Keep knees apart

Ankles turned out and toes turned in

LYING DOWN

Rest between contractions by lying in a forward or sideways position, so tilting the weight of the baby off your spine.

Relax your neck muscles

Lying down *You can relax almost on all fours, but flopped forward onto several pillows, a big floor cushion, or a beanbag to support the weight of your uterus.*

SQUATTING

In the squatting position your pelvis is wide open and the baby's head pressed down. It is good to practice this position for labor, on your own or in a supported squat with the help of your partner.

Practice squatting and leaning *forward onto a chair or onto your partner for support during labor. To improve your balance, you can place a rolled-up towel under your heels to help you tilt.*

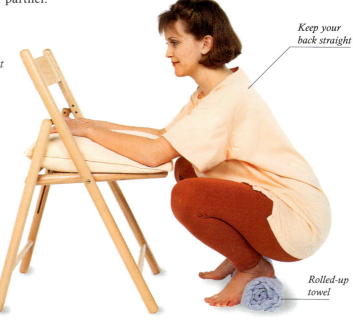

Keep your back straight

Rolled-up towel

Practice a supported squat with your partner, who supports you as you adopt the position. Stand facing each other and grasp forearms. Then your partner bends her knees and leans slightly backward, with one foot in front of the other.

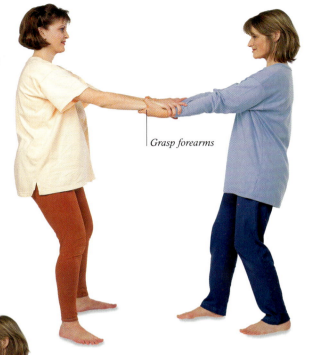

Grasp forearms

With your partner supporting and pulling against you, sink down, allowing your hips, knees, and ankles to give, thus transferring the weight into your lower back and seat bones.

As your partner carries on supporting your weight, she enables you to lengthen up, lean forward, and sink your heels toward the floor, while releasing your hips.

Bend knees

Release hips

HAMMOCK

In some birth centers you will find a small hammock suspended on an adjustable rope from the ceiling for you to use during labor. The beauty of a hammock is that it takes most of your weight and gives you the freedom to swing and rock as you please. If you are having your baby at home, you can hang your hammock on a hook set into a door frame.

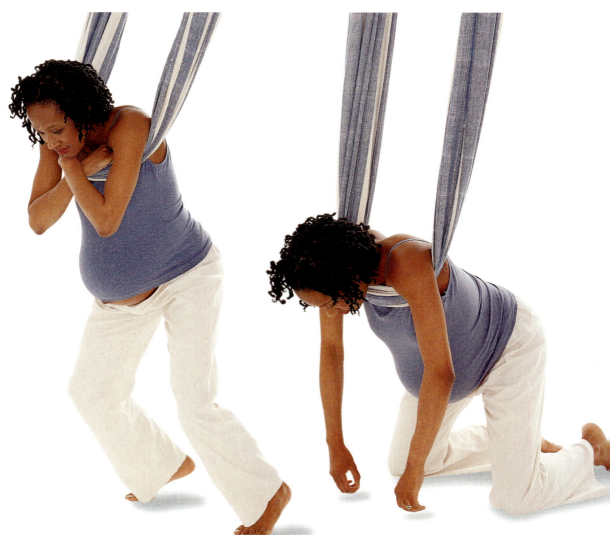

Stand leaning into the *hammock, with your knees slightly bent, allowing the hammock to take your weight. Explore any movements that feel comfortable. Swing gently backward and forward, and rock and circle your pelvis.*

Set the hammock *at a lower level and drop to your knees. Now lean forward into the hammock and let your arms and abdomen hang heavy. Enjoy the feeling of near weightlessness as you rock to and fro.*

The essence of labor is movement. Explore ways in which you can rock, circle, and tilt your pelvis. You can try kneeling, leaning back over your heels, or leaning forward onto a pillow placed on a chair or bed or over the top of the headboard; a knee-chest position with knees placed on either side of your body, rather like a frog; on all fours or squatting, with your back supported. Some of these movements are shown on pages 214–218.

Your aim is to give the baby as much room as possible in your pelvis by keeping your knees well apart and allowing the uterus to tilt forward onto your abdominal wall and away from your spine. In this position the uterus assumes an egg shape, whereas when you are lying flat on your back it tends to be distorted from this natural shape. When you are upright you are also allowing gravity to help the baby down. In all these positions contract only those muscles you need to use to support yourself, and whenever possible use pillows, furniture, or another person to help you.

Some birth centers now have a hammock—a circular strip of strong cloth suspended on a rope from the ceiling. During labor, you stand leaning into the hammock, allowing it to take your weight and give physical support while you enjoy complete freedom to circle and rock your pelvis. If you are having your baby at home and can get a Latin American woven hammock, hang it on a hook set into a door frame in the same way (see opposite).

"IT WAS AWFUL LYING ON MY BACK. I LONGED TO BE UPRIGHT. AS SOON AS I COULD USE THE HAMMOCK I WAS IN CONTROL OF MY LABOR, AND IN CONTROL OF THE PAIN."

You can relieve low backaches in labor, especially common when the baby is in an occipito-posterior position (see page 271), by letting your abdomen hang forward, tilting the baby away from your sacrum. Gently hump your lower back up and let it drop down, or circle your pelvis—whichever feels right for you at the time. This posture is also convenient for back massage and counterpressure, and because the longitudinal axis of the uterus is then in line with the birth canal, it may help the baby to rotate into the correct anterior position. If the baby is lying in a posterior position, you will probably have bearing down sensations before you are fully dilated, and are more likely to be able to control the urge if you try to take some of the pressure off your rectum.

Pressure on the umbilical cord interrupts the flow of blood to the baby. This can cause decelerations of the fetal heart that last after the end of the contractions, and which may be noted if you are having continuous electronic monitoring (see pages 340–344). These decelerations may prompt your doctor to consider a forceps delivery or Cesarean section for fetal distress. If you adopt a position in which your tummy is hanging forward, however, such as on all fours, both the baby and its cord will be tipped away from your spine, and the pressure on the cord may be relieved.

THE BIRTH DANCE
FOR DELIVERY

Explore different positions for birth with your partner
or the people who will be helping you at the birth, so that
everyone has some idea of what to expect. Use a doll,
a ball, even a grapefruit, as a substitute for the baby.

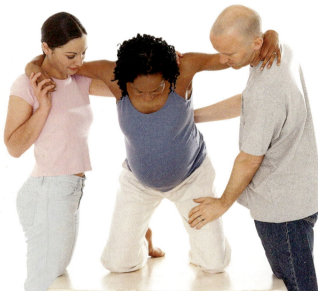

Kneeling opens up the pelvis fully and aids the
baby's descent. You will feel most secure if you
have the support of two helpers, one on each
side of you, while you are rocking and circling.

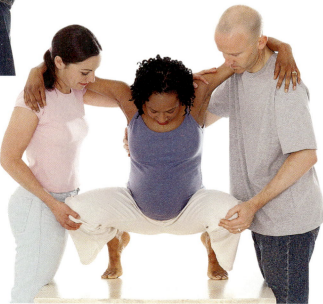

Moving into a squat can also be comfortable.
Again, you will need two helpers who can
support you while you rock and support your
knees when you are bearing down. This is not
a good position for birth if the baby's head is
large, since it can be tough on your tissues.

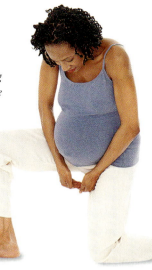

A half-kneeling, half-squatting position is the easiest if you are planning to lift your baby out yourself. Kneel on one knee with the other leg bent, foot flat on the floor. It should give you greater stability than kneeling or squatting, and allows you to guide the baby out.

Kneeling with your body upright and rocking speeds up a very slow second stage. The midwife can deliver your baby from behind and pass her through your legs, or you may actually be able to lift her out yourself.

Kneeling on all fours, with your head down and bottom up, will slow down a second stage that is happening very fast. This position helps you feel more in control, as well as allowing your vaginal tissues time to soften and stretch so that they are less likely to tear as the baby is born. This is also useful in the first stage to help turn a posterior baby, during transition to encourage dilatation of an anterior lip (by slowing down the urge to push), and if the baby's head is large. If the baby's shoulders get stuck (shoulder dystocia), it gives the midwife more room to maneuver.

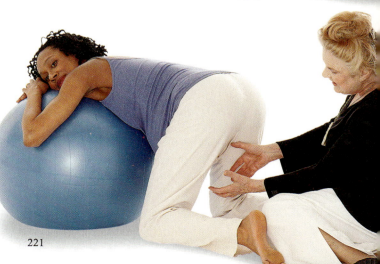

Leaning forward is good if the second stage of labor is fast (because it will slow you down a little), and also if the baby's head is large. The midwife will be able to guide your baby out, and then you can turn around and take the baby into your arms.

Sometimes contractions are inefficient from the very start of labor and do not seem to pick up or, having been effective at first, become weak. In either case it is worth trying a position in which the uterus can most easily form a sphere. It may help to stand facing a wall, with your legs well apart, and lean forward with your hands resting against the wall.

REHEARSING CONTRACTIONS

The experience of labor is difficult to imagine before you have had a baby. Will contractions be unbearably painful or hardly noticeable? Think of them as bigger and bigger hills that you have to climb, each hill with its own peak, until you reach the mountain range at the end of the first stage.

THE ACTION OF THE UTERUS

When the uterus contracts it tightens up, just like any working muscle in the body. Make a tight fist with one hand and raise your arm so that the big muscle on the inside of your upper arm, the biceps, tightens. Feel it with your other hand. You will notice that the biceps has become hard and is sticking out. If a man does the same thing, his biceps may stick out a good deal more than yours because his is probably a bigger muscle. The biceps gets hard as it contracts and also protrudes. This is because the muscle fibers are shortened and thickened. The same thing happens, on a much larger scale, when the uterus contracts in labor. Like your bulging biceps, the uterus bulges forward in your abdomen when you have a really strong and effective contraction. The strong contractions are the most effective of all for helping the baby to be born.

Place your hand just above your pubic-hair line at the very bottom of the abdomen. The cervix lies under this area, and it is here that you are likely to feel the strong, rhythmic pull as it opens—a pull that will feel tightest at the height of each contraction (see page 254).

Contractions are felt mainly as powerful pressure that comes whether or not you want it to. So when you are practicing for them, work with a partner and allow him or her to simulate contractions, deciding when they start, how strong they become, and how long they last. Meet each contraction with a welcoming breath out and use rhythmic breathing right through each one, with a long resting breath out at the end.

Your partner sits beside you so that you have eye contact with each other. He pretends to be your uterus by taking hold of a piece of your flesh, the inner thigh, say, and squeezing it. He will find that grasping a small piece of flesh rather than a big area is the most effective. He should be particularly careful if you have a varicose vein, lifting the flesh up off the leg instead of pressing down into the leg, and avoiding the area around the varicose vein. First he squeezes gently, and then tightens his grip to a strong pinch that lasts for about 15 seconds, after which he gradually releases his hold. The contraction should last about 45 seconds in all. This exercise will help him to be aware of what you are feeling and how you react to stress of this kind, so that he can give you emotional support and encouragement. If you do not want him to do this, because you cannot rely on him to be perceptive and sensitive, omit this method.

In between these mock contractions, talk about the experience. Discuss with him how each contraction felt, and perhaps how he can improve his performance and you can improve your response.

In labor, this rest space between contractions should be used to prepare you for the next one: do not waste time discussing the contraction that has just ended. It is a good idea to change places so that you become your partner's "uterus" and he can experience this firm gripping sensation and learn how to respond to it. This is important for anyone who is going to be with you during labor and wants to help you by breathing with you when and if contractions become difficult.

PRACTICING FOR STRONGER CONTRACTIONS

Switch roles again and imagine that labor is progressing with longer and stronger contractions, each reaching its peak about halfway through. Always remember, however, that contractions vary and that it is no good wishing for a "textbook labor" if your own labor proves to be quite different. Some contractions have their peaks about a third of the way through. Some may even have two peaks. The important thing is that if you go with your uterus, you tune in with it rather like an orchestra responding to a conductor. The conductor in this case is the

> "MY PARTNER WAS VERY RESPONSIVE. I NEVER FELT HE WAS TOO TOUGH ON ME. BUT IT HELPED ME PREPARE FOR STRONG CONTRACTIONS."

uterus. You have to be able to, as it were, "listen" to your uterus in order to react appropriately to it and be in complete harmony with it. For these stronger contractions your partner will need to grip the flesh of your thigh for a minute or a even little longer.

When necessary during these longer contractions, respond by lifting your breathing above the contraction—breathing more shallowly and more quickly (see page 209). Make sure that you relax your shoulders and toes; then, as the contraction becomes slightly less intense, allow your breathing to become slower and fuller.

PUSHING

Bearing down or pushing is often described as an extraordinarily athletic activity, as if you could learn to do it the way you learn to do an aerobic exercise. It should not be like this. It is, rather, a spontaneous welling up of energy that culminates in a triumphant push and an opening of the vagina. You feel mounting excitement. It is as if you are on the edge of a chasm with life at its most elemental surging up from the depths, until every nerve and every pore of your body tingles with urgent desire. You do not have to ask for instructions. You do not have to ask if you can "push now." The creative power in your body is intense and overwhelming.

IMAGINING THE LONGING TO PUSH

First make sure that your bladder is empty. Then rest your hands beneath the lower curve of your abdomen. Take a breath and hold it. Drop your chin forward on your chest and allow the bulge underneath your hands to press downward and forward, so that from inside your abdomen you are pressing your hands out and moving them forward. You probably feel your perineum moving forward, too. Allow the movement to carry right down through you until you feel the tissues of the vagina spreading out, and then rest. Did you get that feeling of something moving forward? When the baby is ready to be born, this movement helps its head to bulge farther down the birth canal. Although it is useful to learn how to do this beforehand by practicing without straining, women who are free to do whatever they feel like have a spontaneous physical and emotional urge to do it anyway when they are really ready to push (see page 260). Now try any of the positions suggested on pages 214–218.

"IT FELT WONDERFUL TO SWING INTO SECOND-STAGE PUSHING. NOW I UNDERSTAND WHAT YOU MEAN BY 'THE BIRTH PASSION.'"

One of the best ways of rehearsing pushing is on the toilet, since we also release pelvic floor muscles for defecation, so they are not put under unusual strain. If you are constipated, as many women are in late pregnancy (see page 135), this movement is an excellent way to encourage spontaneous, easy bowel movements.

Each time you practice you will feel more comfortable in an upright position. This will be an advantage during labor, too, since you are more in control of what is happening, open up more easily for the baby to be born, and can see over the bulge to watch the birth if you want to. Gravity can help you in labor. If you are lying flat, or almost flat, you are pushing the baby uphill, because the uterus is almost at right angles to the vagina (see page 261). In an almost upright position, you can lean on your uterus and press the baby down.

After you have done this gentle pushing a few times, begin to work with your partner. To start, you might like to try sitting. Your partner sits near your head with a pillow over the forearm and supports your head and shoulders with it. This gives you a very wide base of support. With your partner's hands over your lower abdomen, you can both feel what is happening inside. Drop your head forward onto your chest, so that you do not strain with your throat muscles and produce a grunting sound. Take a breath. Lean forward and press from inside steadily out, slowly, gently; a little bit more; let it go; let the breath out and rest. Your partner's hand pressed firmly against your lower abdomen gives you something to press against and will guide you. You will find it is easier to bear down when your baby is actually in the birth canal waiting to be born because you have something to press against. Allow your pelvic floor muscles to bulge forward like a heavy sack of apples. When you have felt the sensation this produces, lift your pelvic floor up again so that it is well toned and not sagging (see page 119). Think of it as smiling.

TRYING OTHER POSITIONS

When you are confident that you have the feeling of pushing with complete release of your pelvic floor muscles, go on to explore other positions that may feel right when you are in labor. Experiment with every type of open position—on a mattress on the floor, on the bed, leaning over or against furniture, using cushions and other kinds of support, cradled by another human body—in which you feel in touch with what is happening and free to let the energy of the uterus sweep through you to give birth. You will soon discover that an almost impossible posture in which to do this is lying flat on your back with your legs in the air in the lithotomy position, which used to be a standard position for the second stage of labor in a hospital birth.

Now, in many hospitals women are encouraged to find any position, and make any movement that is comfortable for them during labor and, if they wish, to give birth on a sheet or mattress on the floor.

WINDOWS INTO THE UTERUS

Apart from the routine urine and blood pressure tests you have every time you go to the doctor or midwife (see pages 48–51), there may be other investigations. Whether they are done at all, or how often they are done, will depend not only on there being some specific reason for them, but also on the part of the country you live in, the hospital or doctor's office you go to, and on your individual provider.

Teaching hospitals have far more high-tech equipment and research projects, so, for example, if you are in a large city hospital you may have ultrasound (see page 229) two or three times during your pregnancy. It is up to you whether or not you accept it.

SCREENING FOR DISABILITY

Screening aims to identify pregnancies in which the risk of abnormality is higher than usual. *Most women whose screening tests reveal possible abnormalities have normal babies.* Screening may be followed by diagnostic tests. These are much more precise.

You have the right to say no to tests. You may have ethical or religious reasons for refusing them or simply not feel happy about having them. You do not have to give a reason. All invasive diagnostic tests that entail entering the uterus bring some risks for the baby. Your doctor should be prepared to explain to you what these are.*

However, every screening and every diagnostic test, even a simple blood test for sugar in the urine, and measurements of blood pressure and weight gain, can be *emotionally* invasive. It may produce conflicting feelings about the baby. On the one hand, there is a tiny being whom you already love and care for. On the other hand, this baby may be damaged and unwanted. If a test raises the question of possible termination of a pregnancy, it is bound to cause anxiety. Even after this anxiety is relieved theoretically by a negative test result, a woman is often left feeling anxious and sometimes can be convinced that there must be something wrong with her baby. She may feel that an initial screening test that produced a positive result must mean that something bad has happened. She may feel that she has not been told the whole truth. All screening and diagnostic tests have side effects, although it is difficult to measure them because they are usually emotional, rather than physical.

MATERNAL SERUM SCREENING

The idea of screening maternal blood for fetal abnormality is simple. Blood is tested for one or more ingredients (alphafetoprotein, human chorionic gonadotrophin [HCG], estriol, and inhibin—different hospitals test different combinations), and results are compared with the expected levels. These vary with the weeks of pregnancy. From this, an estimate can be made of the risk of certain abnormalities in the baby.

The first serum test was for alphafetoprotein (AFP). This is produced in the early phases of pregnancy by the embryo's yolk sac, and later by the fetal liver. When levels of AFP are unusually high, an increased proportion of babies have neural tube defects such as spina bifida (where part of the bony spine is not entirely enclosed) and anencephaly (the absence of part of the brain).

If the AFP level is unusually low, a possible cause is Down's syndrome. Levels of AFP double about every five weeks in the fourth, fifth, and sixth months of pregnancy, but earlier than this are usually low. The best time to test for AFP is between the 15th and 17th week of pregnancy. The result of the serum test should be available in a few days.

"I WAS TERRIBLY WORRIED WHEN I GOT THE NEWS THAT MY AFP LEVEL WAS ABNORMALLY LOW, BUT IT ACTUALLY TURNED OUT THAT MY DATES WERE WRONG."

Nearly all hospitals now offer double screening (AFP and, usually, HCG), triple screening (AFP, HCG, and estriol), and some offer quad screening (AFP, HCG, estriol, and inhibin). In hospitals where an early (12-week) dating ultrasound scan is performed, an abnormal serum result will be discussed in detail with you. But if you did not have an early scan, one can be arranged at this stage to ensure that the test result is not abnormal simply because your dates are wrong (it may turn out that you are more or fewer weeks pregnant than you had thought).

If the results suggest that your baby is at risk of a neural tube defect, a "high resolution" ultrasound scan will be offered to look at the brain and spinal cord. If the results of that scan indicate a high risk (1 in 250 or more of Down's syndrome), you can decide if you want further tests such as amniocentesis (see page 232). With this you run a 1 in 200 risk of miscarrying as a result of the test. As with all medical interventions, it is a matter of achieving a delicate balance between risks, and there is no easy answer.

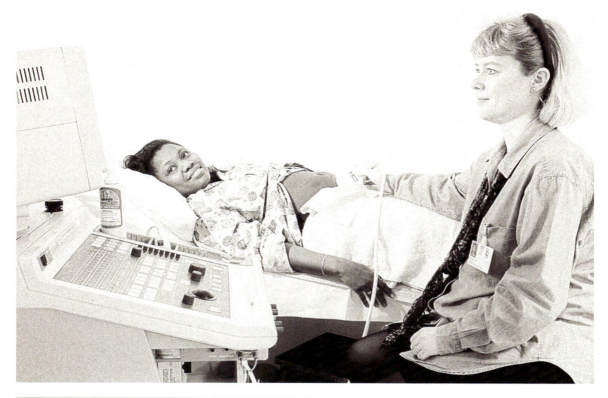

You may be given more than one ultrasound scan or even a series of scans every few weeks during pregnancy (above).

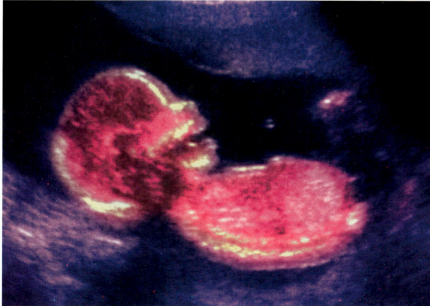

The image on this scan (left) shows the baby's shape clearly, but it is often more difficult to identify the different parts, some of which may be hidden behind the baby's other organs.

ULTRASOUND

Ultrasound (a scan) works on the principle of bouncing very high-frequency sound waves (far higher than the human ear can detect) off solid objects in fluid to produce a pattern of echoes. These are converted into electrical signals that are processed and displayed as a two-dimensional image. It is a method that has been used for many years by the navy to locate submarines in wartime and by fishermen to locate schools of deep-sea fish. Depth sounders in yachts work in a similar way.

USES OF ULTRASOUND

In pregnancy, ultrasound is used to obtain a moving picture of the baby in the uterus. From the end of the second month it is possible to see the tiny fetus kicking, and after 28 weeks breathing movements can be observed. There are a number of reasons why scans are done.

TO CONFIRM PREGNANCY A scan can be used to confirm pregnancy very early on, even before clinical tests are effective: it detects changes in the uterus that cannot yet be revealed by physical examination. From eight weeks it shows the embryo with its heart pulsing. An ultrasound can also detect that you are having twins when you are only eight weeks pregnant.

TO ESTABLISH THE ESTIMATED DATE OF DELIVERY Scans are now used in most hospitals, where you may expect to have them done at least twice during pregnancy. Even in smaller hospitals, it is now unusual not to be scanned at all during your pregnancy.

A scan will possibly be offered at about 12 weeks to find the estimated delivery date. The age of the baby can be established to within seven days (later in pregnancy it is more difficult to be precise because babies of the same age may grow at very different rates). It may be suggested that you be scanned again in the middle and at the end of pregnancy, or even more frequently, at intervals of a few weeks. This is called serial assessment and does not mean that anything is wrong. Only when a scan is used in this way can it give clues about the rate of fetal growth that can be taken seriously.

TO DETECT HANDICAPS At 18–20 weeks, ultrasound can be used to detect certain abnormalities in the fetus, including congenital heart defects, gastrointestinal and kidney malformations, and spina bifida. This is called an anatomic scan. These physical defects can be detected earlier in the pregnancy if the ultrasound probe is inserted into your vagina instead of being placed on top of your abdomen (transvaginal scan). Most babies with major chromosomal abnormalities have extra fluid behind their neck. This is known as increased nuchal fold thickness and can be detected by a scan from 12 weeks.

TO ASSESS FETAL WEIGHT Scans are not good at estimating birth weight, although they can be more accurate with premature babies. Research shows that the mother's guess at her baby's weight is more accurate.*

TO DETECT HOW THE BABY IS LYING If it is important to find out how your baby is lying in the uterus (for example, whether the baby is lying head down or is in the breech position, especially with twins), and the doctor cannot get this information for certain from manual examination, ultrasound can tell this with accuracy. This knowledge may make all the difference to you if, for instance, you want to have your baby at home.

If the baby is lying in a good position, you can proceed with confidence in your plans for a home birth. However, if the baby is lying awkwardly, it might be more sensible to go to the hospital. Either way, you and your doctor can be guided by the information provided by the scan. The scan should not be a condition for your having a home birth. You are free to decline a scan if you wish.

TO ASSESS THE CONDITION AND POSITION OF THE PLACENTA When there is bleeding in late pregnancy, ultrasound can be used to locate the position of the placenta. The danger is that the placenta might be blocking the baby's way out of the uterus (placenta previa, described further on page 139). In fact, a scan done in the first few months of pregnancy often gives the impression that the placenta is lying low on the wall of the uterus, but as the pregnancy progresses and the uterus enlarges and stretches, the placenta usually proves to be in the right place after all. Sometimes a woman worries through the rest of her pregnancy because she is told that she has a low-lying placenta. Occasionally, bleeding in late pregnancy suggests that the roots of the placenta are becoming dislodged with prelabor contractions. The baby's nourishment and oxygen supply would be cut if labor were allowed to proceed. A scan can sometimes show this clearly, and a Cesarean section can be performed to save the baby. Used in this way, or together with amniocentesis (see page 232), an ultrasound scan has undoubted advantages.

> "I FOUND THE SCANS AT SIXTEEN WEEKS AND THIRTY WEEKS REALLY EXCITING BECAUSE THE IMAGES ON THE SCREEN WERE SO CLEARLY EXPLAINED TO ME THAT I COULD EASILY UNDERSTAND THEM."

HOW ULTRASOUND WORKS

You undress, put on a hospital gown, and lie on your back beside the scanner. A water-based gel is spread across your abdomen and then a transducer is slowly passed over it. This picks up echoes from the different planes of your own organs and also the developing baby's tissues, and translates the information into a picture on a screen that looks like a television screen.

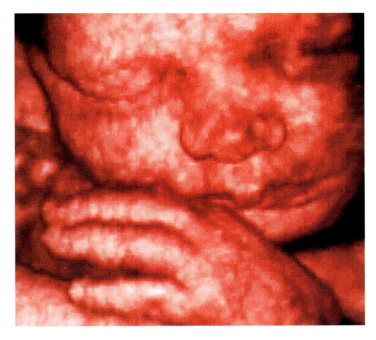

This 3-D image taken from an ultrasound scan at 18–20 weeks of pregnancy reveals the baby's face and hands in extraordinary detail.

A scan in the first few months of pregnancy gains in clarity if your bladder is full and therefore clearly visible, so you will probably be asked to drink a lot of water first and not urinate for an hour or so before the scan. Do not expect to see an immediately recognizable picture of your baby, even in late pregnancy; ask to have the picture interpreted, because it may look more like a map of the moon than a baby, and you may find it difficult to make out the different parts of the body.

Another technique involves the use of a specially designed intravaginal transducer, which is sometimes used in very early pregnancy and for other specific purposes. If you have a transvaginal scan, you will be asked to empty your bladder first.

IS ULTRASOUND SAFE?

As far as we know, ultrasound is safe, certainly much safer than X-rays (see page 110), which earlier provided the only technological method of gaining information about the baby in the uterus. On the other hand, it is known that high-frequency sound waves continued for a long time can damage an adult's hearing. Questions have therefore been raised about effects on the baby's hearing, since, although the sound waves are bounced off the baby for only a short time, the baby may be vulnerable at certain stages of its development. Babies are not born deaf after having ultrasound in the uterus, but no one yet knows if any of them will suffer delayed effects in later life.

Ultrasound has other effects on the body that are not yet fully understood. It generates heat in body tissues, and tiny bubbles inside tissue may dance in reaction to the sound waves. This does not mean that diagnostic ultrasound at the level at which it is normally used in pregnancy is dangerous. But it does imply that we should be asking questions about the likelihood of long-term effects. It is possible that ultrasound could have subtle harmful effects on especially vulnerable babies in the first 12 weeks of pregnancy, when the major organs of the body are being formed.

Babies usually jump around when they are scared. Though we cannot hear the shrill whistle of ultrasound, they can, and it may be stressful for them. In the words of the British Chief Medical Officer of Health, "All ultrasound exposure should be justified and limited to the minimum necessary for the diagnostic purpose. The greatest risk with ultrasound is from inaccurate interpretation of the image, rather than from any physical hazard of the ultrasonic field."*

If you are not at special risk, having ultrasound will not make birth safer or help your baby.* Though everyone may take it for granted that you will have at least one scan, you can say no.

SOME SAFETY MEASURES

It makes sense to expose your baby to ultrasound only when a diagnosis is needed that cannot be made without ultrasound, and when that would result in some change in the kind of care that you are being given. This rules out routine scanning at 16 weeks—now the accepted practice in many countries. It also rules out using ultrasound simply because you would like to see a picture of the baby or to "bond" with the fetus. Many obstetricians are enthusiastic about this and believe that they can make a contribution toward ensuring that babies are well mothered by performing routine ultrasound scans. They do not realize that there are a number of other—better and more intimate—ways of getting to know your baby (see page 238) while it is in the uterus.

The length of time that the baby is exposed to ultrasound should be limited, and when you are discussing what you can see on the screen, ask for the image to be frozen. When the scanner is linked to a video recorder, the examination can be replayed later and there can be full discussion about it without exposing the baby unnecessarily to ultrasound.

AMNIOCENTESIS

Amniocentesis is used to detect abnormalities of the baby's chromosomes (most commonly Down's syndrome and some other genetic abnormalities). The sex of the baby can also be determined by this procedure, which is important in genetic screening because some genetic diseases are sex-linked, which means they affect only one sex.

HOW AMNIOCENTESIS WORKS

A hollow needle is inserted through your abdominal wall into the uterus, where about half a fluid ounce (14 ml) of the amniotic fluid in which the fetus is lying is sucked out. This is fluid that has been swallowed by the fetus and passed out of its body through its mouth or bladder. It is full of cells from the skin and other organs, which, when analyzed, provide information on the baby's chromosomes. The fluid is spun in a centrifuge to separate the cells from the liquid. The cells are left to multiply and then analyzed. Results are available in two to four weeks.

"AMNIOCENTESIS DID FEEL LIKE AN INVASION. THEY TRIED TO BE REASSURING, BUT IT DIDN'T ALTER THE SENSE THAT IT WAS AN ATTACK ON THE BODY."

In the 1950s, when amniocentesis was first invented, mistakes were sometimes made and the needle penetrated placental tissues, causing miscarriage. Now ultrasound is used to locate the placenta, and the risks of damage to the placenta have been reduced. But there still remains a chance that amniocentesis will cause miscarriage. Because of this small but definite risk, there is no point in having it unless there is a well-above-average chance of your baby's being born abnormal. You will have thought carefully about the implications of discovering that something is wrong and

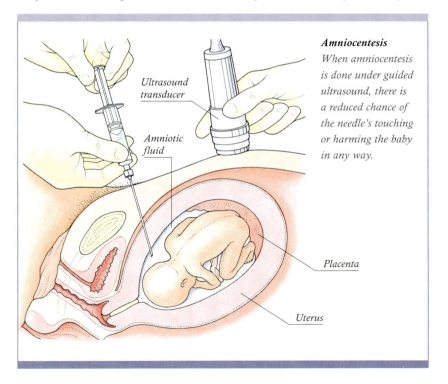

Ultrasound transducer

Amniotic fluid

Amniocentesis
When amniocentesis is done under guided ultrasound, there is a reduced chance of the needle's touching or harming the baby in any way.

Placenta

Uterus

have decided whether you would opt for termination. In some areas, amniocentesis is offered to all women based on their age (over 35, over 37, or over 39), since the chance of some disorders rises with age. Ask to talk to a counselor *before* an invasive diagnostic test. This will help you to reach a decision about whether you want the test. If you do, and an abnormality is revealed, counseling should be immediately available to both parents.

There is a 1 in 200 risk of miscarriage when amniocentesis is performed after 16 weeks. Experiments have been done with amniocentesis as early as 9 weeks, but the miscarriage rate then is between 3 percent and 7 percent, depending on the skill of the operator. Moreover, since less fluid is available at that stage, the lab is unable to grow a cell culture in up to 21 percent of cases, so the amniocentesis has to be done again.*

If amniocentesis is done between the 16th and 18th weeks of pregnancy, when many women have felt the first fetal movement, the decision to terminate a pregnancy is distressing, and the termination is riskier than one performed earlier in pregnancy. The woman needs generous emotional support from her partner and family. Amniocentesis is sometimes performed late in pregnancy if it looks as if the baby may need to be delivered preterm. In such a case, the risks of continuing the pregnancy must be weighed carefully against the risks of delivering a baby with immature lungs. The amniotic fluid can reveal vital information as to whether the fetal lungs are mature, that is, whether they are strong enough for the baby to breathe normally after birth. If the lungs are still immature, corticosteroids can be given to the mother to help mature the lungs, assuming it is safe to delay the delivery. Results of amniocentesis for lung maturity are available immediately.

CHORIONIC VILLUS SAMPLING

Chorionic villus sampling (CVS) entails taking a sample of tissue from the part of the outer membrane around the embryo that will later become the placenta. This is to diagnose whether or not a fetus will have a genetic handicap. One handicap this test cannot detect, however, is spina bifida.

CVS can be carried out before 12 weeks—even as early as 10 weeks—so that an abnormal fetus can be terminated much earlier in pregnancy than it would normally be after an amniocentesis.

But for many women, the risks of CVS outweigh the benefits: there is a high incidence of infection, bleeding, and miscarriage following CVS, and it has also been linked to limb defects. This was discovered not by a medical researcher but by a woman who had CVS and gave birth to a child with deformed

"I DECIDED AGAINST BOTH CVS AND AMNIOCENTESIS. IT WASN'T WORTH THE RISK. THE WAY I LOOK AT IT, A FETUS ISN'T A COMMODITY TO BE INSPECTED. IT'S MY BABY—WHATEVER IT'S LIKE."

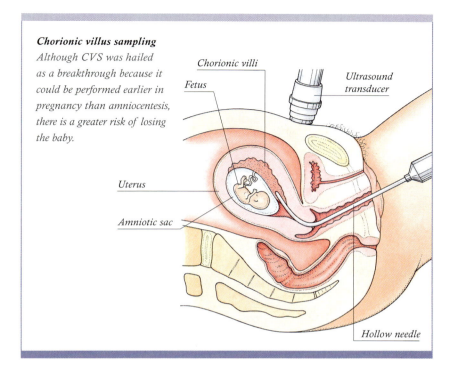

Chorionic villus sampling
Although CVS was hailed as a breakthrough because it could be performed earlier in pregnancy than amniocentesis, there is a greater risk of losing the baby.

Chorionic villi

Fetus

Ultrasound transducer

Uterus

Amniotic sac

Hollow needle

limbs. After meeting another woman whose baby had similar abnormalities after she had CVS at the same hospital, she reported it to a genetic counselor. She was told by doctors that there was no connection. But she continued to ask questions. A study was then conducted, which suggested that there was an association. The earlier the CVS, the more likely a limb deformity will occur, probably as a result of interfering with the blood supply to the limb.* Amniocentesis in the second trimester of pregnancy is safer than CVS. However, for some women, the possibility of discovering and aborting an affected fetus by 12 weeks or so is important enough that they will assume the increased risk. This is particularly true if the fetus is at high risk—for example, a 1 in 4 or 1 in 2 chance—of a genetic disorder.

PERCUTANEOUS UMBILICAL BLOOD SAMPLING

At the end of the 1970s, fetoscopy—photographing the baby with a telescope introduced into the uterus—was the latest technique for finding out exactly what was happening to babies that were known to be at risk. Unfortunately, the risk of miscarriage proved to be as high as 5 to 10 percent. For this reason, fetoscopy has now been superseded by a newer technique called percutaneous umbilical blood sampling (cordocentesis).*

In this process, a very fine needle is passed through the mother's abdomen and uterus into the fetal vein in the umbilical cord, and blood is withdrawn so that it can be tested for disorders and abnormalities. Intrauterine blood transfusions can also be given in this way, and drugs can be injected directly into the baby. Because the fetal vein is fragile in early pregnancy, the technique cannot be performed until after 18 weeks.

Percutaneous umbilical blood sampling is used in some clinics in addition to amniocentesis and ultrasound; it is also used when there is Rh-factor-generated disease (see page 113), in order to diagnose hemophilia in a baby, and to check for metabolic disorders, as well as infections such as toxoplasmosis and rubella.

Dr. Kypros Nicolaides of King's College Hospital, London, estimates that when the method is used by experienced doctors, the risk of losing a baby is only 1 to 2 percent, the same as that for amniocentesis and chorionic villus sampling in that hospital. He emphasized to me that "the greatest risk of any operative technique in pregnancy is always the skill and experience of the operator." This is a technique that should be, and generally is, restricted to a few highly skilled centers.

ETHICAL DILEMMAS

The developing science of prenatal diagnosis presents ethical dilemmas. In many countries it is unregulated. In some countries no counseling is offered. In others, telephone counseling is available. Some firms offer do-it-yourself tests for conditions such as cystic fibrosis—a disorder of the lungs and digestive system. Making decisions about whether or not to have screening, and if so, exactly what to screen for, is becoming increasingly complex. Would you want to know if a child you were bearing, or you yourself, or other members of your family, had an increased risk of having heart trouble in middle age, developing breast cancer at some stage, or getting Alzheimer's in old age? If you did, how great would the risk have to be for you to go through genetic tests? And how great would the risk be for you to decide on termination of a pregnancy? How accurate would tests have to be? Suppose there was nothing you could do to prevent an illness from developing or to treat it effectively if you or your child did get it; would you still want to know? Would you want to have this knowledge if future employment prospects and insurance depended on test results indicating that there was no additional risk?

"I DIDN'T WANT THESE TESTS, BUT I KNEW THAT EVERYONE WOULD BLAME ME IF I HAD AN IMPERFECT BABY THAT I COULD HAVE ABORTED."

The decision to terminate pregnancy is implicit in screening procedures that are now available, such as those for Down's syndrome and neural tube defects. You may feel absolutely sure about what you would want if it turned out that there was a high probability of the baby's having a disability. But now screening is available for conditions that do not produce serious handicaps, which are not life-threatening, and which may develop only in adolescence or later. How can you weigh the pros and cons of such tests? You may want to discuss these issues with your partner, a close friend, or your doctor or midwife, who can put you in touch with a genetic counselor.

The genetic counselor can help you establish your priorities. She will give you the facts and discuss your options. She will not advocate termination, although she will support you if that is what you want. She will not persuade you to go on with a pregnancy, but will support you if that is your choice. It is up to you. You cannot predict your reactions to a positive test result. Even if you are certain that you would not terminate a pregnancy, you may wish to know beforehand that a baby is not going to be perfect, so that you can plan ahead, or you may prefer not to have screening, and to wait and see.

THE LAST FEW WEEKS

Your baby is almost ready to be born. The firm body is
nestled in the cup of your pelvis, and the little arms and legs
are plumper as the last layers of fat form to help the baby's
temperature-control system function efficiently after birth.
Sometimes the baby gains as much as 8 oz (225 g)
in a week at this stage of pregnancy.

PHYSICAL SENSATIONS

You may feel fewer big body movements but an insistent kicking underneath
your ribs on one side or the other. If your abdominal wall is thin, you may
even be able to hold your baby's foot. There may be other strange movements,
perhaps a sudden urgent knocking that continues intermittently for half an
hour or more. This can be so pronounced that you worry that your baby is
having something like an epileptic seizure. But it is definitely not that. The
baby may have hiccups, perhaps from gulping amniotic fluid. Or he may have
lost his thumb, which he was contentedly sucking, and is "rooting" to find it
again, with quick, darting movements of the head from side to side, just as
after birth he will search for the nipple. The baby's head feels like a melon or
coconut pressing through your bulging perineal tissues.

There may also be odd sensations in your vagina, a sharp buzz like a
mild electric shock or a tickle. The baby may be lifting and lowering his
head against your pelvic floor, another movement he will make naturally
after birth too, if put down on his front in an alert state. At times your
baby is drowsy, at other times active—often in the evenings, and just when
you are trying to drift off to sleep.

You may be vulnerable to any suggestion that labor should be induced,
because you are fed up with being pregnant and want to have your baby in
your arms. Unless there are good medical reasons, avoid going down that
route. It will make the birth harder to handle, and you feel shattered afterward.

If you have indigestion, switch to small
meals and avoid eating late in the evening. Sleep
may be patchy. If you can, take daytime naps.
Arrange special treats: a little retail therapy (buy
something for you, not the baby), a day in the
country or by the sea, an aromatherapy massage,
seeing friends, a meal out, or a movie. (Pop a
sanitary pad in your bag in case your waters go.)

Toward the end of
pregnancy it is natural to
feel stage fright as the great
day arrives. Am I expecting
too much of myself? Can
I cope with the pain?

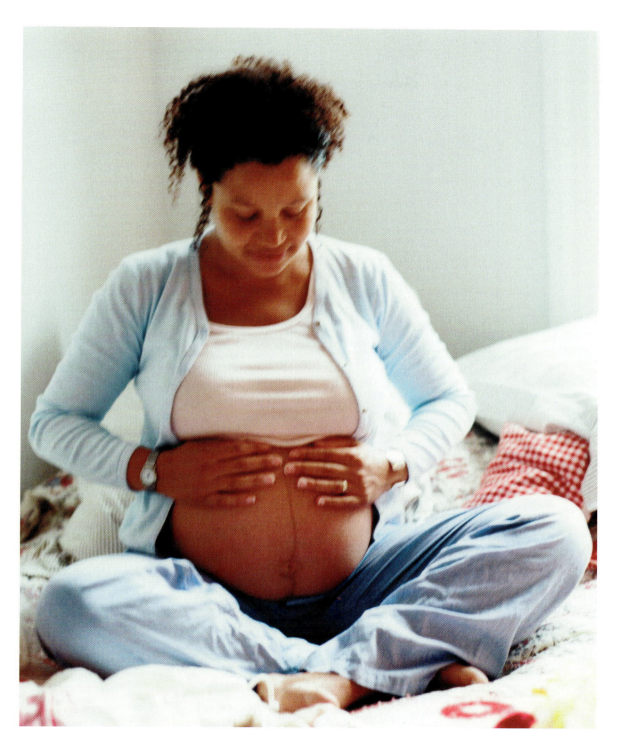

MIXED EMOTIONS

Conflicting emotions are characteristic of these last weeks. You may be tired of being pregnant, but on the other hand the state you are in now is a condition you know and understand, whereas in front of you there is an unknown challenge. So sometimes you want the baby out and long to get on with the labor. But at other times you feel safer as you are and anxious about the future. Some women say that as the birthday draws nearer they feel irritated with the pregnancy. This produces an emotional state that makes them welcome the start of labor. Other women relish these last weeks.

PRENATAL DEPRESSION

It is common to feel low some time in the last six weeks of pregnancy. If you have been practicing and preparing for a natural birth, you may experience a kind of stage fright and be convinced that you are going to forget everything when you are actually in labor. You may also be feeling physically tired and heavy with the weight of your burden.

Depression, though usually short-lived, may suggest a need for more rest. You may feel very different if you lie down to rest in a darkened room in the middle of the day, have some early nights, and adjust your activity to slower, gentler rhythms if possible. If you find yourself becoming depressed, have a talk with your childbirth educator, who, probably a mother herself, will understand what you are feeling.

THINKING AHEAD TO LABOR

You will probably be thinking a great deal about labor in the last few weeks, wondering what it will be like. One thing you can find out is the position your baby is in. Remember to ask when you are being examined. The ideal position for a straightforward labor (and the most common) is head down with the spine in front. Some babies present in different positions, as spine posterior or as breech, for example. The birth may not be so straightforward with the baby in these positions (see pages 270–285).

THE BABY WHO IS PRESENTING AS A POSTERIOR

If your baby is lying head down with its back against your spine, limbs toward your front, it may be either because it is still rather small or because you have such a roomy pelvis that it can still move freely. Women who think they are due but who really have another two weeks or so to go before delivery can have a baby who is still moving like this—sometimes posterior, sometimes anterior. Pre-labor and early-labor contractions usually work to turn the baby into an anterior position in a matter of hours. If your baby seems to have settled in a posterior position, you may find that you can coax it to change during one of its waking periods by very firm hand pressure. The posterior baby is usually lying with the ball of the head on your right side. You want to shift the baby's body around and over toward the left. Treat the baby as if it were a sleeping kitten that you are trying to scoop off the middle of a sofa and move over to the left side. Curve the side of your hand around the most solid section of its bulk and firmly, little by little, edge it over. Keep the fingers of your other hand over your navel. If you are successful the saucer-shaped dip there (the space between the arms and legs of a posterior baby) will become—at least temporarily—a hard, convex curve (the back of a baby in an anterior position). You will be able to detect the change as your navel will probably stick out. Talk to your baby as you move it. This is not simply a clinical exercise, but a bit of maternal persuasion.

Once the baby is stretching the uterus to its utmost, it is a tight fit and you will probably not be able to move it. Wait and see whether first-stage contractions will do it for you, and explore positions and movements that aid rotation while you are in labor.

HELPING A BREECH TO TURN You can try to tip the baby up out of your pelvis yourself by adopting a position with head down and bottom in the air for 15 minutes three times a day (before meals). Some babies turn a somersault once clear of the pelvis—even after 37 weeks.* A knee–chest position, leaning over a firm beanbag on your front with your head on the floor and your hips as high as possible, or lying in this position on a steeply sloping, cushion-padded ironing board propped between the bed and the wall or a solid piece of furniture, offers a range of options—none of them, it must be admitted, very comfortable in late pregnancy! But if you are able to turn the baby, it may make the difference between a vaginal and a Cesarean birth.

THE BABY WHO IS PRESENTING AS A BREECH

Most babies tip head down—in the vertex or cephalic presentation—between the seventh and the eighth month. If your baby is still presenting buttocks first (breech) after 36 weeks, ask if the doctor will try to turn the baby—a procedure known as external version. There is little point in doing it earlier, since the baby often turns back again.*

HOW EXTERNAL VERSION IS DONE You empty your bladder and lie on your back with your knees drawn up. The doctor will probably do an ultrasound scan to find out exactly how the baby is lying and listen to the heart before and after turning the baby. You may be asked to lie on a sloping examining table with your legs up and head down for about a quarter of an hour before the maneuver, so that the baby is encouraged to move clear of the pelvis. Spend this time relaxing deeply. Use abdominal

CHOOSING WHAT TO PACK

Now is the time to think about the comfort things you want available during and after birth. Select a small number of items that you think will be most useful, and gather them together in a lightweight, easily carried case. Choose from the following:

COMFORT AIDS FOR BIRTH	COMFORT AIDS FOR AFTER THE BIRTH
• Cotton pajama top, short nightgown, or baggy T-shirt. • Washcloth. • Two small sponges to be dipped in ice water and used for sponging your face, wetting your lips, and sucking between contractions. • Lip salve or Vaseline for dry lips. • Lavender and other essential oils. • Talc or massage oil. • CD player and CDs. • Swimwear so that your birth partner can come with you under the shower if you wish. • Camera and plenty of film, including fast film for nighttime if you do not want to use a flash/video camera. • Small water spray bottle for moistening your face. • Baby's hot-water bottle or a picnic thermal pack to be heated in water for use as a hot compress in the small of your back, for example, or between your legs. • Rolling pin with cloth tied over it to iron away backache. • Honey to keep your strength up in early labor. • Paper bag to breathe into in case you hyperventilate. • Beautiful object to use as a visual focus if you wish: a painting, photographs, or sculpture. • Nourishing snacks for your birth partner. • Notebook to serve as logbook. • Hairbrush and ribbons or bands if your hair is long; comb. • Books, magazines, playing cards, chess, Scrabble, crosswords. • Herb teas or glucose drinks. • Flexible straws.	• Calendula and hypericum cream from a homeopathic pharmacy, for a sore perineum. • Bottle of witch hazel lotion with which you can soak the sanitary pad next to any stitches. • Sanitary pads (greatest absorbency). • Cotton nightgowns or T-shirts and robe. • Nursing bras. • Toiletry bag, and makeup if you wish. • Earplugs. • List of phone numbers. • Telephone calling card/cellular phone. • Deodorant (you perspire heavily in the first few days after birth). • Baby clothes. • Clothes to wear going home. • Baby seat for the car.

massage to help release your tummy muscles, and use your breathing to help you as well. The uterus often contracts when the doctor's hands are pressing on it, and this makes it more difficult to turn the baby.

When you feel the doctor's hands on your tummy, release and flow toward the touch. Give a long, slow breath out and let your lower tummy bulge out in a great wave as you do so. If the version is successful and the baby turns, walk around for an hour or two so that there is the best chance of fixing the baby head down. Some babies turn back into the breech position. Seven times out of ten, external version at 37 to 39 weeks is successful.* But if the baby tips back again you will have to accept that it prefers this position; discuss with your doctor the sort of delivery you will have (see page 275).

A BIG BABY: SHOULD YOU BE INDUCED?

Unless you have uncontrolled diabetes and are expecting a big baby for that reason, there is no evidence that induction because the baby appears to be large is the best thing to do. Guesses about the baby's weight, even with ultrasound, are often wildly inaccurate. Induction carries few benefits and is likely to result in a more painful labor, more intervention of every kind, and, if it fails, a Cesarean section. A "wait and see" policy is best, perhaps with a plan to induce labor if you go 10 to 12 days overdue. Chances are that you will have started labor spontaneously by then.

BEING "OVERDUE"

If you go *past* the estimated date of delivery you may begin to worry. You are now consigned to the category of the woman who is "overdue," and you probably wonder if your body is going to work properly.

THE ESTIMATED DELIVERY DATE

The date you are given at the beginning of pregnancy for your baby's birth (EDD or EDC) is only an estimate. Studies show that only 5 percent of babies arrive on that day. If you look at the 95 babies out of 100 who do not put in an appearance on the "correct" date, you find that 3 out of 10 babies come before the EDD, and 7 out of 10 come *after* it. This is partly because women's menstrual cycles are of different lengths, and ovulation—and hence conception—occurs at different times within it. But when you reach the end of pregnancy you may not be able to prevent yourself from fixing on the expected

"IT WAS AN ULTIMATUM I WAS NOT GOING TO ACCEPT: TEN DAYS OVER AND YOU WILL BE INDUCED. I POINTED OUT THAT MY MENSTRUAL CYCLE WAS LONG AND I WOULD HAVE OVULATED FIVE DAYS LATER THAN THEY RECKONED."

delivery date as your goal. If it comes and goes and nothing happens, you are likely to become anxious. Each day seems like a week. Unless you plan activity and some fun during this time, your morale will drop to rock bottom. Remind yourself that, although a few babies are born on the day predicted for their birth, 9 out of 10 do appear within 10 days of the EDD. There is nothing abnormal about a baby who is 9 days "late." Many women, however, are made to feel "under sentence of induction" if they go as little as a week past their expected date. Some obstetricians induce labor when the woman goes even a few days beyond, and this is done without further investigation. If your pregnancy is normal and you are in good health, being 10 days "late" is a poor reason for induction.

Whether induction (see pages 334–339) is necessary depends entirely on your baby's well-being toward the end of pregnancy. That, in turn, depends on the condition of the placenta.

THE AGING PLACENTA

At the end of pregnancy the placenta looks like a piece of raw liver about the size of a dinner plate and the thickness of your little finger. Like every other human organ, it has a youth and an old age. An elderly placenta works less well. If labor does not start at the right time (which may be anywhere between two weeks before and two weeks after the estimated date of delivery—and very occasionally later still), the placenta may fail to support the baby in the uterus. The baby is then deprived of nourishment.

This is why there is concern if a pregnancy is prolonged much past the date worked out for the birth. Even so, a baby who is thought to be overdue may prove at birth not to be postmature at all. There are various ways in which the baby's condition can be assessed. Some are tests that doctors do to you; however, probably the most reliable method is one that you can do for yourself (see below).

ELECTRONIC FETAL MONITORING
AND ULTRASOUND

Ultrasound may be used to check the flow of blood through the umbilical blood vessels (Doppler flow studies) and the volume of amniotic fluid. Electronic fetal monitoring (called a nonstress test) can reveal whether the baby's heartbeat shows the usual variations when the baby is active and at rest. If the baby's heartbeat is normal, induction may be harmful. However, even if the results are normal, these tests cannot reliably predict how well the baby will be in 48 hours.

Another test that can be carried out is a biophysical profile (BPP). This is a specialized sonogram that evaluates the baby's condition by four to six different criteria, which are scored 2 for normal, 1 for less than normal, and 0 for not present. These criteria include, for example, fetal movement and fetal breathing (movement of the diaphragm). A total score, such as 8 out of a possible 8, 10, or 12, is given.

FETAL MOVEMENT RECORDING

One of the most accurate ways of knowing if a baby is doing well while still inside the uterus is something you can do for yourself. This is to note the baby's movements. In the last weeks of pregnancy, until it engages, the baby usually wriggles, dips and turns, bangs and kicks, and moves like a porpoise from side to side in great sweeps of activity that you can see through your clothing. Once it has engaged it often moves less because it is a rather tight fit inside the uterus. Even so, a vigorous baby moves even after it has gone down into the pelvis, though movements then tend to be just the knocks from knees and feet. You feel as if you have a rolling coconut in your groin or just behind your pubis (the head turning), and later the buzzing sensation of the engaged head bouncing against the pelvic floor muscles (see page 238).

You may not be aware of most of these movements while you are busy, but as soon as you sit down to rest, or lie down hoping to sleep, you cannot help noticing them. They are a good sign that your baby is healthy. Studies of fetal activity show that every baby has its own individual pattern of waking and sleeping inside the uterus, and by late pregnancy you have probably noticed what your baby's pattern is. Sometimes you may be wide awake and expect to feel a kick; and if nothing happens it can be disconcerting. The baby is probably fast asleep. If you have had alcohol or taken sleeping pills, your baby will be affected by them, too.

Mothers vary in the extent to which they observe fetal movements. Sometimes this is related to the amount of amniotic fluid, since fluid cushions movements. If you are preoccupied and concentrating hard on something, you may also be less aware of fetal activity. If you are still working outside the home, or busy inside it, there may be too much going on for you to notice fetal movements. Each woman's experience of movements is fairly consistent if her baby is thriving in the uterus, bearing in mind that the nature of movements changes after the baby has engaged. If it is thought that your baby may be "at risk" (usually because your tummy has not gotten bigger over time or because you are "overdue"), use your sensitive awareness of your baby's movements, created over nine months of pregnancy, to keep a check on its well-being.

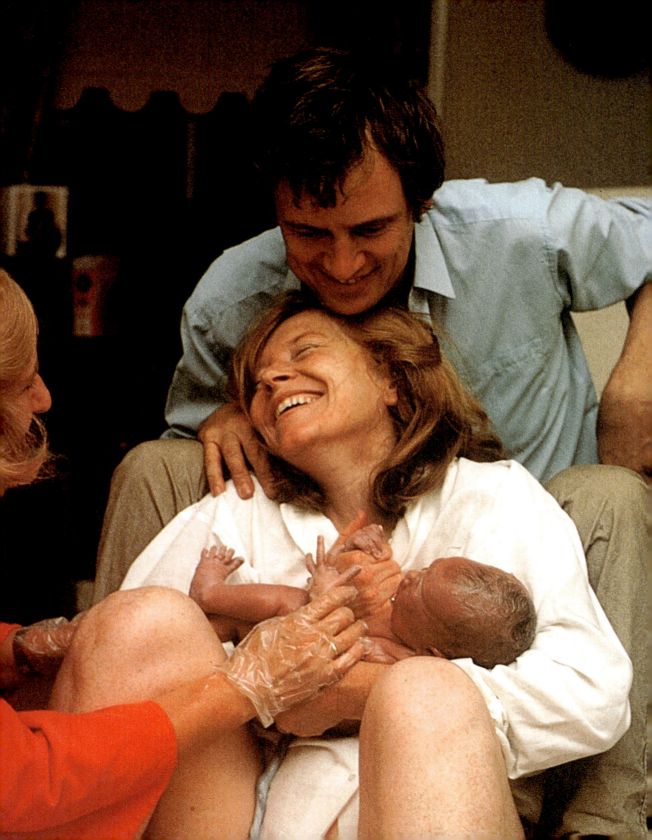

THE EXPERIENCE *of* BIRTH

248 | WHAT HAPPENS IN LABOR

270 | DIFFERENT KINDS OF LABOR

286 | GIVING SUPPORT IN LABOR

304 | DEALING WITH PAIN

324 | TOWARD THE MEDICAL CONTROL OF BIRTH

356 | GENTLE BIRTH

WHAT HAPPENS IN LABOR

Textbooks describe three distinct stages of labor, but many women do not think of birth in this way. For them, labor is an overwhelming and dramatic experience that does not fall into neat stages. To explore the feelings and physical sensations of birth, we need not only medical terms but also those that express the personal experience of birth.

Language shapes the way we think. It is never neutral. The language that is used by men about women's bodies—especially their genitals—is often degrading. In some languages, the only words available for parts of women's bodies express disgust. In Swedish, German, and Dutch, for example, a nipple is a "breast wart." In Polish and Swedish, the vaginal labia are called the "shame lips" and the pubic symphysis is the "shame bone." In Japanese, pubic hair is the "shame hair." Terminology like this must make it difficult for women to feel positive about their bodies, in particular the organs involved in childbirth, which are associated with a sense of shame and pollution.

Today, the language that is used about childbirth imposes a medical view of birth. This does not mean that you should not understand medical terminology, but it is important to find words for your own experience of pregnancy and birth, too, both the negative and positive aspects of it.

Women in the childbirth movement have been working to create a language of birth that is not medically dominated. They have invented or adapted words like "rushes" for uterine contractions and "visualization" for the mental pictures that help a woman to adjust to the sensations of birth. Some have analyzed the inappropriate and often sterile or destructive language that is employed by obstetricians, and sometimes nurses and midwives, too, to describe the birth process.

The medical model of birth incorporates an image of the pregnant woman as an ambulant pelvis. For a woman having her first baby, this pelvis is "untried." During labor she becomes a "contracting uterus," and the birth process is an equation among the "powers," the "pelvis," and the "passenger," for the baby is seen as an inert passenger moving through the skeletal structure. Metaphors of war and conflict are often employed. Obstetricians talk about "the aggressive management of ruptured membranes," "the oxytocin challenge test," "a trial of labor," and "the trigger factor for labor," and as the baby is about to be born, its head "hits the pelvic floor." Midwives sometimes urge a woman to push by telling her to "get angry with her body" or even to be "angry with the baby." A woman may be made to feel that she is being blamed for failing to function effectively: she is in "false labor." Her cervix is "incompetent," "sloppy," or "rigid." There is "failure to progress" because her uterus is "lazy" or the fundus is "boggy." Some terms, such as "elderly primigravida," and "abortion" when used to mean miscarriage, have all but disappeared from the medical vocabulary because they were so obviously offensive. But there are plenty still around.

In this chapter, as we explore the feelings of birth and the ways in which you can adapt to your physical sensations, I will use medical words when necessary but also richer language that expresses the full range of a woman's experience during childbirth.

THE STAGES OF LABOR

There are three stages of labor. During the first stage, the cervix is being drawn up into the main body of the uterus and dilating (opening). In the second, the baby is pressed down through the birth canal; this stage culminates in the birth. During the third, the placenta and membranes are sloughed off the lining of the uterus and expelled.

It is important to add, however, that for many women labor is an extraordinary emotional experience, and you are certainly not sitting around thinking in terms of stages. There is no fanfare of trumpets to tell you when the first stage is under way or when the second stage has started. Some women have a clear physiological message, such as the breaking of the waters and sudden strong, regular contractions, that leaves them in no doubt that labor has begun, and when they reach the end of the first stage they know with equal certainty that they are now in the second stage and have to push. For a great many women, however, the different stages of labor shade over into each other. The experience is rarely as tidy and compartmentalized as birth books seem to suggest, and the third stage may even pass completely unnoticed as you hold your newborn baby in your arms and marvel at the fact that you are finally able to see him.

THE BABY SIGNALS THAT IT IS
READY TO BE BORN

The *baby* initiates labor by sending endocrine signals to the placenta to produce enzymes that stimulate production of estrogen. These signals consist of catecholamines (see page 360). Simultaneously, the same hormonal signals help the baby's vital organs to mature. If labor is induced artificially, the timing may not be right either for the uterus to work most effectively or for the baby to be ready for life.

THE BUILDUP TO LABOR

Labor starts with the gradual softening and ripening of the cervix at the base of the uterus. This can take many days, or can happen overnight, especially if you have had a baby before. Once the cervix is soft and stretchy, contractions—which are occurring anyway in late pregnancy—draw it up bit by bit, so that it changes from a long canal hanging in your vagina to being a dip in the bottom of the uterus.

You are not considered to be in labor while all this is happening. Your labor has not started in medical terms until you are having regular contractions that are effectively dilating the cervix; it is work that has to be done before the cervix can open wide. Usually this means you are at least 3 cm dilated (see page 254) before you are considered to be in labor. Many women already have a partially dilated cervix by the time they begin to realize that they are having contractions.

It is obviously more pleasant for you if your body is working for you while you are shopping, eating, sleeping, and seeing friends. So carry on with normal living for as long as is comfortable.

THE FIRST SIGNS OF LABOR

Three things can indicate that labor has started or is about to start: you see a show, the waters break, or contractions begin.

A SHOW This is the bloodstained mucous discharge that appears when the cervix is beginning to stretch. Until the start of labor, this mucus has acted as a gelatinous plug in the cervix, sealing off the uterus. Its appearance is a good sign that there is some definite activity around the cervix. But it can come out two or three weeks before you actually go into labor and contractions are established, or it may appear when your labor is so far advanced that you may not notice it. So, although you can take it as an encouraging sign, do not rush off to the hospital. Go on with your everyday activities or, if it is night, have a hot milk drink and go back to sleep.

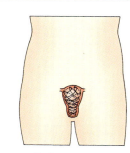

Early pregnancy

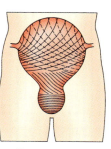

Late pregnancy

Muscle bundles

The uterus is composed of spiral muscle bundles that in early pregnancy start to unfold into an open-latticework formation at the top of the uterus. If you think of the uterus as a clock, the muscles are spaced out most between 9 and 3—that is, over the fundus of the uterus. By the end of the pregnancy, these bundles of muscle have unfolded much more and are stretched lengthwise.

THE BAG OF WATERS BREAKS When the membranes surrounding the baby have been pressed down like a wedge in front of its presenting part (usually the head) and pressure has built up, the bag pops. It may do this suddenly with a rush of water or, more likely, with a slow trickle of water. You may not be sure whether the bag of waters has burst or you are wetting your pants. If you are not sure, forget it (if you can) and carry on as usual, unless you are still several weeks away from your EDD, in which case you should call the doctor or midwife. If it is more than three weeks before your baby is due, it may be best to be in a place where special care is ready for the baby at delivery.

You will probably have been told to call the hospital or your doctor or midwife if the waters break and you lose a lot of water at once. This is because, if labor is slow (taking 24 hours or more from the rupture of the membranes), there is a chance of infection. If labor starts within 24 hours, however, there is no increase in risk of infection.*

The other concern is that if the baby's head does not fit neatly into the cervix, the waters might sweep the cord down through the cervix (prolapsed cord). This results in blockage of the oxygen supply to the baby. So if you know that your baby is breech before you go into labor, or that the head is still high, be ready to go to the hospital if the waters break. Although a prolapsed cord is rare, it is serious. Quick action, which could include a Cesarean, may be needed to save the baby's life.

Obstetricians may wish to stimulate the uterus once the membranes have ruptured. If your baby's head is well down, it is a good idea to give nature a chance. There is an 85 percent chance that contractions will start naturally within 24 hours. Many obstetricians will allow more than 24 hours if all is well with the baby and you let them know that you really wish to start labor naturally if possible. Involve yourself in some gentle activity or get a good night's sleep. Say "no, thank you" to vaginal examinations. They increase the risk of infection. Say "no, thank you" to any offer of induction before at least 24 hours have passed. Research shows that induction leads to longer labors, greater need for painkilling drugs, more operative vaginal deliveries, and more Cesarean sections.*

You do not have to worry about having to go through a "dry" labor, with the baby traveling down an unlubricated birth canal, because there is no such thing. Your amniotic fluid is completely reformed every three hours. Actually, a "wet" labor is more likely and can be uncomfortable, since continual leaking during labor is cold and unpleasant. Wear a sanitary pad and change it frequently. If you are in a bathtub or birth pool, you will not notice any leaking, so you will be much more comfortable.

> **"THE WATERS WENT WITH A WHOOSH—THAT WAS EXCITING. I WAS IN THE MIDDLE OF BAKING SOME BREAD AND THERE WERE LOADS OF OTHER THINGS I HAD PLANNED TO DO BEFORE LABOR STARTED, SO I GOT A MOVE ON!"**

USING GRAVITY TO HELP YOUR LABOR

If you stay more or less upright in labor and continue to
move around, the downward force of gravity will help
to push the baby out. Your contractions will be more
effective, too, and less painful than if you were lying down.

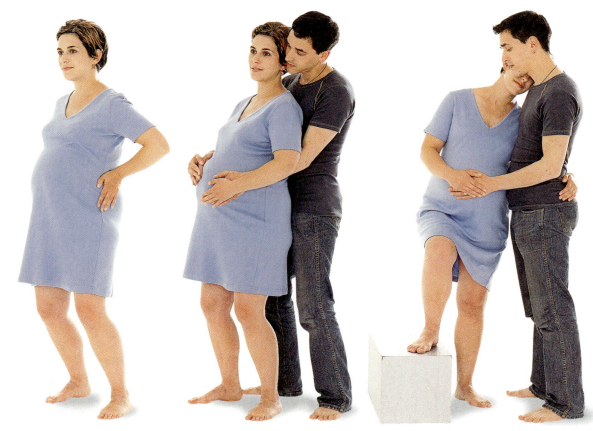

Rock your pelvis backward and
forward and make slow, circling
movements, imagining that you
are doing a dance.

Try a supported dance—in a
standing position, supported by
your partner from behind, move
together in a slow dance.

Move into a lunge, with as firm
support as possible from your
partner and one foot raised on
a chair, stool, or low table.

Or try bending forward leaning over a bed or windowsill, and rock your pelvis while your partner applies counterpressure to the small of your back.

A kneeling position, supported by a bed, a chair, or a pile of firm cushions, may become more comfortable than standing.

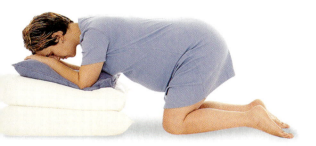

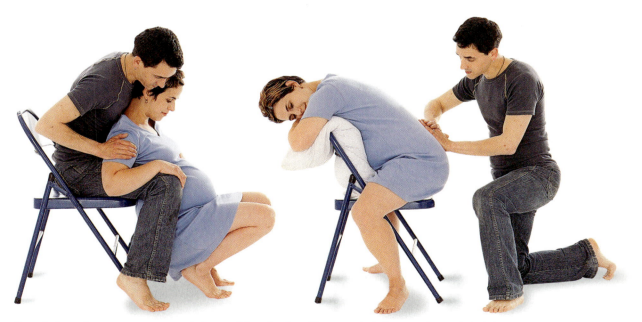

Crouch down between your partner's legs and lean back against him, using his knees for support. Now you can rock or rotate your pelvis with greater ease.

Sit on a chair leaning forward slightly over its back, with your partner behind you giving firm counterpressure with both hands placed on the small of your back.

CONTRACTIONS START Contractions generally feel like a tight elastic belt slung under your tummy and around into the small of your back, being drawn tighter, gripping for 15 to 20 seconds, and then being released. This sensation occurs again after 10 minutes or even sooner. They might be the Braxton Hicks "rehearsal" contractions that some women experience in the last three weeks or so of pregnancy. These tend to be called "false" labor. All this means is that you thought you were in labor, with good reason, but were not. These practice contractions are useful because they are softening your cervix, getting ready for it to open later on.

To be fairly sure about being in labor, time contractions over a period of 30 minutes or an hour. Note the interval between the start of one and the start of the next, and note the length of each. Contractions need to come closer and closer together and to last longer (40 seconds or more) before you can be confident that labor is established.

During contractions, muscle fibers of the uterus tighten, pressing in and down on the center and producing an upward pull on the cervix. When the baby's head is pressed down by a contraction, the muscles and fibrous tissues of the cervix are drawn apart. In a straightforward labor most of the physical sensations caused by contractions come from this area in and around the cervix, apart from a hardening and swelling felt at the top of the uterus.

Once contractions are going well, they have a regular rhythm and last longer and longer, while the interval between them is reduced. You may feel contractions as firm squeezes that make you want to gasp, like hot sunlight pouring through your pelvis, or rushing ocean waves.

THE FIRST STAGE

The hormonal changes that the baby has started now stimulate the beginning of a remarkable process. The uterus produces prostaglandins and, as a result, contractions that you have been having in late pregnancy become bigger and come closer together. So the contractions of early labor may feel

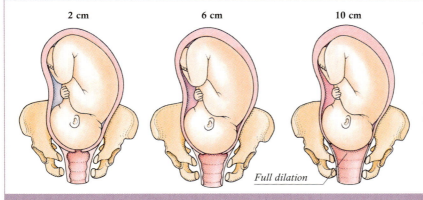

2 cm   6 cm   10 cm

Full dilation

Dilatation of the cervix
The cervix has to be 10 cm dilated (widened) before the uterus can press the baby out. The time taken to reach full dilatation varies enormously: some women are 3 cm dilated before they realize they are in labor, some take many hours to reach 5 cm.

similar to Braxton Hicks contractions, but are heftier and more regular. These more efficient contractions press the baby's presenting part down to the base of the lower segment of the uterus and against the cervix. This then becomes progressively stretched and thinned out as the muscle fibers are pulled up into the upper segment. This stretching of the cervix triggers the production of oxytocin from the posterior pituitary gland. This stimulates the uterus into a steady rhythm of contractions. Labor is now under way!

MOVING AROUND IN LABOR

Going to bed in the first stage of labor and becoming more or less immobile is not a good idea. It can slow down labor or interfere with its starting effectively because the presenting part may not be pressed down against your cervix. When you are upright and moving around, gravity helps you: everything is being pressed down.

It was not until the end of the 18th century in Europe that women began to lie down in order to give birth. Before that time, they walked around during much of labor, used birth stools to sit on, or sat up in bed or on a chair. Birth stools were designed like horseshoes with the open part at the front, and were low on the ground so that the woman squatted. As a result, she was in a physiologically excellent position for childbirth.

Mauriceau, the obstetrician to the French court, introduced the lying-down position, and it soon caught on because people sought to imitate the manners of the court. When forceps were first introduced, obstetricians found that they were easier to use on a woman who was lying flat. Still later, the lithotomy position (first devised for surgery on gallstones), in which the patient lies on her back with her legs fixed to raised stirrups, was introduced. This highly artificial posture is uncomfortable for the woman, pressing her uterus against the big blood vessels in the lower part of the body. This interferes with her circulation, causing hypotension (low blood pressure), and also with the production of urine. It can cause distress to the fetus, too.

Research on the effect of different positions in the first stage of labor* has shown that most women prefer to be up and around, not lying in bed, and that contractions are stronger and labor shorter with the woman in an upright position. The uterus is working nearly twice as efficiently to dilate the cervix. Keep walking around between contractions. Try pelvic rocking and circling as if you were belly dancing—through contractions, too, if it feels good. If dilatation is taking a long time, soak in a deep, warm bath or squat on a low stool under the shower.

WHEN TO GO TO THE HOSPITAL

Unless you feel strongly that you need to be in the hospital during this time, or your doctor or midwife has advised that there is a special reason that you should come in as soon as there are any signs of labor starting, it is best to stay at home and carry on as usual. This is partly because of the psychological effect of going to the hospital, being admitted and prepared, and getting into bed. If you have only just begun labor, all this can stop it entirely. There are many women who have rushed to the hospital with contractions that are still more than five minutes apart, and who have then gone out of labor and have either had to wait around with their morale dropping steadily or have had an intravenous oxytocin drip inserted in an arm vein to stimulate the uterus into action. Remember to eat and drink. Labor may last a long time, and both you and your birth companion are going to need strength.

Knowing that contractions will be coming once every two minutes and last about one minute or longer just before the baby is born may give you some perspective on your labor when it is just starting. Having contractions every five minutes can be tiring, and some women experience this for 12 hours or more, usually when the baby is in a slightly awkward position, facing the mother's front instead of her back (see page 271). But the baby cannot possibly be born when contractions are coming this far apart, so if you are happier at home, stay there. Keep a careful record of what is happening, time contractions now and again, and be ready to go to the hospital as soon as membranes rupture or contractions come more often than every five minutes. Bear in mind the distance from your home to the hospital and the difficulty of getting there.

If you are going in your own car, it is a good idea to do a trial run beforehand at rush hour to see how long it can take and to be sure that you know the way, even in deep snow, hail, or fog, and also any shortcuts. Your partner should drive steadily, but not fast, and should certainly not brake suddenly at corners or at lights. Decide early what you will need to make the journey comfortable and whether you would prefer to be in the front or back seat.

ADMISSION PROCEDURES

When you get to the hospital, a nurse will take you to a room where you will be "prepped" for labor. She will ask you questions about how labor started, if the waters have broken, and, if so, when, how often contractions are coming, and so on. She will do some things you are already familiar with, such as requesting a urine sample, checking your blood pressure, feeling the position of the baby through your abdominal wall, and listening to the fetal heart. She or a doctor will feel through your vagina and into your cervix to find out if you have started dilating. If you are already partially dilated, he or she may break the waters (see page 327). This is done routinely in many hospitals at 3–4 cm dilatation, and sometimes even before this phase has been reached. *If you want your membranes to remain intact until they rupture spontaneously, you can say so before your internal examination.*

Sometimes you may not be admitted. A hospital is not the right place to be if you are not in labor, and you may choose to go home if you feel you would be better off for the time being in familiar surroundings. You may need to come back in only a few hours, but that does not mean that the decision to go home was the wrong one.

It used to be hospital practice to shave a woman's perineum, and in some hospitals every perineum was required to be as bald as a hard-boiled egg. Even today some attendants like the hair surrounding the vagina to be clipped short. Women have spoken out strongly against the unnecessary, uncomfortable, and degrading practice of perineal shaving; research has also shown that it is entirely useless in preventing infection and, however carefully done, always results in some injury to the skin.

Some nurses still give an enema to empty the lower bowel, but there is really no point in doing this unless a woman is very constipated. In the hours before labor starts, most women tend to have loose movements, and the lower bowel is cleared naturally.

After you have been examined, you may be asked to don a hospital gown; it is usually done up at the back, but if you hope to have your baby at the breast immediately following birth you will find it easier to wear it with the opening at the front. Many women prefer their own clothes. Select something made of cotton rather than a synthetic fabric, since hospitals are often overheated. Whatever you wear should be short and loose so that you can move around freely. An external or internal fetal monitor may be attached to assess your baby's heart rate and response to contractions, as well as the strength of the uterine contractions. It is routine practice in many hospitals to do an "admission trace" of the fetal heart sounds for 20 or 30 minutes. Research shows that there is no value in this, so you can say that you do not want it.

In some hospitals your partner may be asked to wait outside while you are admitted, but most take it for granted that a couple will want to stay together. It can seem like a very long time to be separated, and if your partner has been helping you cope with contractions until now, it is good to go on having the same kind of support. It also gives the nurse or doctor a chance to talk to you both, which means that they are meeting you not as an isolated patient but in your relationship with someone who is important in your life. If you have chosen to have a doula, friend, or relative with you, they should also be able to stay. Labor is not a good time in which to have people coming and going. You will be able to relax, knowing that you are with someone who understands you and is giving continuous emotional support.

A doctor may come into the room at intervals to assess progress or to discuss your case. If you have any questions, take this opportunity to ask him or her. If you are planning a birth without drugs, want to walk around in labor, or have any other wishes, remind the doctor or midwife of these and ask if they have been or can be noted on your chart.

COUNTDOWN FOR BIRTH AT HOME

If you are having your baby at home, plan ahead. When you think you are in labor, start to prepare for the birth. Put a plastic sheet (a shower curtain also works well) on the bed or over the carpet. If the bed is not already at right angles to the wall, move it to this position. Put out things that the midwife has asked you to have ready on a small table or, better still, a cart, arranged on a clean towel, and cover them with another piece of cloth. Arrange the lighting so that the midwife can direct some light onto your perineum for the birth and so that other lights can be dimmed or turned out. Put the baby's clothes out and a change of clothes for yourself. Boiling water is used mostly for making coffee or tea.

Turn your mind to what you are going to eat and drink for the next three days and also what you want to offer visitors. You will have been wise to have stocked up your food cupboard and freezer well in advance.

Call the midwife to let her know that you may be needing her later, and pin all important phone numbers within easy reach by the telephone. The midwife will call to check how you are doing and encourage you to contact her whenever you wish.

TRANSITION

Toward the end of the first stage, when you are between 8 and 10 cm dilated, you are in transition. For most women, the very end of the first stage is both stormy and challenging. Contractions follow each other relentlessly, with hardly a pause between, and they tend to be arrhythmic, with sharp peaks and sometimes with more than one peak to each contraction. The buildup of energy with each may be so sudden and tumultuous that there is no time for slow breathing. You must adapt right away and may need to breathe more lightly and quickly if you are to soar over the top of the peaks with your breathing. The length of contractions may demand total concentration and determination, and you need strong emotional support and unfailing encouragement.

At the same time, other physiological signs may occur that can be unsettling, until you remember that they are indications of progress, and that if you are aware of three or more of them, you are likely to be 8 cm dilated and in transition. Feeling hot, then cold, then hot again, your cheeks flushed and your eyes shining bright, suggests that you are in transition. So does a fit of hiccups or belching, or you may feel nauseous and actually vomit. Perhaps your legs feel icy cold and begin to shake uncontrollably. The surest sign is feeling that you have a large grapefruit pressing against your anus or that you want to empty your bowels. You have a catch in your throat that stops your easy, rhythmic breathing, or you involuntarily hold your breath or start to grunt. You may suddenly feel that it is all too much hard work and that you would like to forget all about having a baby. Or you may become irritable with everyone and hypercritical of the help your partner is giving.

Not all women experience these physiological signs, but a sufficient proportion of them do to make it a good idea for your partner to memorize them, so that at the right moment he or she can say: "I think you are in transition." You may have forgotten that you are having a baby by this time and are simply concentrating on the work of handling each contraction as it comes. You are also likely to feel that you are not making any progress and have lost all sense of time. You may get an urge to push, but continue with your breathing, and do not hold your breath until you absolutely must.

"MY CERVIX WAS COMPLETELY DILATED, BUT I HAD NO STRONG URGE TO PUSH. THE MIDWIFE SAID, 'JUST TAKE THINGS EASY. THE BABY HAS PLENTY OF ROOM, SO DON'T PUSH UNNECESSARILY.'"

Pushing for a long time against an incompletely dilated cervix can make it puffy and swollen, so that the opening closes rather than opens wider. You may be asked not to push until you simply cannot avoid it. This is sensible, because you can then be certain that your body is ready for it. You will enjoy the experience of surrendering to the great sweeps of energy that come with the contractions that follow in a way you cannot if you are pushing simply because someone has told you to do so.

THE "PREMATURE PUSHING URGE"

Sometimes when a woman is about 7 cm dilated, the pressure of the baby's head stimulates stretch receptors in the pelvic floor muscles. Her breath is caught and she begins to grunt. She feels increased pressure against her rectum and, as this builds up, she cannot help pushing. If she is ordered not to push she gets confused, irritable, angry—sometimes even panic-stricken. She often starts to overbreathe and hyperventilate in an attempt to control the urge. If you have to push, you have to push! If this happens to you, get into a forward-leaning or all fours position to take some pressure off your rectum, push only when you must, and continue breathing.

Transition may be very brief—just a few contractions—or it may last over an hour. It is likely to last longer if the baby is in an occipito-posterior position (see page 270). The cervix has to dilate to 10 cm before the baby can be pressed down through the opening. At full dilatation (10 cm or the width of the palm of a large man's hand including the thumb joint), the cervix is open enough for the baby's head, its largest part, to ease through. The baby has spaces known as fontanels between its skull-bones, which can close up as the baby slides down the birth canal, thus shaping its head to make the journey much less arduous, even for a big baby. This is the reason that, especially in first labors, the baby's head is molded. This shaping gradually disappears in the first week or so after birth (see page 376).

THE SECOND STAGE

This is the most exciting stage. During the first stage, the cervix has thinned out and opened. At the end of the first stage, it is open to 10 cm, making the uterus and vagina one birth canal. Contractions ease the baby's head down farther, and there is often a lull before the active second stage.

THE "REST AND BE THANKFUL" PHASE

Women are sometimes wrongly told to start pushing as soon as the cervix is fully dilated. This does not shorten the second stage. With the first baby, the second stage may take one or two hours. With the second or subsequent baby, it may take only ten minutes. If a woman does not have an overwhelming urge to push, it is usually because the baby's head has not yet fully rotated into the best position for birth. If she starts straining to push the baby out, or is told that she ought to push, it may not be what her uterus wants to do. *Forceful bearing down pushes the head down too soon and results in deep transverse arrest.* That is, the baby gets stuck.* The woman has wasted all her energy in this harmful activity and may not be able to push energetically when the time is right. Sometimes she has lost the synchronization between her uterus and her actions and never gets the desire to start pushing again. Many forceps deliveries and vacuum extractions are performed for this reason.

Focus on the idea of *opening up* for the baby to come out. Wait to push until you cannot avoid doing so, or until the baby's head can be seen on your perineum. If you experience a pause at the onset of the second stage of labor, trust your body and enjoy this "rest and be thankful" phase.

PUSHING Then follows a wonderful time when you can push. The second stage is often described as if it were sheer, grinding hard work, but you will *want* to do it. You will probably have an overpowering urge to bear down and press the baby through the birth canal. This is passionate, intense, thrilling, and often completely irresistible, and for some women it is close to overwhelming sexual excitement. Pushing is not something you decide to do rationally, but a force that sweeps through your body and culminates in the birth of your baby. Let your body take over.

There are a few women who do not feel much urge to bear down. Sometimes women who have had other babies do not experience a strong pushing urge. The mother seems not to need to do much bearing down because the baby is going to be born very easily anyway.

There are three to five urges to bear down with each second-stage contraction, although sometimes we talk about these contractions as if they were all push. Frantic pushing results in desperate straining to press the baby just a little bit farther. This is not necessary, because surges of desire to bear down come with each contraction, and it is important to go naturally with each as it comes. Allow yourself to hold your breath, bear down, and open up with the surge, which usually lasts five or six seconds,

JOURNEY THROUGH THE PELVIS

About 80 percent of women have well-rounded pelvises that are good for childbirth. Problems may be encountered if your pelvis is narrow: an android pelvis, for instance, is shaped like a triangle at the brim, which is hard for the baby to negotiate. Even when the pelvic shape is not ideal, the uterus works to press the baby into a neat package that, given time, can often make the journey easily.

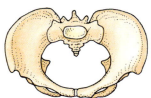

Usual female pelvis

Basically, the baby consists of two balls that move against each other. The ball with the larger diameter is the baby's head. The other ball is the baby's trunk with the limbs well tucked in. The action of a uterus that is contracting well molds the baby into the right shape for the journey down the birth canal.

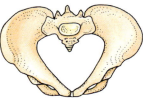

Android pelvis

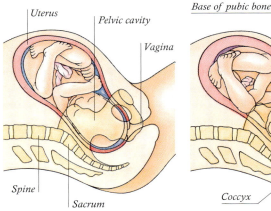

Uterus
Pelvic cavity
Vagina
Spine
Sacrum

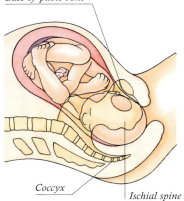

Base of pubic bone
Coccyx
Ischial spine

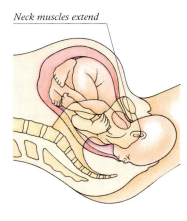

Neck muscles extend

The baby has to pass through *what is almost a right angle between the vagina and the uterus. Among several bones that may hold up its progress is the sacrum, which forms part of the pelvic brim. Once the head is below the brim, it is in the pelvic cavity.*

Having negotiated the brim, the *baby moves to the pelvic outlet. This is bordered by the pubic bone at the front, and the ischial spines, two projections on the side walls of the pelvis. The coccyx at the back slips out of the way as the head comes through.*

The pressure of good, powerful *contractions eases the baby's head down. As the head comes through the steep curve at the beginning of the vagina, the muscles at the back of the neck extend. This is why the baby is usually facing backward as it is born.*

no longer. Only you can know when these surges are there. Some people think it is a good idea for a woman to hold her breath for as long as she possibly can and only then is she really working hard. However, directed pushing, prolonged breath-holding, and sustained bearing down is not only exhausting for the mother but can also be dangerous for the baby, because it reduces the oxygen content of the blood.* So trust your spontaneous feelings and do what comes naturally.

YOUR BABY'S HEAD APPEARS

When the top of your baby's head can be seen for the first time, it looks like a wrinkled walnut in the vagina, not like a baby at all. Your partner will probably see this before you, and will be able to tell you the color of the baby's hair. Then there comes a time when the widest part of the baby's head is at the birth opening and does not go back in between contractions. You feel stretched to your utmost. At this moment of "crowning," it is important not to go on pushing, even though you feel very much like it. Otherwise the perineal tissue could tear. The doctor or midwife may perform an episiotomy if they think you are going to tear (see page 331). If you want to avoid having one, say so, and before the head crowns, start to *breathe* the baby out instead of pushing it out (see page 208). The midwife or doctor will check to see that the cord is free of the neck.

> "IT WAS JUST AS I WANTED IT TO BE. THEY LEFT ME TO DO WHAT MY BODY TOLD ME. I COULD FEEL HIS HEAD FILLING ME, AND THEN IT SLID OUT, SMOOTH AND SWEET."

The baby's head slips under your pubic bone and extends, the chin lifting off its chest. As the head emerges, damp and sticky with mucus, it is often violet or purple. This is nothing to worry about: the child has not yet taken that first great gasp of air that will oxygenate its blood.

The baby may be covered in vernix, a creamy substance that coats the baby's skin in the uterus and makes it look as if it has been spread with cottage cheese. The head has been molded by the journey down the birth canal, so it may be odd, pointed, or bumpy and asymmetrical, and the forehead may recede and the baby be almost chinless. The nose is often flattened, and there are little red marks between the eyes and on the eyelids.

The shoulders are still turned sideways inside you. Once the head is free, it turns to come in line with the shoulders. You may need another push for the shoulders. The doctor or midwife may press the baby's head down so that the shoulder nearer your front slides out first. Tell them if you would prefer them not to. A shoulder slides out next. At last the whole body slithers out and your baby is born!

There is often a great gush of water, and the baby may be already breathing and crying, limbs lashing, and face puckered up with what looks like rage. The lower end of the body seems very small in comparison with the head end, apart from the genitals, which often look extraordinarily large. All this is normal. If the baby is not yet breathing, attendants suck out the respiratory tract, hold the child's head downward, and may give oxygen. If you are propped or upright, you can reach your baby, provided that he or she is lying over your thigh, between your legs, or on your tummy, and you may want to take your baby in your arms.

THE THIRD STAGE

Although you may not feel the contractions, your uterus continues to contract after the birth of the baby. This makes the placenta separate from its lining, since the placenta cannot contract. As the uterus squeezes down into a firm, hard ball, the placental mass is automatically peeled off. The sinuses in which the placental blood vessels were rooted are closed by the tight squeezing of the uterus, and these contractions also prevent excessive bleeding from the uterine wall.

When the placenta has detached itself, the midwife or doctor may pull on the cord (see page 333). Take a breath, hold it, and bear down at the same time to help this process. You can ask that instead of having cord traction, you can push and do it by yourself.

There is a squelchy, slippery feeling as the placenta slides out. It is then carefully examined to make sure that every part is there. Pieces of placenta left inside the uterus could cause unnecessary bleeding, pain, and infection in the postpartum period. Although the placenta looks like a large piece of raw liver, it was the tree of life for your baby. It has a rough side, which was against the wall of the uterus, a smooth side, which lay toward the baby like a soft, velvety cushion, and a network of blood vessels that provided your baby with its life-support system.

If you need suturing (the technical term for stitching) it is done under local anesthetic and may take a long time, sometimes as long as an hour, since the underlying layers of muscle must be correctly aligned. You should be able to keep your baby in your arms or near enough to touch.

The midwife will help you to put on an ice pack, to reduce perineal swelling, and a sanitary pad, since there will be some bleeding now and for several days. The length of time during which there is a bloodstained vaginal discharge (lochia) varies greatly among women. Some new mothers bleed for just a few days, others for as long as five or six weeks.

BEING TOGETHER

In many hospitals staff tidy up at this point. They dry your baby's skin, give you a wash, change your gown, shorten the cord, and reclamp it. But practice is changing fast, and many midwives now give the parents a quiet time with their baby immediately following the birth, only doing the basic essentials and leaving the couple alone for an hour or so to start to get to know their baby. Being together should always come first.

A HOME BIRTH

Pauline chose a home birth for a number of reasons. In conversations with friends who had recently become parents, she found that several of the fathers had not felt fully included in their babies' hospital births. Her partner, Clifton, was eager to take an active part in their baby's birth, and she wanted to be sure that he would be able to do so.

Pauline knew that she would feel more confident and relaxed in familiar surroundings and would be able to move around as much as she wished. Just as important, she felt that it would be best for her baby to be born into a calm home environment, which she herself controlled.

Pauline is 7 cm dilated by the time she calls her midwife, Nicky. Over the months of her pregnancy, she has come to regard Nicky as a friend as well as her midwife.

Clifton lies beside Pauline on the bed, giving her encouragement and loving support. When she kneels by the bed, Nicky holds a heating pad on her lower back to relieve her backache.

Nicky tells her, "Make as much sound as you want but keep the tones low." Pauline says this really helped. "I felt in control all the time. I felt safe, and I had my own space."

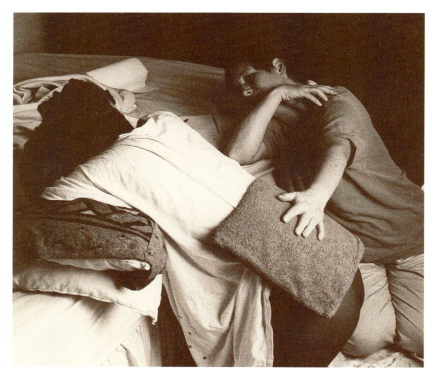

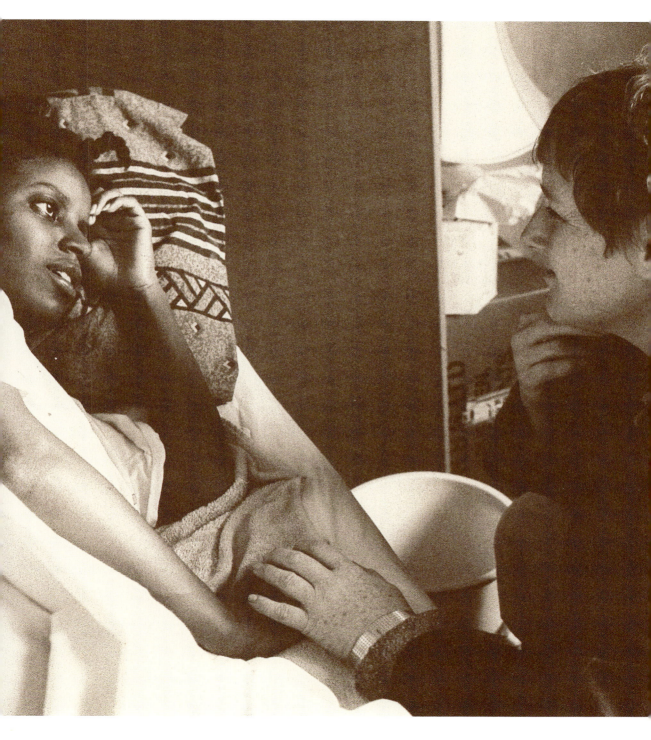

Pauline moves around, keeping her pelvis and knees loose, sometimes on the bed, sometimes off it, whenever she feels she wants to. She tells Clifton exactly where she needs to be massaged, or when she simply needs to have firm pressure from his hand.

Contractions come closer and closer together and get stronger and longer until there is a new one every two minutes that lasts about a minute. After each there is a brief lull, during which she relaxes completely, before the next huge contraction wave sweeps through her.

Suddenly it feels as if she is caught in crosscurrents as the contractions follow each other with hardly a pause between them. Her breath is caught involuntarily. She cannot possibly go on breathing steadily. As she holds her breath, she has an irresistible desire to push. She is in the second stage!

The baby is born still inside the bag of waters. Nicky says, "Pauline was brilliant! Completely focused on the task at hand." She tells her, "It's coming now. It's lovely—well done!" and then she prepares her for not pushing with the next contraction to enable the baby to be born gently.

Then in the space of one contraction, the baby's head advances, inside the membranes; the head slides out facing the mother's back and rotates to align with the shoulders, which are still inside. Next a shoulder and arm slip out, and are followed by the other shoulder; then finally the whole body emerges.

A glistening, transparent veil of membrane envelops the baby. Supporting the baby's back, the midwife takes the membrane off the baby's head so that she can take her first breath. Nicky rests the baby between Pauline's legs, and Pauline exclaims, "Oh, it's a girl!"

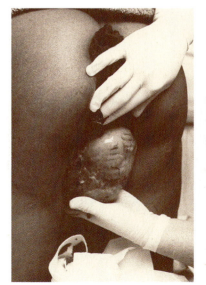 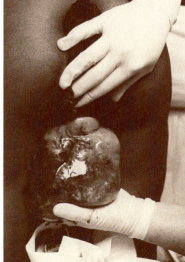 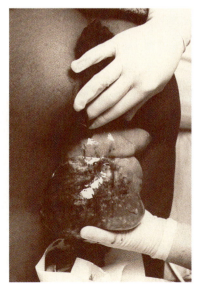

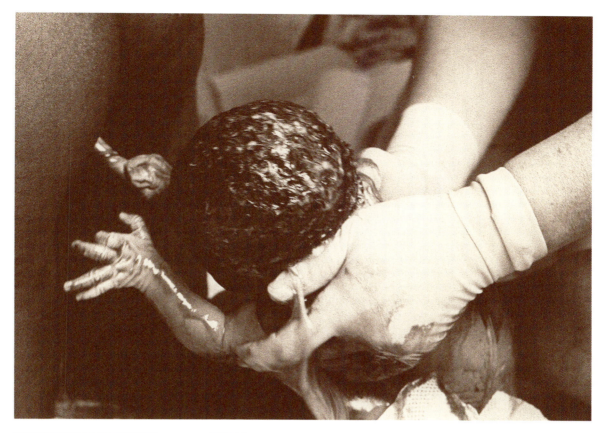

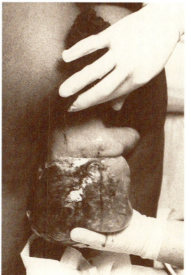
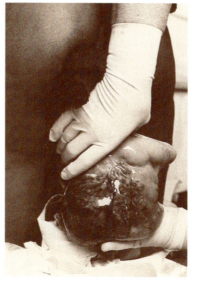
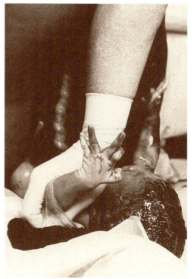

The baby cries and is a perfect color. Pauline picks up her daughter and cradles her in her arms, the cord still uncut. After all her striving to bring this child to birth she is radiant.

Everyone is laughing and admiring this beautiful new baby. Pauline is still bleeding quite heavily, so Nicky gives her a quick injection of syntocinon in order to stimulate the uterus to contract. Then she clamps and severs the cord.

When the baby's searching mouth indicates that she is ready to suck, her mother offers her the breast, and after nuzzling and licking as she explores this new sensation, she latches on. The parents share together the miracle of birth in an atmosphere of timelessness and peace. These are moments that they will never forget.

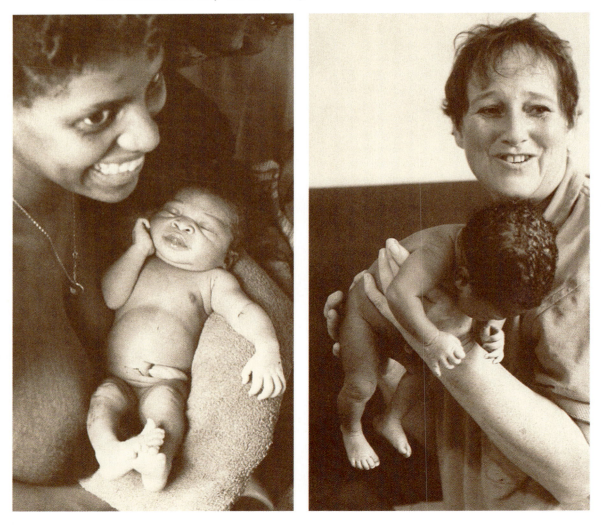

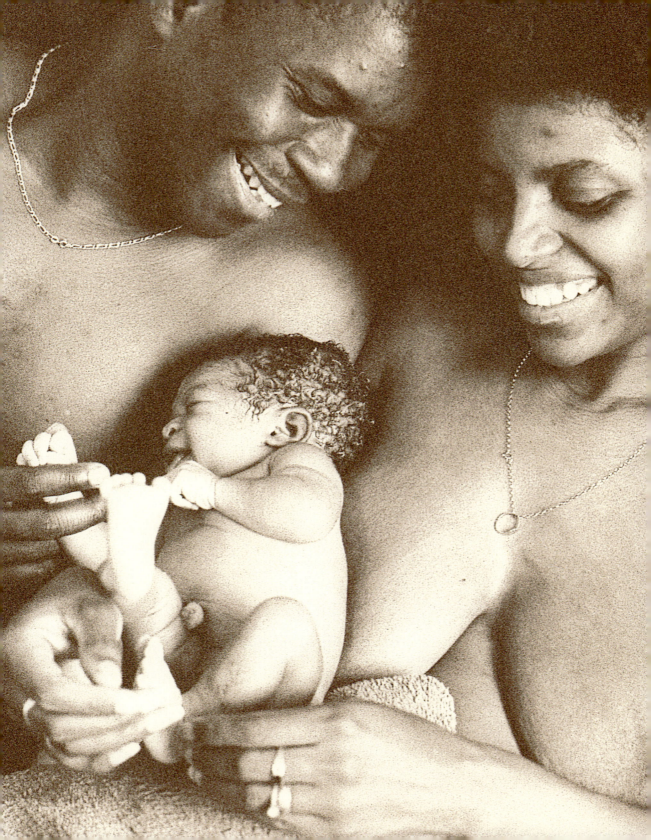

DIFFERENT KINDS OF LABOR

However much other people may advise you not to have any preconceptions about your labor and just to be ready for whatever comes, it is difficult not to have some, because it is almost impossible to prepare yourself to cope with a situation that you have not imagined in advance.

So it is useful to think ahead to the major variations on the theme of childbirth that you might confront. However, it is still vital to keep in the forefront of your mind the normal, rhythmic, and harmonious pattern of a straightforward labor. Otherwise all the medical technicalities may seem quite bewildering, and you may interpret each uncomfortable physical sign as an indication that something has gone wrong. This section looks at some different types of labor, all of which can throw you unless you understand what is happening.

LABOR WITH A POSTERIOR BABY

When the back of the baby's head presses against your sacrum, the baby is in an occipito-posterior position. Most women have some backaches in labor, but women with posterior babies may have them all the time, so that the labor can be described as a "back labor." Few women with posterior babies do not have backaches, which can be the most tiring and stressful thing about a labor—especially if, as is often the case when the baby is posterior, it continues *between* contractions as well as during them.

Another characteristic of labor with a posterior baby is that it starts very slowly, often over a period of several days, and contractions are felt as one big one followed by a feeble one. Plan for morale-boosting activity during a long first stage. Do not go into the hospital too soon. A walk in the park or the country is better. Eat and keep up your strength in early labor and drink plenty of fluids, remembering to empty your bladder regularly. Your partner also needs stamina to keep you going by giving you total attention during difficult contractions.

If the baby is posterior, there are some good reasons that the membranes should not be ruptured artificially. It is much easier for the baby to rotate if it is still floating free. When membranes are ruptured, the baby often drops down into the pelvis in a posterior position and is fixed rather like a cork stuck in a bottle.

PRESENTATIONS FOR BIRTH

When the baby is lying head down and curled into a neat ball (occipito anterior), the uterus can usually work well to open the cervix and press the baby down into the birth canal to be born. There are other positions that the baby may adopt, and these can sometimes lead to problems during labor and giving birth.

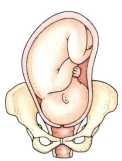

Right occipito anterior

This position is a common presentation for labor.

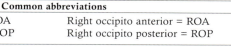

Common abbreviations	
Left occipito anterior = LOA	Right occipito anterior = ROA
Left occipito posterior = LOP	Right occipito posterior = ROP

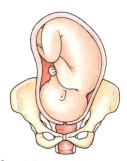

Left occipito anterior

The most usual presentation is with the baby facing to the left.

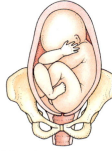

Full breech presentation

With this position the baby is able to flex during labor.

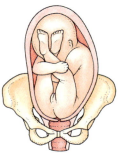

Frank breech presentation

This type of presentation makes flexion difficult.

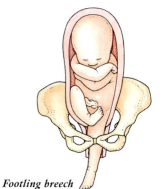

Footling breech

In this type of presentation the baby's foot is born before the rest of the body.

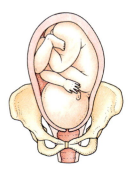

Left occipito posterior

This position can cause backaches in labor.

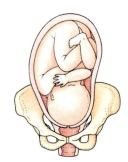

Right occipito posterior

More common than LOP, this also causes backaches in labor.

The baby will probably rotate at the very end of the first stage or at the onset of the second, and it is plain sailing from then on. About 5 percent of posteriors do not rotate, and the hard work has to be continued in the second stage; you may need obstetric help (see pages 346–355) to deliver the baby. But chances are that the baby will swivel around by itself and then complete the journey down your birth canal with ease.

WAYS OF DEALING WITH A BACK LABOR

You may find that some of the things described on the following pages are helpful in the first stage of a back labor.

HEAT A hot-water bottle wrapped in a towel, or a hot compress (a washcloth or small towel wrung out in really hot water), applied to where you feel most pain may bring relief. A hot shower with the water pulsing on your back also helps.

COLD Use a packet of frozen peas or corn from the freezer wrapped in a cloth, or crushed ice in a knotted plastic bag, to numb pain and relieve muscle spasms.

CHANGES OF POSITION Keep upright and moving around. In this way you tip the baby down to press through the pelvis and birth canal instead of into the small of your back. Crouching, leaning forward, leaning forward with one foot placed on a chair beside you, kneeling, squatting, getting onto all fours, and lying on your side with your back well rounded, your head and shoulders curved forward, and a pillow between your legs may all be positions in which pain is eased. They may encourage rotation of the baby's head. Research has shown that an all-fours position helps babies to rotate from posterior to anterior. It can be combined with pelvic rocking. Seventy-five percent of posterior babies turn when women adopt a hands-and-knees position. But babies do not turn when women sit upright.*

MOVEMENT If you want to get a tight ring off your finger, you do not just pull it. You wiggle it. In the same way, you can help your baby's head rotate by rocking your pelvis forward and backward, from side to side, by circling it, doing these movements with one foot up on a stool or chair, going up and down stairs, rocking from foot to foot, walking slowly with big strides, and doing a birth dance. Spontaneous movements that feel right not only relieve pain but also help the baby's head rotate.

PRESSURE Ask your partner to provide firm pressure, either right over the place where your pelvis joins your spine, or to the left or right of this if pain is more to the side. He should use the heel of one hand, with the other resting over it, and press his body weight down through his arm. Or you may prefer the feel of knuckles.

RELIEVING A BACK LABOR

One of the greatest threats to morale in childbirth is having constant backaches. Practice the techniques below with your partner. They will help you to take the edge off back pain in labor and find the energy to cope with it.

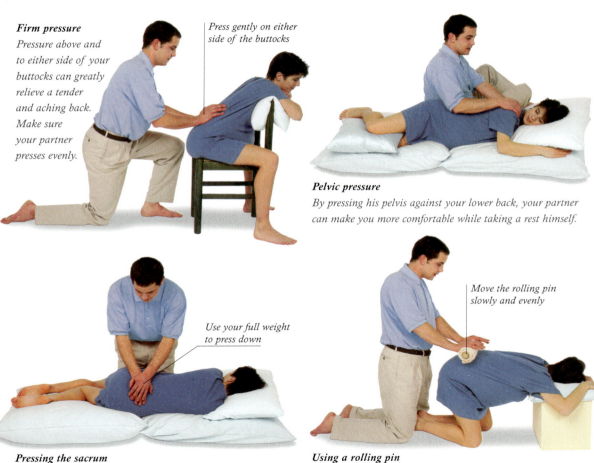

Firm pressure
Pressure above and to either side of your buttocks can greatly relieve a tender and aching back. Make sure your partner presses evenly.

Press gently on either side of the buttocks

Pelvic pressure
By pressing his pelvis against your lower back, your partner can make you more comfortable while taking a rest himself.

Use your full weight to press down

Pressing the sacrum
Your partner can apply firm pressure to your sacrum by leaning over and allowing his full weight to pass down through his arms.

Move the rolling pin slowly and evenly

Using a rolling pin
Your partner can also roll a rolling pin wrapped in a warm towel slowly and evenly over your lower back.

Stimulus on pressure points may help you handle the pain more effectively. One place where deep pressure of a thumb or finger may feel good is on your bottom, level with the top of the slit between your buttocks and a little more than a palm's width out toward the leg on each side. Experiment to find the spot: it feels tender, but pressure on it is satisfying. If you are in a position in which you are tilted forward, your partner can apply pressure to the spot on both of your buttocks at once.

If you are on your side, your partner will be able to reach only one pressure point, but even this may help.

PRESSURE POINTS Your partner can exert pressure on parts of the body far away from where you are feeling pain, but where a strong stimulus can offer almost miraculous relief. Known as *shiatsu* or acupressure, this can be particularly effective in childbirth when used on the feet. One pressure point is just below the center of the ball of the foot. Another is between the fleshy pads under the big toe and next toe. Your partner holds one foot firmly, exerting very strong pressure with a finger or thumb on the chosen spot, providing light counterpressure with the rest of the hand over the top of the foot.

> "IT WAS EXTRAORDINARY HOW PRESSURE ON THE BALLS OF MY FEET RELIEVED PAIN DURING LABOR. THE PAIN RECEDED INTO THE DISTANCE, AND INSTEAD I FELT EXHILARATED AND IN AN ODD WAY COULD ENJOY THE CONTRACTION."

There are acupressure points on the buttocks, too. Kneel forward over the seat of a chair or lie three-quarters over on your side so that your partner can "map" places on your buttocks where it feels good to have strong, steady pressure. Your partner may try pressing just under the curve of the buttocks, and beneath the bony pelvis at either side of the buttocks. Another place where pressure can be effective is on the inside wrist, between the tendons. Care should be taken to press only with the fleshy pad of a finger or thumb—not with the

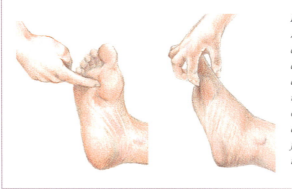

Footwork

Applying pressure to certain parts of the feet can relieve pain from contractions. One spot is just below the center of the ball of the foot; another is between the fleshy pads under the big toe and the next one.

nails. It is surprising how strong the pressure from finger and thumb can be on the right spot, and in all these places continuous pressure will produce a tingling, buzzing sensation. Acupressure for up to 10 seconds at a time followed by a pause, and then repeated in a steady rhythm, can provide effective pain relief during powerful contractions, whether they are felt in your front or back, and wherever the pain is centered.

MASSAGE Massage may feel better than pressure, or feel good alternated with pressure. The massage that suits most women best is firm, slow, and steady, moving the flesh and muscle on the bone. You can use powder, cornstarch, or massage oil to avoid skin irritation, and your partner should have some hand cream if massage is to be applied for a long time.

Another effective way of giving massage is to use a rolling pin. Knot a washcloth or hot compress around it to get more grip. Your partner can sit on the bed with his pelvis against your lower spine and lean back against you, too. This provides welcome rest for someone who after several hours of working to relieve a backache may develop back pain himself!

IMMERSION IN WATER A birth pool or deep bathtub is enormously helpful in back labor and may take away pain entirely. You don't have to lie back in the water. Try a hands-and-knees or floating squat position instead. Not only is warm water comforting and relaxing, but it enables you to move smoothly and easily. If you leave your head loose, you can change position frequently without any strain, one movement flowing into another in a slow, luxurious water dance.

LABOR WITH A BREECH BABY

A Cesarean may be safer for a breech baby than labor.* If your baby is presenting as breech in the last weeks of pregnancy, evidence suggests that it should be turned, manually rolling it around by external version (see page 241) until it is head down.* But some babies can't be turned, and some flip back.

Labor with a breech baby may start with the waters leaking. This is because the baby's bottom does not fit the opening cervix as well as the oval of the crown of the head, so part of the bag of waters becomes wedged between the baby's bottom and your cervix. Call the doctor if this happens and the baby is not yet engaged. The risk is that the cord might slide down and be caught between the baby and the cervix, so that the oxygen supply to the baby is cut off.

If the waters do not break, keep walking around through the first stage, until they break spontaneously. If a breech baby is left in its bag of waters, there is less chance of pressure on the cord.

After the waters are gone, the best positions are on all fours or your side. You may have a backache and, if so, your partner could exert pressure with the knuckles in the small of your back.

BIRTH DANCE IN WATER

It is easy to move in water and you will probably do so
quite spontaneously. But it helps to explore in advance
different movements for birth, with the people who
will be helping you at the time.

KNEELING SLIDE

Kneel forward, *grasping the rim of
the pool with your arms extended.
Slide to and fro, lifting your head
and bending your arms as you pull
forward and extending your arms
as you slide backward.*

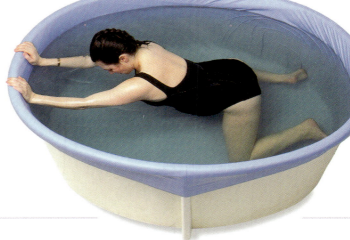

SQUATTING AND FORWARD SLIDE

Squat in the water *with your arms and shoulders supported by
the rim of the pool, feet well apart so that your pelvis is at its
widest. Slide down with your legs extended, and back up to a
squatting position again.*

At the height of a contraction it may feel good to drop your head into the water and blow out.

Lift your head as you pull forward and slide back with your arms extended.

SQUATTING AND BACKWARD SLIDE

Squat in the center of the pool, knees wide apart, arms extended and holding the rim of the pool. Drop your body forward and extend your legs behind you. Grasp your partner at waist level, while he supports your upper arms.

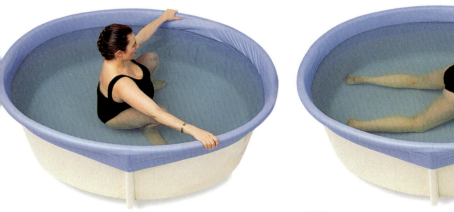

FORWARD AND BACKWARD SLIDE ON FRONT

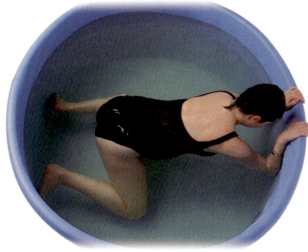

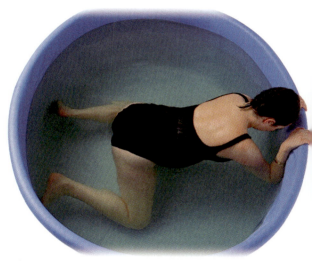

Kneel in the water *with your arms supported by the rim of the pool. Keep your knees well apart so that your pelvis is at its widest.*

Then slide down *in the water with your legs extended. Push with your feet against the side of the pool to get back up to a kneeling position again.*

SUPPORTED KNEEL

Kneel leaning forward, *knees wide apart, with the rim of the pool under your arms. In this position the cervix is tilted forward, which is helpful during the second stage of labor.*

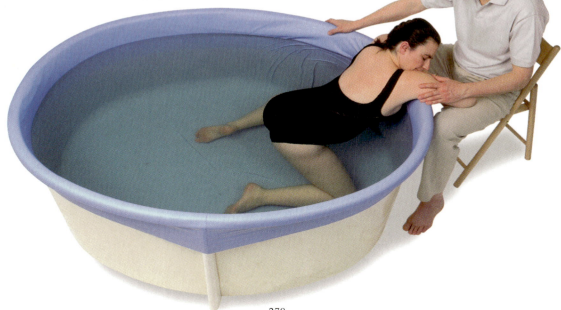

FORWARD AND BACKWARD SLIDE ON BACK

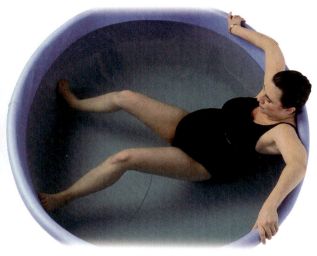 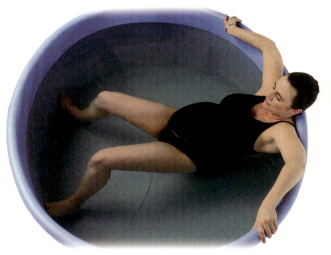

With arms spread wide and supported by the pool rim, sit with your legs across the width of the pool so that your feet are resting on the opposite side.

Slide forward and backward, using your feet against the side of the pool to propel you. Padding behind your neck may make you more comfortable.

HEAD-CRADLED FLOAT

Lie back in the water with your head cradled in your partner's hands. He should use a light touch, so that you can still move your head quite freely as and when you wish.

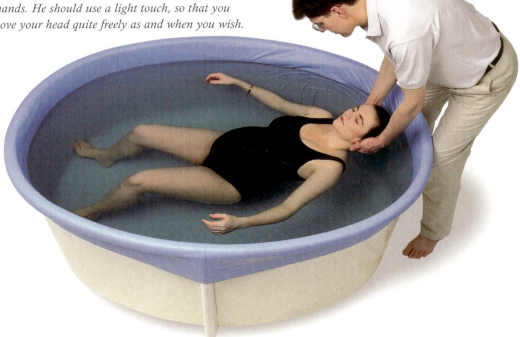

THE SECOND STAGE OF A BREECH LABOR

You may be moved to the operating room before the second stage starts, in case you need an emergency Cesarean section. If you want your partner to stay with you, make this clear.

Many doctors prefer to deliver breech babies with the woman in the lithotomy position (see page 255), since they have most control over the birth this way. But you will probably be more comfortable squatting, on all fours, dangling, standing, or standing and bending your knees during contractions.

Let the second stage proceed with no voluntary exertion until the body is born and the head about to slip out, so that the body is born on contraction waves only. (It may be easiest to do this if you are on all fours.) Concentrate on total release: breathe, rather than push, the baby out. If it has both feet up by its head, the doctor or midwife may slip a gloved hand in to draw down a leg and turn the baby into a "footling" (see page 271). Relax and breathe as this is done. Once a foot is down, the baby can take the curve of the birth canal more smoothly, since its legs are no longer splinting its spine.

If you are not having an epidural (see page 319), local anesthetic is injected into your perineum if an episiotomy is to be done (see pages 331–333), before the baby's head is delivered. It takes one or two minutes to be effective. Most obstetricians do a large episiotomy with a breech so that the head can be delivered unimpeded. But if you give birth with breathing

STANDARD BREECH BIRTH

Breech babies can be born vaginally as long as the pelvic outlet
is wide enough for the head to pass through.

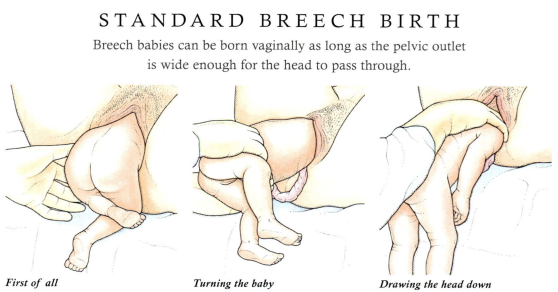

First of all
The buttocks are usually delivered first, and are followed by the baby's legs.

Turning the baby
The baby turns so that the shoulders can emerge as easily as possible.

Drawing the head down
The baby's weight draws the head down and its legs are lifted to deliver the head.

BREECH BIRTH IN THE SQUATTING POSITION

If you stay more or less upright in early labor and continue to move around, the downward force of gravity will help to push the baby out. You can kneel on all fours, dangle, stand and bend your knees, or squat supported by a helper—whatever feels most comfortable. Your contractions will be more effective, too, and less painful than if you were lying down.

Backaches are common during a breech labor, and massage is particularly effective. Ask your partner to apply pressure above and to either side of your buttocks. This can greatly relieve the pain of a tender and aching back.

In the second stage, a supported squat is a good position for delivery. You do not need to push until the body has emerged, and the head is ready to slip out.

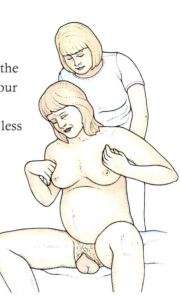

The mother is supported by her helper standing behind her. The baby's buttocks emerge first.

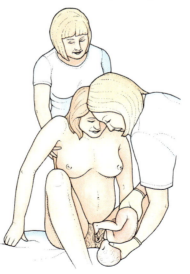

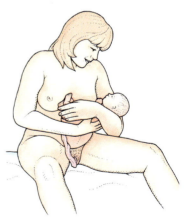

After the baby's buttocks, the rest of the body and legs are born and are caught gently by the midwife as they emerge.

The baby simply uncurls and drops into the midwife's hands. The baby's body is supported as the head is born.

The mother can then sit back and take her baby into her arms in the moments after birth and see him face-to-face.

instead of pushing, your tissues may fan out well and an episiotomy may not be necessary. Since there is unlikely to be an opportunity for discussion at the end, when things will be happening fast, talk about this earlier on in your labor (between contractions).

The head is delivered using hands or forceps to cradle it. You will be asked to push for the head and will probably need to bear down only once.

Sometimes women help to deliver their breech babies by leaning forward and lifting the baby's legs up, while the midwife controls delivery of the head and supports a shoulder. I first saw this done by mistake when a helpful midwife told a first-time mother to put her hands down and touch her baby while its head was still inside her. The mother was so excited that she held the baby's legs, lifted them, and as she did so the head slipped out.

Epidural anesthesia (see page 319) is often used for breech deliveries and has largely replaced general anesthesia. It means that you only feel a pulling sensation, are awake and aware, and can hold your baby as soon as it is breathing well. An increased number of obstetricians routinely do Cesarean sections (see page 348) for all breeches. Discuss this with your obstetrician.

When thinking ahead to the kind of birth you will have for your breech baby, it is important to remember that the pelvis is not a rigid, confined space. During pregnancy, joints relax, bones move more freely on each other, and the pelvis actually expands to make more room for the baby. Moreover, both the width and the size of the opening from front to back are increased in 28 percent of women when they switch from lying down to a squatting position.*

In Dr. Michel Odent's practice, most women with breech babies have vaginal births. He likes the woman to be upright: "Our only intervention will be to insist on the supported squatting position for delivery, since it is the most mechanically efficient. It . . . is the best way to minimize the delay between the delivery of the baby's umbilicus and the baby's head. . . . We would never risk a breech delivery with the mother in a dorsal or semi-seated position."* If the first stage goes well without any intervention, a woman has every chance of a vaginal birth. But if first-stage contractions are inefficient yet painful, and dilatation does not progress, a Cesarean section is decided on.

SHORT, SHARP LABOR

It is wrong to assume, as some textbooks do, that a short labor is bad for the baby. In many apparently short labors, the cervix is dilating gently (see page 254) over a period of days before the woman realizes she is in labor. Some short labors can be delightful. But however easy it might be physically, a violent precipitate labor is emotionally demanding and may leave you feeling drained and shocked.

If, from start to finish, your labor lasts less than an hour or two, you need a great deal of active help from your partner, as well as his emotional support. It is like starting at the very end of the first stage. Your partner needs to concentrate with you, and it may help to maintain eye contact and breathe with you. A partner who becomes anxious or excited may hyperventilate if everything is happening quickly. So remind each other to keep the breathing butterfly-light over contraction peaks.

When you feel the baby pressing like a grapefruit against your anus, it may be easiest to avoid pushing if you turn on your side with your knees drawn up, or onto all fours. Whatever position you choose, push only when you have to and for as short a time as you can. Open your mouth, drop your jaw, and relax your lips. Continue breathing in and out through a relaxed mouth, and concentrate on releasing all the tissues around your vagina as they fan out and open wide.

If the baby is coming very fast in the second stage you will probably need to blow as well as breathe quickly. If you feel as if you really must push, blow as if you were extinguishing a candle flame to reduce the intensity of the push (see page 212). You will not stop the push altogether, because the expulsive power of the uterus is there whatever you do, but you can limit it. Some women feel after a labor of this kind that they want the baby inside them again. They wish that they could go back to the beginning, because everything happened so fast that they cannot make sense of it. Some even feel "cheated." If this is so with you, talk through each event of labor with your partner, fitting the pieces together, and reliving the birth in your thoughts until you can see its shape.

LONG-DRAWN-OUT LABOR

A lengthy labor is psychologically taxing and physically exhausting. You need constant, confident emotional support from someone who knows you well and will not leave you. Unfortunately, a prolonged labor tends to make a partner anxious, unsure of his role, and often feeling that he ought to leave it all to the professionals.

A long-drawn-out labor can seem prolonged for two reasons: first, you may be unable to differentiate clearly between the lead-in to labor proper—the "latent" phase—and active labor.

"THROUGHOUT THE ENTIRE LABOR I WAS CONSCIOUS THAT I COULD ONLY GO WITH THE CONTRACTIONS. I FELT IT WAS LIKE RUNNING IN A MARATHON."

Second, active labor may be prolonged because contractions are faint and infrequent, or because they are not achieving dilatation of the cervix.

Psychological support from your partner and midwife, accurate information, and a chance to rest are vitally important. Even if contractions seem to be ineffective and dilatation is slow until you reach 4 cm, everything may coordinate suddenly so that from then on labor goes like a bomb. Over 90 percent of women having a lengthy latent phase go on to have a normal labor and birth if given the chance.* So do not assume that if labor takes several days to start, it is going to be like that all the way through. Take relaxing hot baths, sleep or rest in different beds if possible, so that you have a change of scenery, and take up different positions. There may be a couch, an easy chair, or a blanket to lie on as a change from your bed. Do not go into the hospital until you think you would feel happier there. Even if you have a long first stage, the second stage may be completely normal.

The progress of labor is assessed in terms of the rate of dilation of the cervix (see pages 254–256). Provided that the baby is all right and its heart tones are regular, *slow dilation at the onset of labor does not harm the baby*, however tiring you are finding it. Slow dilation in the early phase is not the same as complete lack of progress over several hours once active labor has started (that is, after the cervix has dilated about 3 cm).

Remember that it is difficult to be accurate about dilation. You may be examined by someone who says you are 5 cm dilated, but an hour later someone else says you are only 4 cm or perhaps 5 cm dilated, when by then the first person would have determined you to be 6 cm dilated.

WAYS OF DEALING WITH A LONG LABOR

In the hospital it is often difficult to walk around and alternate periods of rest with sessions of activity. But if you can, it is the best natural way of helping a uterus that is contracting ineffectually to work more efficiently.

Be sure to drink enough fluids, since you can forget to drink and become dehydrated. You may be given an intravenous "cocktail" of dextrose solution to keep up your strength and ensure that you do not become dried out. If this is the case, get into an upright position beforehand so that you are not stuck lying down with an intravenous drip in your arm. If you have to stay in bed, take up positions in which the long axis of the uterus is in line with the birth canal. Do this by kneeling or squatting. It is one of the most effective noninvasive actions you can take. Do so *before* taking drugs for pain relief (see pages 317–318), having an epidural (see page 319), or accepting hormone acceleration of labor (see page 339).

"I WALKED, ROCKED ON ALL FOURS, KNELT. I COULD MOVE AROUND AS I WISHED. I SPENT MOST OF THE TIME WALKING AND SWINGING MY PELVIS."

Sometimes fear or anxiety seems to prevent a uterus from functioning well. If physical difficulties have been ruled out, work together with your partner on facing up to any worries that may be on your mind. Both of you together can create a psychologically positive atmosphere by concentrating on the reality of the baby who is coming to birth and on the visual image of the cervix opening up. In New Guinea, when labor is long-drawn-out the woman is urged to confess any hidden anger she may feel, because it is thought that labor will proceed smoothly and easily once she has gotten rid of negative feelings she is bottling up.

The general obstetric term for a long-drawn-out labor is "failure to progress." Unfortunately, it is one of the main reasons that Cesarean sections are carried out. In the words of two obstetricians, "In many cases, failure to progress is really failure to wait."* It is only common sense that, however hard the uterus is working, it cannot push the baby out unless your cervix is soft and opening up. In most long-drawn-out labors, the cervix simply needs more time to soften and open up.

HOW SLOW IS TOO SLOW?

In the U.S., the most common reason for a Cesarean is the diagnosis of dystocia—prolonged labor. Thirty-eight percent of Cesareans are done for this reason. Another 20 percent of labors are augmented with intravenous oxytocin in its synthetic form (pitocin) for the same reason. As a result, women suffer more infection, bleeding, and a longer hospital stay—and many are left with the feeling that their bodies have failed them.

Two studies, covering 4,000 women who were cared for by midwives, have shown that a long labor does not necessarily mean that anything is wrong. Some women's bodies just work that way.* These women had support from family members, kept active, breathed through contractions, ate and drank if they wanted to, used massage, showers, and baths, had intermittent (not continuous) fetal monitoring, and used nonpharmacological methods of pain relief. The active phase of the first stage (from 4 cm dilation) was, on average, nearly eight hours for first babies, and five and a half for other births. The second stage lasted 54 minutes for first babies and 18 minutes for other births. This is twice as long as the standard time allowed in U.S. hospitals.

Professor Leah Albers and the other authors of these studies suggest that when things go wrong with a long labor it may be because of the way women are cared for in a medicalized birth system that imposes numerous vaginal examinations, pitocin augmentation, epidurals, and operative deliveries. They conclude that labor is still normal if dilation is only 0.3–0.5 cm per hour. If everyone is patient and has confidence in the mother's body, the mother is more likely to deliver normally in her own good time.

DYSFUNCTIONAL LABOR

One thing that may hold up labor is incoordinate uterine action. Unfortunately, it is possible to have massive contractions and yet for the upper segment of the uterus not to be able to draw up and pull open the lower section. It is as if one part of the uterus is working against another part. With this kind of labor, floating or crouching in a birth pool or in a deep bath, with lights dimmed, might help.

If there is still no progress, an epidural and augmentation of labor with a pitocin intravenous drip may be the answer. The obstetrician usually decides on augmentation because an epidural has the effect of prolonging labor. If you choose an epidural, you will have time for a rest and then, if you wish, the anesthetic can be allowed to wear off a little so that you can push the baby out yourself.

GIVING SUPPORT
IN LABOR

It is now accepted that fathers are in the birth room and that couples often want to be together. There is still some way to go before many hospitals are as welcoming to several companions, or to a woman partner, as they are to the baby's father. You should be able to choose exactly whom you want with you for this important experience in your life.

If the baby's father cannot be with you at the birth, or if you feel that he is not the right person to help, you may want another person, such as a paid doula—a woman who gives one-to-one support in childbirth and works harmoniously alongside the midwife, focusing only on your needs—or a woman friend or relation, instead of or with the father. In many cultures, it is not acceptable for the husband to be present. In others, women appreciate having their partners there to know that they can rely on them and that they are loved, and they gain strength from this. In the past, women have always been supported by other women. A woman should not be deprived of companionship because her male partner cannot offer the support she needs, or she does not want him with her, or because religious or cultural tradition prohibits it.

Research has shown that the presence of an experienced doula or other woman reduces the need for pain-relieving drugs, shortens labor, makes birth an easier and happier experience, cuts the Cesarean rate, and results in fewer babies' needing intensive care.*

Whoever is going to support you at the birth, it is important to learn in advance exactly how to help most effectively. Childbirth classes can be useful in teaching how to give emotional and physical support, explore the emotional aspects of birth, and understand the stresses felt by a birth partner. Massage, help with breathing, and all the different techniques (see pages 180–185 and pages 189–200) learned in classes for couples may be really useful. Or, on the other hand, they may not. You may not want your partner to do anything at all but just give you quiet encouragement. You may want to be held but not touched. Some fathers, especially anxious ones, get too busy and do not realize that a woman needs her own space. This becomes intrusive at times and can have a negative effect on the progress of labor.

THE FATHER AT THE BIRTH

The man who knows how to help is in a much better position than one who is merely invited into the birth room but has no idea of what is going on. It is not just a question of holding his partner's hand, although this can be a way of giving emotional support, but of being able to judge where and when she needs guidance and encouragement with relaxation. He has also learned how to breathe "over" the contractions so that he can breathe with his partner at times when she needs extra support. He knows how to rub her back and do gentle, light massage over her lower abdomen when the uterus is opening up, and how to apply firm pressure to her shoulders, arms, and legs.

"MY PARTNER AND I WERE SHOWN TO OUR LABOR/DELIVERY ROOM AND IT WAS MADE OUR OWN BY A MIDWIFE KNOCKING AND WAITING TO BE ASKED TO ENTER. THERE WAS NO BREEZING IN AND OUT."

But it is one thing to learn how to give your partner support in the relaxed atmosphere of a childbirth class, where couples are working together, with much discussion interspersed with laughter, and quite another to put that into practice in a large, impersonal hospital. Confronted with figures in white or green whom he has never met before, whose names he does not know, in a strange, clinical environment, the father can feel out of place and lacking in confidence.

This is why it is a good idea for him, as well as for his partner, to have toured the hospital, and especially the birth room, beforehand. Women sometimes say that it was when they were approached with some unfamiliar piece of equipment that they began to tense up, and that if they had known what it looked like and how it worked, it would have been easier to remain relaxed. Also, men who have been giving good support to their partners before a piece of apparatus of this kind is used sometimes give up, since they feel that the machinery is controlling the labor.

This is understandable, because when an intravenous drip stand or monitoring equipment is brought to the bed, it is difficult for the man to get close to his partner, and a monitoring belt that fits around her abdomen may make it impossible for him to massage that area. He may feel that experts and machinery have taken over.

THE SUPPORT YOU CAN GIVE

The most important thing for a companion helping a woman during the long first stage of labor is to be relaxed. This is difficult in an exciting situation, but any anxiety is immediately communicated to her. If labor is different from what you expected, that can worry you more than it does the woman, who is enveloped in the force sweeping through her and who may shut out irrelevant stimuli. You may be made anxious by the doctor's tone of voice, a midwife's remark to a colleague, or by the (quite normal)

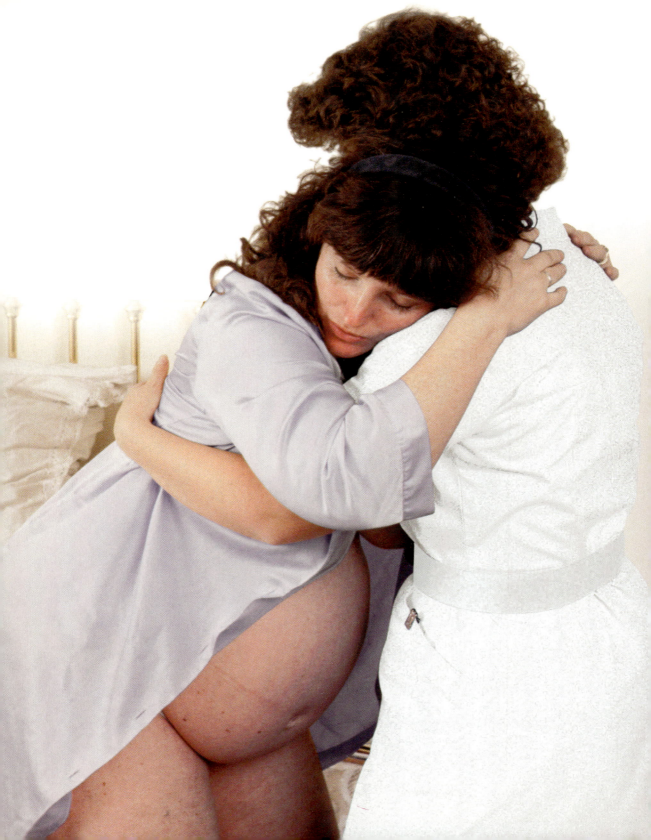

appearance of bloodstained mucus during a contraction. Ask for information, because if you are in doubt about anything, it is better to find out early rather than late. Speak slowly and quietly. Move slowly and deliberately. Touch your partner without haste, resting a relaxed hand on her body and, when you lift your hand away, do so slowly. If you are massaging her, stroke very slowly.

DISTRACTIONS IN THE BIRTH ROOM

When helping your partner to achieve focused concentration on what is happening in her body during contractions, never break that concentration by chatting with anyone else, watching a machine, or allowing yourself to be distracted by what is going on around you. As well as causing the woman in labor to become anxious and tense up, modern equipment can often be so fascinating that you may become so involved with watching a monitor, for example, that the woman takes second place and feels that emotional support has been withdrawn. Do not forget that, however sophisticated the machinery, it is the woman who is having the baby. Once labor is well under way, your attention should be focused entirely on her, and encouragement by word, touch, or look should be given with every single contraction.

On the hospital's side, too, an induced or speeded-up and monitored labor becomes an interesting clinical exercise. Nurses, doctors, and students may come in to watch. Teaching may go on at the bedside. Discussions about the equipment sometimes take place while the woman is busy with a contraction and would appreciate silence so that she can concentrate better. Although you cannot insist that everyone be quiet during contractions, you can indicate politely by your own silence and attention to her that you are not available for conversation, and encourage her to enter a "circle of solitude" with you and the baby coming to birth.

Occasionally machines break down and technicians arrive. This is very distracting for the woman in labor. Fortunately, she is not dependent on the monitor or other pieces of equipment to have her baby.

POSITIVE SUPPORT DURING CONTRACTIONS

Give your partner your full and undivided attention. Be on the same level, not towering over her. Use eye contact to give her emotional support. If she is coping well, she may like to close her eyes and handle contractions without looking at anybody, but if the going gets hard, suggest that she open her eyes and that you go through it together. This will be of special help at the end of the first stage, after her cervix is 6 cm dilated.

The late first stage, *with contractions coming every two minutes, may feel like a whirlwind.*

Everything that you say should be positive. Do not say "You're not relaxed here" or "Your shoulders are tightening." Say "Your feet are beautifully relaxed. Do the same with your hands," or give her positive suggestions such as "Pull your shoulders down and now let them go." When she is doing well, tell her so. This helps most as contractions reach their peak. It can be useful to hold her shoulder firmly during big contractions, and if she has practiced relaxation techniques that help her flow out toward your touch (see pages 190–200), these will keep her shoulders loose and thus prevent her from hyperventilating. Between contractions, talk to her about where she likes to be held. It may help her work with her contraction if you describe to her what is happening as the uterus goes into action: "You are opening up wider and wider. Your cervix is being pulled up and open, and the baby's head is pressing down." Ruth Wilf, an experienced American midwife, suggests that if the woman seems out of touch with her body, the support person should quietly discuss with her, between contractions, any negative thoughts she may be having. This gives you something to work on during the next contraction. Create an image for the next one—the baby pressing down, the cervix opening up. The woman may be able to suggest other things you can do (or not do) to help her focus her concentration.

UNDERSTANDING LABOR'S PROGRESS

The woman also needs information on what is about to be done by her birth attendants. Being in labor can be disorienting. Fear of the unknown is the main reason why women panic, and a request for pain-relieving drugs is usually one for reassurance. A woman may be distressed because she does not realize the progress she is making. She loses all sense of time, and each contraction is so enveloping that she cannot see the pattern of her labor. If the waters have not broken by the time contractions are coming every two minutes, you can be fairly sure that they will break soon. If she does not want to have an amniotomy (see page 327), make this clear. If she has one, prepare her for the renewed strength of contractions after it. In the second stage, remind her that the hot, throbbing, tingling feeling is a sign that the baby is about to be born and will soon be in her arms.

> "I COULDN'T HAVE DONE IT WITHOUT MY PARTNER. I REALLY NEEDED HIS STRENGTH, ESPECIALLY SINCE IT TOOK ME A LONG TIME TO PUSH THE BABY OUT."

Know when to be quiet. Talk when it helps, but keep quiet during the times when she may need other forms of emotional and physical support. Facial expression, gesture, touch, and massage can be just as important as conversation. One of the best ways of helping is to rest a hand on her shoulder with the other hand at her wrist as she goes through the contraction. If she has a backache, she will welcome firm pressure or massage over the sacrum, or slightly to one side of it (see page 198).

HOW TO HELP WITH BREATHING

Breathe with your partner through difficult contractions. Do not wait until she is tense to start the breathing. Begin with a relaxed breath out together. Keep closely in rhythm with her own breathing at the beginning of the contraction so that there is a partnership. Do not impose a radically different level or rate of breathing on her, or it will become a fight between her breathing and yours. If she starts to drag through the contraction with heavy breaths, this is the time to try to differentiate your breathing from hers.

Help her enjoy complete relaxation between contractions. This is especially important in stressful labors, since otherwise she carries tension from one contraction to the next and the effect is cumulative. When she is relaxed, you can talk together about how to meet the next contraction. When you speak about the uterus or cervix, remember it is "your" uterus and "your" cervix, just as it is also "your" or "our" baby. Any words used during contractions should be simple, rhythmic, and repetitive.

COPING WITH PAIN

Labor companions are often unsure whether or not they should mention the word "pain." For some it is taboo. It is imperative to acknowledge pain when it exists and not to pretend that it is not there. To do so is to deny a woman the validity of her own experience and to say in effect: "You aren't feeling what you think you are feeling, and if you are, there must be something wrong with you or with your labor." If she tells you it hurts, agree and say, "I understand" or "Yes, I realize that." It might be the moment to add, "Your uterus is working very hard" or "The baby is pressing down," and also to help her see the pattern of her labor. If she is more than 6 or 7 cm dilated, she is now at the most difficult part of labor.

"WE DIDN'T PLAN ON MY HUSBAND BEING THERE FOR THE BIRTH. BUT THE DOCTOR TOOK IT FOR GRANTED HE WOULD COME INTO THE ROOM. HE WAS DELIGHTED AND AFTERWARD COULDN'T STOP TALKING ABOUT IT!"

Show her with your hand how far she is dilated. Help her change position, freshen her up with a face wash, brush her hair, and use massage to help her. Give her your total, undivided attention. Emotional support of this kind can often take the place of drugs for pain relief.

The most undermining thing that you can possibly do is to encourage her to start feeling sorry for herself. The woman who is told by her helper, "I can't bear to see you in such pain," or words to that effect, is actually being deprived of emotional support. Even the expression on a helper's face can give that message, sometimes even more clearly than words could do. We would not think much of someone who leaned over the side of an ocean liner and called to the person in the water, "It looks terrible down there. The waves are so huge and, poor thing, you look as if you are drowning. Do you want an injection?" Yet this is the equivalent of the sympathy and the offer of "something to take away the pain" that some attendants offer to a woman in labor. The woman who has prepared herself wants help to enable her to cope with the mountainous waves, rather than the offer of a drunken stupor or sensation-free childbirth. If she wants drugs for pain relief, this should always be entirely her own decision. If she does ask for narcotics or an epidural, she should do so freely, certainly not because she has been persuaded or coerced.

STAYING TOGETHER

If you feel queasy or that you must take a break, tell your partner you will be back in a moment and stroll out. Women especially need support when they are being examined, when drugs for pain relief are offered, or when there is any intervention, and to go out then is the worst time. This is one point in labor when the woman can herself speak up and state her preferences. She could say, "I'd very much like my partner to stay, please. Don't send him away. I really need him," or "I don't think I'll be relaxed if my friend goes out." She could add, "She's learned about what happens and understands it pretty well. She's being a wonderful support!"

START–STOP LABOR

Some labors seem to come to a halt for a time, and a woman may be stuck at 4 cm dilatation or more for several hours. This is a sign for a change of activity. Lying flat on one's back is not a good position for labor, from either the woman's or the baby's point of view. When she is lying on her left side or is upright the blood flows freely to the placenta, allowing more oxygen and nutrients to get through to the baby than when flat on her back, and it is also easier to cope with backaches.

It is not a good idea to lie still for long periods, so suggest that she may like to roll over onto the other side occasionally or to sit up. If she is sitting, supported by four or five pillows, there is not the same problem of decreased blood flow to the placenta. It is also fine if she wants to squat, kneel, stand, or adopt any of the many positions that women spontaneously choose in labor (see pages 214–218). But the variety of possible positions is very much limited if intravenous drips and machinery are in use.

If labor comes to a stop, encourage her to get up and move around. If she is already walking around, suggest a bath or a shower, perhaps a back massage, and then rest in bed with hot-water bottles placed around the areas where she aches. Jamaican midwives give the woman a sponge-down and then wrap her in hot towels and offer a drink of hot thyme or mixed-spice tea when labor fails to progress. Perhaps we could learn something from this.

A full bladder can cause unnecessary pain. It used to be thought that it could hold up labor, but there is no evidence to support this. For her own comfort, remind the woman to empty her bladder every hour and a half, or more often if she feels the need. If progress is slow, help her feel that her natural pace is the right pace. Each labor is different, and having a baby is not a competition to see who can do it fastest. Especially when labor is long, affirm your confidence in her body rhythms. Between 8 and 10 cm dilatation she may feel lost and tossed in the turmoil of contractions following each other almost without a break. Keep eye contact and breathe with her through each contraction. Letting her know that you trust her own natural rhythms is nowhere more important than at this point. Her legs may feel cold and begin to shake, and you can help by firmly massaging the inside of her thighs.

THE LULL

There is often an apparent pause in labor for 20 minutes or more when the woman's cervix is just about fully dilated. She may have no urge to push, and feel no contractions, yet her attendants are alert for the start of the second stage. They expect action, but nothing seems to be happening. They may worry that the uterus is not going to do its job of pushing the baby out, and some try to get her to push even though she does not feel like it, so that she gets exhausted. They may also call for pitocin to stimulate contractions.

"IT IS NOT A QUESTION OF BEING THERE JUST FOR HER SAKE, BUT FOR YOUR OWN. YOU DON'T KNOW WHAT YOU'RE MISSING IF YOU ARE NOT AT THE BIRTH."

If the woman feels rushed and that there are anxious eyes upon her, she gets tense and anxious herself. Reassure her that there is all the time in the world. This is a normal part of the unfolding birth process—the "rest and be thankful" phase when the baby's head is still not deep in the pelvis. The head usually drops lower naturally if she can rest and refresh herself.

Help her stand up, and perhaps take a shower, offer her a sponge bath, and put some music on. She may want to walk around, gently rocking and circling her pelvis, enjoying slow belly dancing movements. You can stand cradling her body against yours as she does so, holding her shoulders, elbows, or wrists, and move with her. After half an hour or so— occasionally an hour or more—contractions pick up, and with renewed energy and excitement she enters the expulsive stage.

SUPPORT IN THE SECOND STAGE

When the woman begins to push the baby out, she can be in any position that feels comfortable to her: held firmly in your arms or cradled by your body, or with something solid to grasp or over which she can lean. She needs to be free to round her back, roll her shoulders forward, and rest her chin on her chest during contractions. You can help by providing physical support if she wants it and, perhaps, by reminding her to keep her head forward at the height of each pushing urge (without making any attempt to force it forward). From time to time give, her a sip of water or juice through a flexible straw, or ice cubes to suck.

Do not say "push." Say "open up" instead. Straining wastes energy and results in uncoordinated expulsive efforts. If you suggest she does not push at all unless she feels she has to, she will push in the right way at the right time.

Avoid clock-watching. It can be as disastrous to have one eye on the clock as it would be if you were watching the clock while trying to make love. A birthing woman needs to feel secure in a world without time or standards of performance, simply able to be herself and experience the intensity of what her body is telling her to do. If the pushing urge is strong and difficult to control, and it looks as if everything is happening too fast, help her to lie on her side or get down on all fours, as this may reduce the impulse. Encourage her to put her hands down and feel even before any part of the baby's head is slipping through the vagina. If you see that the crown is moving forward, but she is still holding her breath, say quietly, "Breathe." She should breathe out and go on breathing in and out with a dropped jaw.

SHARING IN THE BIRTH

Many women are anxious that they might be too small. Reassure your partner that there is room, and her feelings of openness and flexibility will help to make room. The power of suggestion is so great that each word and phrase used can affect her ability to work with her body.

When you are with a woman in childbirth, you share with her a journey into the unknown. The helper is like the lookout on a yacht sailing at night, watching for the coastline and helping to steer her through. She needs your constant presence—to be left alone is the most frightening thing of all. Giving support in labor needs vigilance, skill, patience, an understanding of a woman's rhythms, her responses to stress, an awareness of what she is thinking, how she is feeling at each moment, and your complete commitment to this task. It demands endurance and courage. It can be hard, exhausting work. But yours, too, is the excitement, the deep satisfaction, and the joy when a child is born.

SURPRISE BIRTH

If you are alone with a woman who is about to give birth unaided, the most important thing is to stay calm and give her quiet and confident support. Drop your shoulders and relax! Tell her she is doing well. Hold her in your arms and help her feel secure.

MAKING THE WOMAN COMFORTABLE

If the room is cold, heat it. The baby will need a warm environment after birth. If you can, place a pile of newspapers or a plastic sheet or tablecloth under the mother. She may like to sit or kneel on a firm cushion or beanbag. Cover whatever she is on with a sheet if there is one available. Find some big towels, a blanket, or something else warm to wrap the baby in. Offer her sips of water if her mouth is dry. Put pillows or some firm support behind her back, shoulders, and head to allow her to sit up, kneel, or squat comfortably or for her to lean over, unless she prefers some other position. Her own feelings about this are likely to be right. If traces of feces appear at her anus, wipe with cotton balls or toilet paper out and away from the vagina. Wash your hands and scrub your nails thoroughly.

If she is pushing, gently remind her to "open up" and not to hold her breath or push unless she feels she needs to. Just before the head crowns, suggest that she pant, so that from then on she breathes the baby out instead of pushing it out. She can then push gently between the contractions if the birth is slow.

If a loop of cord is around the baby's neck as its head slides out, hook a finger around it and lift it carefully over the head. Be careful not to pull the baby or the cord, since this may detach the placenta from the wall of the uterus. If a membrane is over the baby's face, lift it off. Either you or she can then catch the baby. Lift the baby up onto the mother's upper thigh or tummy, with the head slightly down so that any mucus can drain away safely.

AFTER THE BIRTH

Cover the mother and baby with a coat or blanket, or, better still, a comforter, which is both light and warm. Put a bowl between her legs to receive the placenta. There is no need to cut the cord. Enjoy the peace as you admire the baby together and wait for the placenta. Make her comfortable. She may be shivery and like a hot-water bottle and a cup of tea. Let the baby nuzzle close to her breast, and when it is ready to suck, lift it to the breast so that the nipple is well back in the mouth.

If you are in a car, away from any help or home comforts, there is no need to do anything about the placenta or cord. However, if you have a plastic bag or some newspaper, you can wrap the placenta in it and keep it at the same level as the baby.

If you are at home, boil shoelaces or soft string for tying the cord, and scissors for cutting it. If the placenta does not come after about 20 minutes, ask the mother to kneel and give long, slow blows out. It may slip out then. Never pull on the cord. Put a bowl under her buttocks and pour warm water between her legs. She can keep her uterus contracting and reduce bleeding from the placental site by massaging it firmly and putting the baby to the breast.

Tie the cord about 4 in (10 cm) and again about 6 in (15 cm) from the baby, and cut with a pair of sterilized scissors or a new razor blade between the ties. Check that there is no bleeding from the cord stump. If there is, make another tie nearer the baby.

The greatest heat loss from a newborn baby is from its head, so cover the head. Keep mother and baby cuddled together and cover both of them. When birth comes by surprise it is unlikely that anything will go wrong. This is nature at its most efficient.

A WATER BIRTH

Jane's third baby was born underwater. She decided to give birth at home with a midwife who was experienced with water birth, and to rent a birth pool. When she sank into the water, she experienced instant pain relief.

The birth went smoothly, and she breathed the baby's head out by herself while the midwife watched and waited. The cord was loosely around the baby's neck, and her midwife unwound it underwater and lifted the baby to the surface. They waited for the cord to stop pulsating and then Stewart cut it. Jane squatted and pushed out the placenta while still in the pool. Her midwife said, "It was such magic, being there!"

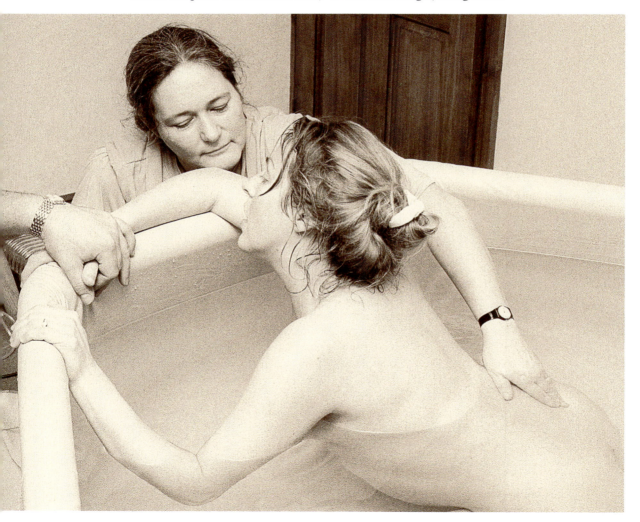

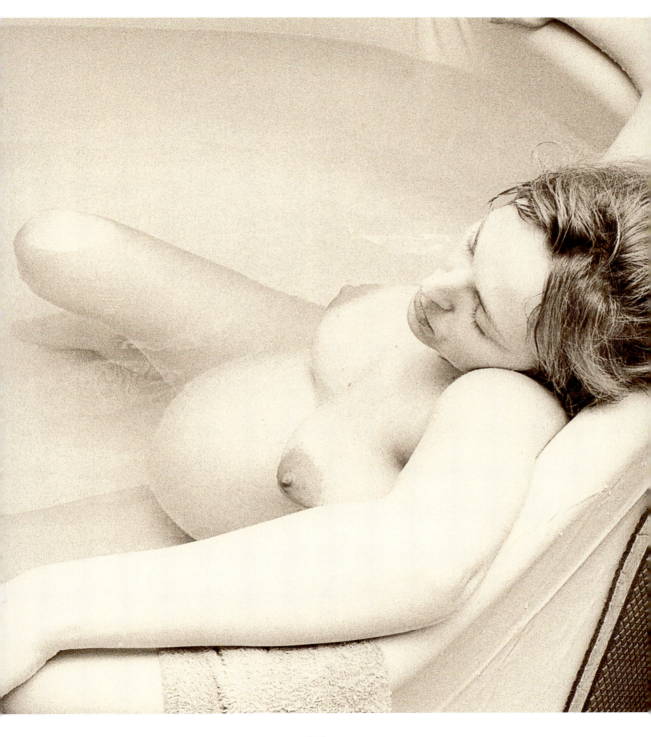

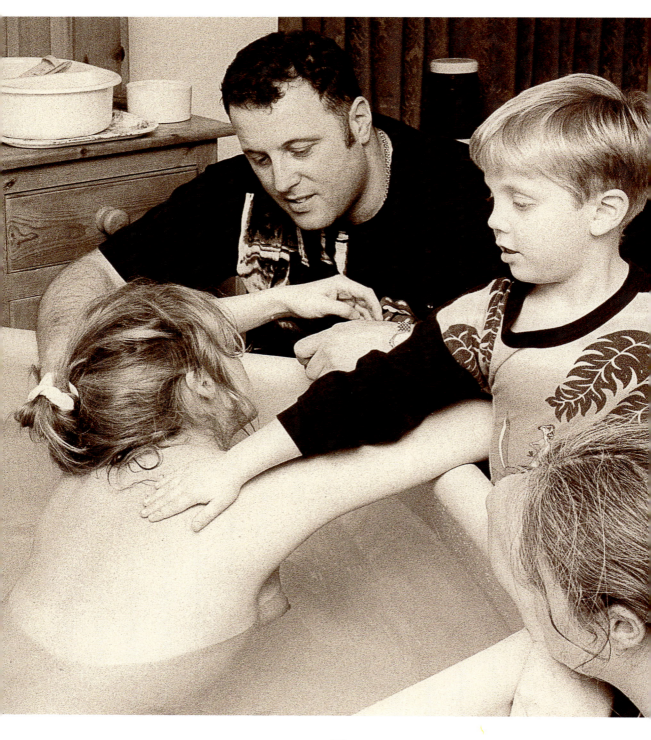

When a woman labors in a birth pool in a calm and peaceful atmosphere, other family members are quite naturally included. Children can do things to help: pressing a damp washcloth against the woman's brow, stroking her shoulders—or just giving her a hug.

For everyone, the presence of children contributes to the normality of the birth experience. Children who share in the experience of birth in a loving environment where there is no fear learn that birth is an important transition in the life of the family, witness the power of a woman's body in the act of creation, and celebrate the birth of a new brother or sister.

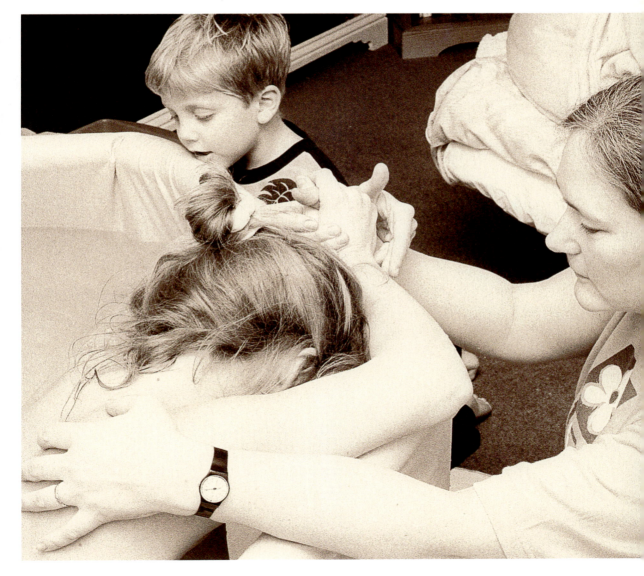

It is easy to move in water, and a woman often switches between forward-leaning and other upright positions without even thinking about it, because it feels right at the time. This movement helps the rotation and descent of the baby's head.

One position a woman may like to adopt as she pushes the baby down is a supported squat, her upper back against the side of the pool and her partner's arms under her shoulders. It is important that he not press on nerves under her arms and that he hold her securely without gripping her. Her knees are spread wide so that her pelvis is open. She feels her pelvic floor muscles and the tissues of her perineum fanning out as the baby presses through, until at last the top of the head can be seen glistening in her vagina.

Then she has another passionate urge to push and the head begins to slide forward. The midwife watches, leaving the baby to uncurl naturally, her hands poised to support the body as it emerges. Gently, carefully, intermittently pushing and breathing, the mother eases the head out. Only one more push, the shoulders are free, and the whole body slides out.

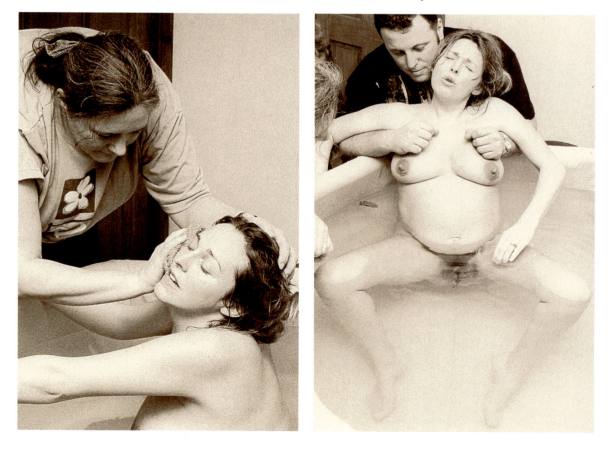

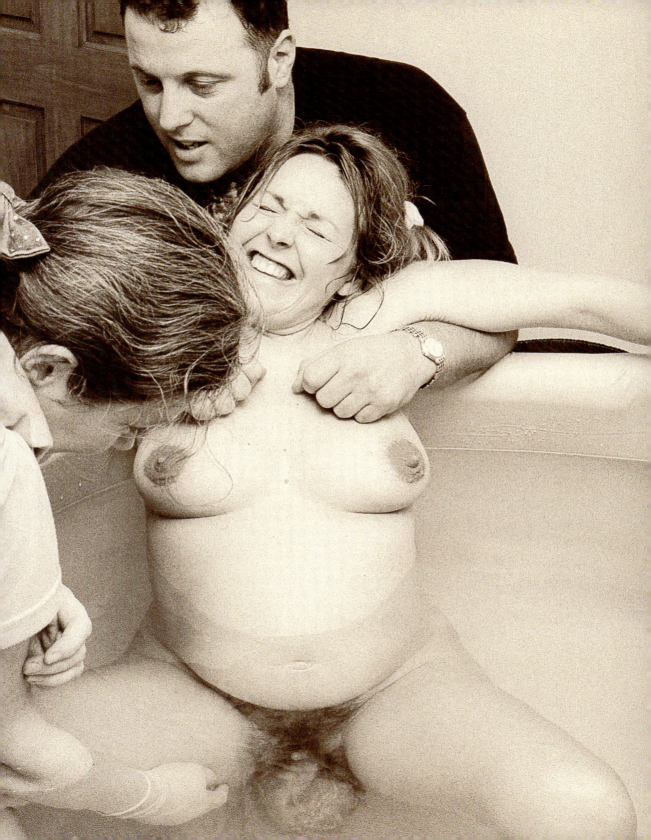

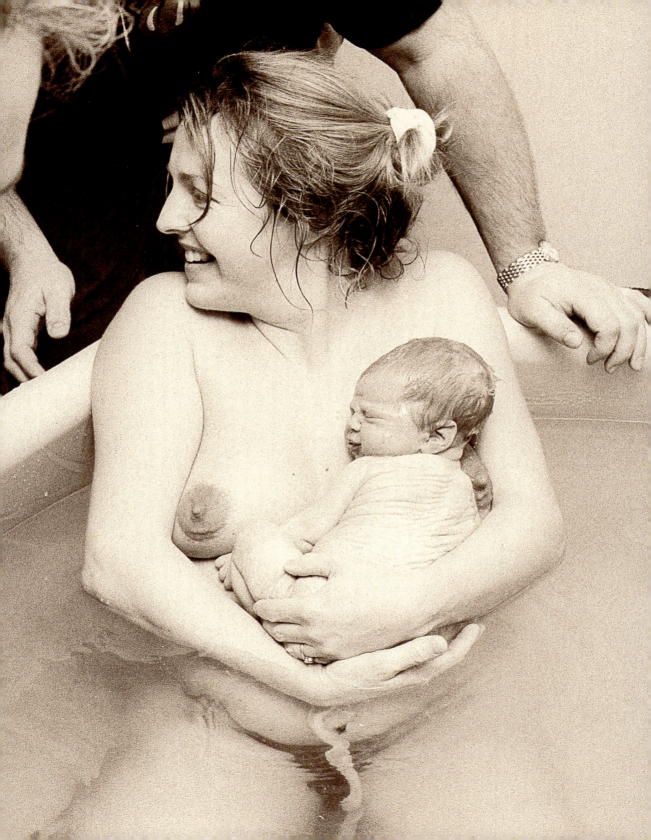

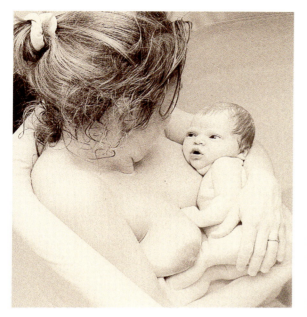

The baby is lifted gently from the water immediately into the mother's arms, either by the midwife or by the mother herself. The cord is not clamped and cut until it has ceased to pulsate, thus enabling the baby to receive the blood that rightfully belongs to her.

The room is warm, so there is no hurry to cover the baby, and Jane can cuddle her and put her to the breast when she starts rooting. Because the lights are dimmed, the baby opens her eyes, looks up, and is fascinated by the sight of her mother's face.

With eyes wide open, in the quiet, alert state that often follows birth, this baby gazes at her two brothers, who welcome her with delight. As her mother cradles her in her arms, they start the first of many "conversations" together and join in the dance of interaction that forms the basis of all later socialization.

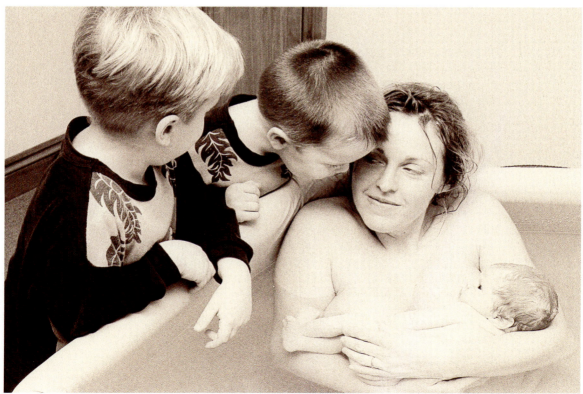

DEALING WITH PAIN

Many women who are pregnant for the first time fear that pain is going to be overpowering. They may never have experienced pain that tested their inner resources and feel ignorant of the kind of pain that they are likely to face.

The three statements that follow express what many first-time mothers feel:

"I've got a very low pain threshold. I can't stand going to the dentist, so I can't think what labor is going to be like!"

"The idea of the pain really worries me. I've never really experienced severe pain, and I can't imagine what it's like to be in pain for hours and hours and hours."

"What is labor pain like? I mean, is it like breaking your arm or a bad headache or period pains or indigestion—or what? If I knew what it was going to be like I could face it better."

PUTTING PAIN IN CONTEXT

People often think that pain is just a matter of a "high" or "low" pain threshold. There are very few women who think that they have a high threshold and can bear pain well. In fact, the idea of a pain threshold being like a wall, with some of us possessing high walls and others low ones, is a myth.

It is now known that the pain sensation threshold is the same in all human beings.* In one research study in the United States, members of Italian, Jewish, Irish, and other ethnic groups were given electric shocks ranging from mild to fairly strong, and every single person said pain occurred at exactly the same point. Yet obviously we do not all *react* to pain in the same way, because it depends on what is going on in our minds. There are times when a pain, which you once bore easily, becomes too much to take and you cannot stand it anymore. A toothache that you can handle without difficulty when you are busy and preoccupied can be absolutely shattering when you go to bed, lie down, and try to sleep. So you cannot judge the degree of pain simply by watching how an individual reacts in a laboratory situation.

People may see a pain-producing stimulus as a test of their power to *endure* pain, and may not always be ready to admit to being hurt. In the Sudan, for instance, a young man who cannot bear pain loses social esteem and is unlikely to find a girl to marry him. As in many cultures, the ability to bear pain stoically is part of a code of values.

In every society, there are cultural stress points, situations that are seen as threatening and thus predispose people to feel pain. When we know what makes people anxious, we can begin to understand these stress points. Pain is further complicated by the fact that in many societies some painful stimuli may be linked with pleasure. In lovemaking, for example, slightly painful stimulation may be sexually exciting. The borderline between pleasure and pain can be indistinct.

The context within which pain occurs is important. As an experiment,* electric shocks were given to test people first when they were feeling relaxed and cheerful, and then when they had been made to feel anxious. The electric shocks were felt as much less painful when the subjects were cheerful. In another study,* as many as 35 percent of a doctor's patients experienced marked pain relief when given a placebo, an inactive substance that they were told was a painkiller. It has also been found that the degree of pain tolerated bears a direct relation to the rate of increase in pain, rather than to the level of pain reached.* A person experiencing a pain stimulus that gets worse rapidly feels it more than someone experiencing just as strong a stimulus that takes longer to reach the same point. It helps to have time to *adapt* to pain.

This may have particular relevance to very rapid labor, especially an induced labor (see page 334), when the pace is more than a woman can cope with. We sometimes talk about labor as if a long labor were difficult and a short one easy. But speed alone can give no indication at all of how a woman experiences her labor.

Pain perception involves not only a recording of the stimulus by the brain, but also a judgment as to its significance and its place in the scheme of things—the meaning of the total situation in which the stimulus occurs. The experience of pain in labor is profoundly influenced by the values of the society in which the woman grew up and everything that she learned about birth when she was a child.

So labor pain is partly a product of personal and social values about the meaning of childbirth. The way we eat, sleep, empty our bowels, make love, have babies, and die makes these experiences more than simple biological acts. They all express ideas about good and evil, beauty and ugliness, the pure and the polluting, what is healthy and what is diseased, and what is normal and what is abnormal.

SOME PHYSICAL CAUSES OF BIRTH PAIN

As the first stage of labor progresses, nerve fibers that record pain are stimulated because the muscles of the uterus are squeezed tightly. A similar thing happens if you contract a muscle in your leg or arm very tightly and hold it taut for a minute or so. The uterus is the largest muscle in your body, so it is not surprising that this squeezing hurts. Pain of this kind is a sign that you are having good, strong contractions.

When the uterus contracts firmly, the flow of oxygenated blood into the muscle and of deoxygenated blood out of it is slowed down until the contraction is over. So there is a temporary buildup of waste products, which are released again in the interval between the contractions. Relaxing and taking complete breaths as soon as each contraction is over enables you to provide fresh oxygen for this hardworking muscle so that it can function effectively.

As the cervix is stretched to make space for the baby to pass through, localized pain is felt at the place where the cervix is dilating. This pain, at the very bottom of your abdomen, is common in straightforward labors and a good sign that your cervix is opening.

When pelvic ligaments and joints are stretched as the bony pelvis spreads wide and the baby descends, nerve fibers that run through them are stimulated, resulting in pain as your body opens up. This pain from ligaments, though difficult to handle, is a sign that your body is working well.

A baby who is not curled up, head down, in a neat ball with its chin tucked into its chest, takes longer to pass through the cervix and down the birth canal, and the pressure produced by the back of its head sticking into the small of the mother's back, or the unflexed head pushing down through soft tissues, causes pain. This also happens sometimes if the baby is very big. As contractions become stronger and more frequent they usually have the effect of rolling the baby around and down into a better position. So this pain may disappear entirely once the way is clear and you can push. You help your baby to rotate by being upright or on all fours. Upright positions such as standing, kneeling, or squatting enable you to use gravity. An all-fours position lets the baby drop away from your spine so that it turns more easily against your springy abdominal wall.

"THE BACKACHE WAS BAD, BUT I KEPT THINKING OF WHAT YOU SAID, 'THE BABY IS OPENING THE GATE,' AND SUDDENLY HER HEAD TURNED AND FROM THEN ON IT WAS EASY."

PAIN RELIEF IN OTHER CULTURES

There are two myths about the ways in which women in traditional cultures give birth. One is that labor is always horrific and dangerous, but that women do not cry out because of strong taboos against showing that they are in pain. The other is that women all have completely painless births, and just squat down in the fields and have their babies before getting back to work again. The truth is probably somewhere in between the two extremes. In many traditional cultures, healthy women have straightforward labors while other, malnourished women suffer a great deal.

Most cultures have methods of relieving pain in childbirth, so there is obvious recognition that it exists. But the ways in which pain is relieved and labor made more comfortable are radically different in the technological Western countries. We can give complete relief from pain and remove all sensation from the waist down with regional anesthesia. This is what an epidural does (see page 319). We have other forms of pain relief that partially remove pain or that eradicate the memory of it. We rely on pharmacological substances to do this for us. Herbal medicines are used in traditional cultures, and some of them have narcotic or mood-altering properties, just like modern drugs, although it is much more difficult to prepare the right dose when you are using plants. There are also other kinds of help that are favored in these countries and that used to be employed in the West. They include religious and magic rites, counterstimulation, massage, hot and cold compresses, changes in position, and emotional support from others sharing the experience with the woman in labor. These supporters hold her, stroke her, rock her back and forth, and live through the birth with her.

Much of what is done by birth attendants in other cultures provides simple, practical help based on the handed-down experiences of generations of women. It has a psychosomatic effect, too, helping the baby to be born by positively influencing the mind of the woman in labor. This kind of practical help is forgotten or misunderstood in our modern hospitals. Yet there are advantages in coping without drugs, because all powerful drugs have side effects, and they all go through the mother's bloodstream to her baby.

IMAGINING YOUR LABOR IN ADVANCE

It is a good idea to work out how you might like to be helped to be more comfortable, and how to use your mind to help your body through relaxation, focused concentration, and ideas and mental images that produce a harmonious pattern between what is going on inside your uterus and the way you think about it. You may find that all this is difficult to conceptualize before you have your first baby.

Trying to master your body or run away from sensations can actually produce pain, because you become tense and chemical messages are sent instantaneously into your bloodstream that

"MY MIND WAS FULL OF SEA IMAGES. IT WAS AS IF I WAS AN ISLAND WITH WAVES RUSHING AND SWIRLING AND OPENING MY BODY IN READINESS FOR BIRTH."

affect your whole metabolism. This causes changes in skin and muscle tone, blood pressure and heart rate, breathing, and digestion. Psychosomatic factors can even change the action of the uterus itself in ways we do not yet fully understand. A woman who is very anxious may have a long labor because her uterus does not work efficiently or stops contracting.

WHAT LABOR FEELS LIKE

In a normal labor, pain is quite different from the pain of breaking a leg, for example, or being injured. The physical feelings produced by a strongly contracting uterus are powerful and challenging. They involve a combination of sensations—a very tight squeeze, a pulling open of tissues, and the firm, downward pressure of the solid ball of the baby's head through a passage that is being slowly stretched wide. In movies you sometimes see a pregnant woman suddenly double up, her hands clasped over the top of her abdomen. Labor has started! But it never happens like this in reality. Instead, there is a sensation of being gripped by tightening muscles low down in your abdomen or in the small of your back. All the sensations are at hip level. Nor is the feeling a sudden one. A contraction has a wavelike shape, building up to a crest and then subsiding and disappearing until the next contraction. There is a rest period between them, often lasting a minute or more, even in the stormy late first stage. As contractions get stronger, longer, and closer together, the tightening may extend right around your body, so that it feels more like

> "I KNOW SOME MIDWIVES CALL THEM 'RUSHES.' THAT'S EXACTLY HOW THEY WERE FOR ME. EVERY CONTRACTION BROUGHT A RUSH OF ENERGY."

a circle of thick, wide elastic across your pelvis that is being steadily drawn in, held firm, and then slowly released again. Or you may be conscious of expansion during contractions and aware of the top of the uterus spreading and rising, tilting forward in your abdomen, while the great muscle squeezes its lower part open and presses the baby down.

PAIN WITH A PURPOSE

Feelings during labor may be painful, but it is pain with a purpose and different from the pain of injury. Contractions are not painful in themselves, and in fact the uterus contracts strongly and rhythmically at intervals in the second half of pregnancy, usually without causing any pain. It is the peak of the contraction, when the muscle is working hardest and is making most progress, that is most likely to be perceived as painful, and this may last as long as 30 seconds or as little as 15 seconds.

The idea of a pain that is *qualitatively* different from other kinds of pain is difficult to accept for anyone who has not experienced it. Yet sheer physical effort, like that involved in running a race or climbing a mountain, produces that kind of "functional" pain, the ache of muscles that are working very hard. If the athlete thought only of pain instead of about winning the race, she would give up. If the mountaineer thought that her aching muscles were the sign of some dreadful physical injury instead of the natural result of working them so hard, she would forget all about her goal and lose the feeling of triumph when she reaches the summit.

Pain in labor is the by-product of the body's creative activity. Contractions are *not* pains. They are tightenings that may be painful, especially when they are being most effective. There is an art in approaching each new contraction, in thinking "Splendid! Here's another one!" and later, as you approach the end of the first stage, when they are at their strongest, "Oh, this is a really good one!"

When you are in the thick of labor, your whole self is involved. It is almost impossible to think about other things or to hold a part of yourself back. The intensity of labor can be frightening, especially for the unprepared woman who does not know what to expect, or for one who wants to keep it all at the level of a learned skill, doing her exercises in the same way as she might carry out a three-point turn in a driving test. This is why preparation merely for handling contractions is never enough. You also need to prepare yourself mentally and emotionally for the overwhelming sensations and feelings of labor.

MOVEMENT

One of the best ways of handling pain is to move. Walk around, and when a contraction comes, lean on your partner or against furniture, and rock or circle your pelvis as you "go with the flow" of the contraction.

Your partner can join you in a slow birth dance. You lead—your partner follows. You may want to place your hands behind your partner's neck, fingers interlaced, and rest your head against her chest or shoulder. Or it may feel best to have your arms dropped and relaxed. Let your partner's arms encircle you, and her strong hands give counter pressure in the small of your back.

You can move this way in a kneeling position, too. Or it may feel good to put one foot up on a chair, and move in a lunge position. It is easy to sway and rock your pelvis when you are on your hands and knees, too. An all-fours position like this often relieves pain. Explore some of the movements suggested on pages 214–218.

BREATHING

When we are in pain, our breathing usually changes. We hold our breath, gasp, or breathe in and out rapidly with a cry. The result is underbreathing or overbreathing, both of which, over time, alter the balance of blood gases and make it harder to cope with pain.

Birth pain comes and goes in waves, gradually building up to the peak of the contraction, then subsiding and disappearing. In most labors, it continues for some hours and comes at regular intervals.

Breathing in panic becomes part of a vicious circle. The reaction to pain causes more pain, and as a woman gets increasingly tense and tired, the pain gets worse. Her panicky breathing begins to affect people close by and makes them anxious, too. She picks up their concern and becomes more and more agitated. No wonder that the only way out of this circle of pain and distress seems to be an epidural.

Backache, also common in labor, is not rhythmic. It tends to be there all the time, getting more severe at the height of contractions. In reaction to back pain, breathing can become constricted, or breath is pumped in and out rapidly in gasps, and this makes the pain worse.

Smooth, rhythmic breathing is a way to handle pain. Focus on the breath out and avoid gulping in air. Use the greeting breath and the resting breath described on page 208 with each contraction. As pain peaks, blow out, or give a long, deep groan on the breath out. Keep the pitch low, as if it were going down into your pelvis. Rehearse the breathing pattern suggested on pages 208–209 to manage your pain.

HYPNOSIS

Some women find hypnosis an effective method of relieving pain in labor. It has the great advantage over chemical anesthetics of not reducing the baby's oxygen intake or making the woman feel drugged and drowsy. In fact, about a quarter of women who have had hypnosis in childbirth say that they experienced no pain, but results vary, and most women who have hypnosis choose chemical pain relief as well.

The common belief that hypnosis involves some magic trickery and that you can be made to do anything the hypnotist wishes is way off base. Hypnosis is a state of increased suggestibility induced by deep relaxation and concentration.

With hypnosis, some women become immune to pain and may have a forceps delivery or be stitched up after an episiotomy without a local anesthetic. Two out of every hundred women can be so deeply hypnotized that they could even have a Cesarean section without feeling any pain.*

If you plan to have hypnosis in childbirth you are usually trained in progressive relaxation to remove anxiety and are helped to think positively about childbirth. You can also be taught to use autohypnosis; the hypnotist suggests that you will be able put yourself to sleep and wake up when you wish. After the birth, the doctor may suggest that in the future you be hypnotized only by someone for a therapeutic purpose, so that you need not be afraid of being put into a trance by anyone using hypnosis for their own purposes, or for fun.

It could be claimed that all good childbirth classes teach autohypnosis. Thinking ahead to labor constructively when you are deeply relaxed is equivalent to using the power of suggestion. Whether or not you decide to try hypnosis, you can use autosuggestion and positive fantasies about labor and your beautiful baby to prepare yourself for childbirth, in the knowledge that this is completely safe.

ACUPUNCTURE

Another way of reducing pain in childbirth is by acupuncture. It derives from a system of beliefs about the human body completely different from that of Western medicine. Hair-fine needles are used to stimulate 12 lines of energy called "channels" flowing beneath the skin. This energy keeps the blood circulating, warms the body, and combats illness. Acupuncture is used prenatally, for example to relieve nausea and vomiting, cure constipation, encourage a breech baby to turn, and to start labor. Acupuncturists sometimes use moxibustion, the burning of a small pellet of mugwort at certain parts of the body, to turn the baby. In labor, electroacupuncture may be used at points in the ear for analgesia, and with this technique the woman herself can control the degree of stimulation.* In Beijing today, acupuncture is performed in preference to epidural anesthesia for 98 percent of Cesarean sections.* It is also sometimes combined with small quantities of drugs.

The advantages of acupuncture are that it is noninvasive, easily administered by someone trained in the method, instantly reversible, and babies are in better condition at birth than after Demerol has been given. Some studies show that acupuncture shortens the first stage for women having a first baby. Women say that they feel more in control than when they have taken drugs for pain relief.*

TRANSCUTANEOUS ELECTRONIC NERVE STIMULATION (TENS)

With TENS, which is being offered in some hospitals, a pulsed wave of variable intensity is passed through electrodes attached to the skin surface. This stimulates the production of natural pain-relieving substances in the body (endorphins and enkephalins). You operate a switch like a retractable ballpoint or two dials as you feel a contraction build up. There is a tingling sensation when it is switched on. The electrode pads are usually stuck on your back but can also be used on the abdomen or in the groin. The disadvantage of TENS is that it cannot be used in water.

REFLEXOLOGY

Similar to shiatsu, reflexology is a form of acupressure. It consists of manual pressure on reflex points in the feet, hands, and face to stimulate subcutaneous nerve endings. The belief is that it causes the brain to release natural endorphins and other chemicals that help to reduce pain. In childbirth, reflexology involves massage and gentle pressure on the feet.

AROMATHERAPY

At its simplest level, aromatherapy is a matter of breathing in pleasant smells that help you feel good about yourself. It provides you with a positive sensory environment for birth. This is useful if you are having your baby in a hospital, where it can erase any unpleasant hospital smells. Doctors and midwives can relax and enjoy it, too. The essences used are highly concentrated, and molecules that can cross into the bloodstream may reach the baby. Since we demand rigorous trials of drugs, most of which are derived from plants anyway, research into the effects of aromatherapy is important, too. Plant essences stimulate sensory cells in the nose, which send chemical messages to the limbic area of the brain, which cause neurochemicals to be released into the bloodstream. These essences are energizing—imagine smelling an orange, a lemon, eucalyptus, or a sprig of rosemary—or relaxing—imagine breathing in lavender, sweet geranium, or the scent of an old-fashioned rose. Essential oils also stimulate the production of endorphins, the body's natural analgesics, which are similar to morphine, so that you are less likely to need drugs for pain relief.*

You can put drops of essential oil on a pillow, handkerchief, or hot, damp washcloth and keep it close to you. They can also be mixed with a vegetable or nut oil (soy, jojoba, apricot kernel, wheat germ, sunflower, almond, and avocado are all good) and massaged into the skin. They can be added in concentrated form, or mixed with a dispersal oil or milk, to the water of a bathtub or birth pool, so that you are enveloped in their scent. You can use them in a warm footbath. Oils can be heated up using an electric teakettle.

"THE OBSTETRICIAN CAME INTO THE ROOM AND ASKED, 'WHAT'S THE WONDERFUL SMELL? OH, I LIKE THAT!' THE AROMATHERAPY MADE A RELAXING ATMOSPHERE THAT WE ALL ENJOYED."

As you inhale essential oils, notice how your face becomes softer and your breathing slower and fuller. The breathing of fear, anxiety, or panic is rapid and jerky. When you are relaxed and confident, breathing is rhythmic, and each breath is complete, with a slight pause between the breath in and the breath out, and another between the breath out and the breath in. During pregnancy you can experiment with essential oils to discover which ones work best for you and enable you to breathe easily, and which refresh and reinvigorate you and help any tension flow out of your body.

Lavender can be put directly on the skin. It can be mixed with one or two other essences, such as chamomile, sweet geranium, cedarwood, frankincense, myrrh, jasmine, neroli, rosewood, rosemary, peppermint (but do not use peppermint if you are also taking homeopathic medication), melissa, or mandarin. Some essential oils are overpowering if you use more than one or two drops, so sniff the bottles first before you concoct your recipe to make sure that it is well balanced. Some good combinations—all relaxing—are lavender and orange; lemongrass and orange; geranium and orange; ylang-ylang, sandalwood, and jasmine. Rose, neroli (very expensive), and sandalwood in jojoba oil can be massaged into your forehead, face, and neck.

Clary sage should not be used in pregnancy, since it can stimulate uterine contractions. This is why it may be helpful if the cervix is dilating very slowly in labor, the introductory phases of labor are lasting a long time, or you are two weeks past your due date and want to give gentle encouragement to your uterus to start contracting.

A reliable source of where to find aromatherapy oils and advice can be found on page 427.

HOMEOPATHY

Unlike conventional medical treatments, homeopathy aims to treat the whole person, including the mental and emotional states that have an adverse effect on physical well-being. There are 2,500 homeopathic remedies, many derived from plants, but others from metal (gold, silver), animal products (cow's milk, snake venom), allergens (pollen, house dust), and drug extracts (aspirin). The principle behind the remedies is that like is treated with like, but in minute quantities. The more diluted a remedy, the more effective it is.

A homeopathic labor pack might consist of ¼-oz (7-g) bottles of the following remedies:

• Arnica (leopard's bane) at 30c. It helps reduce bleeding and bruising.

• Hypericum (Saint-John's-wort). This promotes healing of the skin and can be taken with Arnica (leopard's bane), starting when labor begins and continuing for at least five days.

• Staphisagria (stavesacre) at 2 tsp (10 ml). This is said to be a remedy for trauma to the urethra, and also a treatment for postnatal "blues."

• Hypericum and calendula (pot marigold) can be combined in a 2-tsp (10-ml) tincture, which helps to soothe and heal skin that has been bruised or grazed. Mix ten drops with 1½ tbsp (20 ml) of sterile, cooled water and stroke it on wherever you feel sore.*

When you go to a homeopathic practitioner, the case history will take about an hour. This readiness to listen may be one element in the success of homeopathy. On the other hand, there are homeopathic veterinarians, so results cannot all be chalked up to the placebo effect. In the U.S., homeopathy is considered very alternative and is rarely covered by standard insurance. Some states license various practitioners, but most do not, so there are no standards or prescribed education for these practitioners.

BACH FLOWER REMEDIES

These remedies, another form of homeopathy, treat emotional states, not physical conditions. They can be used in pregnancy and during labor as antidotes to stress, fear, and lack of confidence. Tinctures are available in homeopathic dilutions, and the plant essences are preserved in brandy. There are 38 remedies for different emotional states, such as depression, shock, apprehension, and irritability, and because emotions are often complicated, they are often used in combination. The general "rescue remedy" is recommended for those "distressed by startling experiences."

IMMERSION IN WATER

You already know how soaking in a warm bath can relieve pain, whether you have experienced backaches, aching muscles from strenuous exercise or a state of physical tension, or menstrual pain. Being immersed in water can be comforting in labor. Lying in warm water increases venous pressure so that veins return blood to the heart more efficiently. It also enhances cardiac action and slows the pulse rate. Total relaxation in the warmth and comfort of a bath helps the uterus to contract more effectively. But it does more than this. Water both counteracts the force of gravity and any pressure a woman may feel against her back and buttocks, and also reduces pressure felt from inside the body, so there is a further pain-relieving effect.*

Sometimes pain is so much reduced and dilation proceeds so fast as a woman surrenders herself to the water that the baby slips out while she is still enjoying the bath. This is quite safe, since the baby takes a breath only when lifted clear of the water, and for a few minutes after delivery blood is still pulsating through the cord, thus providing the baby with oxygen. After the baby has left your body, the midwife will rest a finger on the cord so that she can feel the blood pulsating through it. You may like to do this, too.

WATER BIRTH

If you would like to use water in labor and birth, discuss it with your doctor or midwife.* Some hospitals are not happy about births taking place underwater but encourage it for labor. Some obstetricians have expressed concern about cross-infection, particularly with HIV, from using birth pools. There is no reason that birth in water should make cross-infection more likely than birth on land. In some hospitals, women with high blood pressure, those whose membranes rupture at the start of labor, or who are carrying twins or a breech baby, are not allowed to use water. But you can stand under a shower and have a powerful jet of water directed against your back. If you have drugs for pain relief you should not give birth under water because they may affect the baby's breathing.

Using a birth pool is now well-established practice in hospital and home births.* It is no longer considered an "alternative" but is a readily available option. Half of all the women who use water in labor go on to give birth in the pool, too. They enjoy the freedom of movement, the way that water relieves pain, and the peaceful atmosphere provided by a birth pool when attendants watch and wait without interfering. They often believe that water provides a more gentle transition to life for the baby, who has been floating in amniotic fluid for nine months.

In a water birth, the baby should never be left under the water but should be lifted immediately into the mother's arms. You know how cold you can feel after getting out of a bath. The baby quickly becomes chilled, too, so the room should be warm, and you and the baby should be wrapped immediately in big, warm bath towels.

It is probably unwise to decide in advance that you are definitely going to give birth in water. A woman for whom floating in water feels blissful late in the first stage of labor may want to get out of the water and have her feet firmly on the ground once the second stage starts. Do whatever feels right at the time.

THE SAFETY OF WATER BIRTH

A major pediatric study of over 4,000 babies born in water reveals that water birth is not dangerous.* A healthy newborn does not breathe underwater.* Babies breathe inside the uterus, although it is fluid rather than air that passes in and out of their lungs. Before labor starts, the baby stops this breathing, probably because of hormone changes and a rise in the level of prostaglandin E2. This hormonal inhibition of breathing continues while the cord remains untied because blood containing prostaglandins is still flowing through the cord into the baby for several minutes.

Amniotic fluid is warm. In fact, the baby's temperature is slightly higher than the mother's. Very hot water may reduce oxygen in the blood flowing to the baby. Water in the pool should therefore be at body temperature. A healthy baby born into water at approximately blood heat does not breathe it in.

The effort, hard work, and all the squeezing and activity of labor bring about a normal reduction of oxygen in the baby's blood (hypoxemia). The result is that the baby makes no attempt to inhale water. Only if a baby is very short of oxygen (hypoxia) is gasping stimulated.

The waves of huge contractions are easier to ride if you are immersed in water.

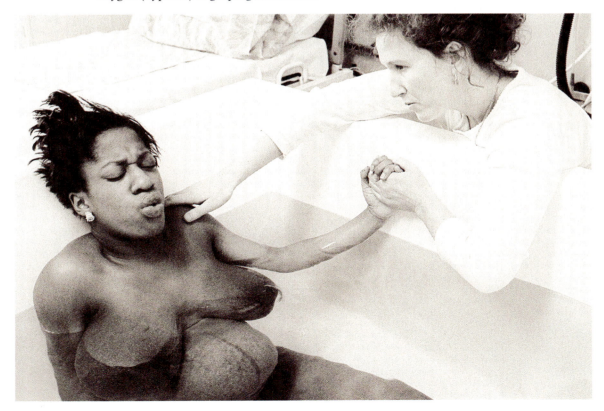

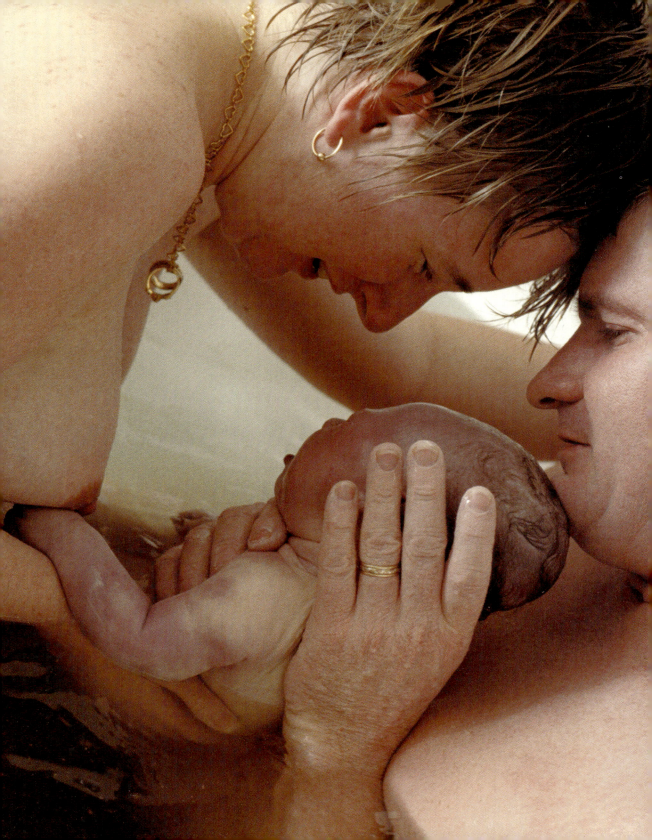

There are powerful chemoreceptors at the entrance to the baby's larynx that enable it to taste and discriminate between things that should be breathed and things that should be swallowed. A baby born into water is much more likely to swallow water than breathe it in. On the other hand, one born into salt water may breathe it in, because saline is similar to amniotic fluid. We do not know if this is harmful or beneficial, and research needs to be done.

A baby's head should not be delivered above the level of the water and then dunked. This might happen if there is insufficient water in the pool to cover your pelvis or if you grip the sides of the pool with your arms and push your pelvis up. If you give birth in water, ensure that it covers your tummy, and keep your shoulders and upper arms relaxed so that you do not tilt your perineum up out of the water.

DRUGS FOR PAIN RELIEF

A variety of pain-relieving drugs is available, and different drugs suit different women. It is important to understand what can be used and how each type works so that you can make an informed decision as to whether you want a drug and, if so, which kind. Whether or not you have drugs—and how much you have—is up to you. As one obstetric anesthetist has stated: "The only arbiter of pain is—or should be—the patient. A stereotyped prescription cannot cope with individual variations in response to pain."*

All drugs for pain relief pass through the mother's bloodstream to the baby. They all affect the baby—some more than others. None of them does the baby any good. When considering whether to accept drugs, bear in mind that some forms of anesthesia and analgesia can interfere with your first meeting with the baby.

ANALGESICS

OPIOIDS Drugs most widely used for analgesia (taking the edge off pain) in labor are opioids, such as Demerol. This is usually injected intravenously and the onset of pain relief is rapid (within a few minutes), wearing off within three to four hours. Some women like them and say they helped them cope with painful contractions by making them feel relaxed and slightly drunk. Others hate opioid drugs and call them "stupefying." They say they were woozy and out of control. Some women even hallucinate. Blood pressure may plummet, producing pins and needles, faintness, and disorientation.

A common side effect of opioids is nausea. One or two women out of every ten vomit when they are given pethidine. It is sometimes combined with an antihistamine to prevent nausea, but this tends to make you even sleepier. Opioids can sometimes depress respiration, and it is wise to avoid them if you are giving birth to a preterm baby.

The baby is brought gently to the surface with a loving welcome.

317

Demerol also drugs the baby, who may be knocked out at birth. Large amounts will be present in the baby if Demerol is injected within five hours before the birth, and especially if it is given three hours before delivery. This is when contractions are strongest and you may want drugs for pain relief. If injected within 45 minutes of the birth, however, Demerol is unlikely to have built up in the baby's tissues. The snag is that you will probably not want Demerol in the second stage because you will be working hard to get the baby out. Some hospitals provide patient-controlled analgesia by a computerized syringe, allowing you to pump in the drug as you need it. Women tend to use less Demerol when giving it to themselves than when it is injected by caregivers.

Some research suggests that opiate or barbiturate drugs used in childbirth may be imprinted on the baby, increasing the risk of addiction later in life. Swedish researchers recommend that methods of pain relief that avoid passage of large amounts of drugs across the placenta should be preferred.*

NUBAIN AND STADOL Nubain (nalbuphine) and Stadol (butorphanol) are also commonly used. These are stronger synthetic narcotics, which are combined with a narcotic antagonist intended to decrease the respiratory depression of both mother and baby.

PHENERGAN AND VISTARIL These are also antihistamines and are often combined with a narcotic to relieve nausea and decrease the dose of narcotic needed. They do cross to the baby and may slow reflexes for many hours, interfering with breast-feeding.

GAS AND OXYGEN (Entonox) is used in Great Britain, but not in the U.S. It is a mixture of 50 percent nitrous oxygen and 50 percent oxygen, from a machine that you use yourself. If you use it only through the first half of each contraction, it gives pain relief over the peak of the contraction. It is cleared from the baby's system with the first breaths it takes at birth.

The analgesic effects, which are not enough for some women, occur within 15 to 30 seconds and last for up to a minute. Timing is important. In the words of one woman: "As I felt the very start of the contraction I took three full breaths of gas and oxygen in and out through my open mouth. I remembered to make them really slow. . . . Then as the contraction got bigger I dropped the mask and went into quick breathing. It was fantastic."

LOCAL AND REGIONAL ANESTHETICS

Local anesthetics can also cross the placenta. They are least likely to affect the baby when injected into the area around the vagina and the perineum. This is done before an episiotomy (see page 331) and before a forceps delivery (see page 346) if other anesthesia has not been given. When local anesthetics are used to bathe nerves that cover a large area of the body, they are called *regional* anesthetics.

PUDENDAL BLOCK is an injection numbing the nerves in the perineum given at any time after full dilatation, and is often used before an episiotomy or a forceps or vacuum extraction.

EPIDURAL ANESTHESIA is injected into the space just outside the dura, the outer membrane around the spinal cord. Replenishing injections or a continuous drip of anesthetic are given through a fine plastic tube, which is left in place. The continuous drip allows the anesthetist to use a lower concentration of the drug, which reduces undesirable side effects. An epidural may be given with you sitting up and curled forward, or lying on your left side curled into a ball—a difficult position when you are in strong labor. An epidural takes about half an hour to set up.

An epidural can provide complete pain relief and is used as an anesthetic for Cesarean section. It removes sensation from the waist, or sometimes from your navel, down, either completely or partially, while allowing you to stay conscious. For a painful, prolonged labor it can seem to be the perfect answer. Many women say how marvelous the epidural was, but it is important that it is your own choice—no one should be put under pressure to have one.

An epidural should not be given if you have low blood pressure, are taking anticoagulants such as Warfarin to avoid blood clots, or have a skin infection where the needle is to be introduced, or if you have severe preeclampsia. An epidural tends to prolong labor, so stimulation of the uterus with an oxytocin intravenous drip is often necessary. It is also important to

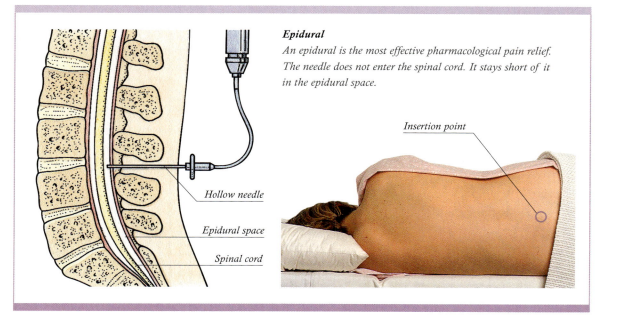

Epidural

An epidural is the most effective pharmacological pain relief. The needle does not enter the spinal cord. It stays short of it in the epidural space.

Insertion point

Hollow needle

Epidural space

Spinal cord

remember that epidurals do not always work. It may be difficult to inject into the right place, or the anesthetic may work on one side only, so that you feel contractions occurring in only half your body, which can be disconcerting. The anesthetist can try to adjust the placement of the epidural so that finally you can get good pain relief.

"I HAD TO LOOK AT THE MACHINE TO SEE WHEN I WAS HAVING A CONTRACTION.... I DID WANT TO FEEL HIM SLIDE OUT, AND NOT FEELING THAT WAS TERRIBLY DISAPPOINTING."

The anesthetic is similar to that used by dentists, and you feel it like liquid ice numbing your tummy, bottom, and legs. Even though it anesthetizes only part of you, it must be given by a skilled anesthetist, and under sterile conditions. If by mistake the anesthetist punctures the dura, you may end up getting a complete spinal. You are more heavily anesthetized, and a common side effect is a bad headache that can last a week or more after the birth.

SHOULD YOU HAVE AN EPIDURAL?

An epidural lowers blood pressure, sometimes drastically, so that other drugs may have to be given to raise your blood pressure again. This happens to one woman in eight, although the drop may be slight.* Because of this, an epidural is sometimes offered to a woman whose blood pressure is already high, even though she may not be having a painful labor. If your blood pressure suddenly drops, you feel sick and faint and may vomit. This sudden lowering of blood pressure affects the baby too, since the oxygen-bearing blood supply is pumping more weakly and slowly through the placenta. If your blood pressure drops and causes fetal distress, you will be given an oxygen mask to get more oxygen to the baby.

Epidural techniques and drug dosages vary in different countries. In many countries, a continuous infusion pump is almost always used and the dose of bupivacaine is kept low, to reduce side effects. But because drug cocktails are often given, there are new side effects from these other drugs.

To reduce the risk of a sudden drop in blood pressure, intravenous fluids are given very fast before the epidural. This increases your blood volume. If blood pressure drops significantly, another drug is given to raise the blood pressure. Excessive intravenous fluids can sometimes cause postpartum swelling.

Having an epidural may start a chain of procedures that you did not bargain for. Because an epidural makes labor last longer, you may have oxytocin to augment labor and you will have continuous fetal monitoring. There is an increased risk of ending up with a Cesarean section.* This appears to be greatest if a woman has the epidural before she has reached 5 cm dilation. Because you have no feeling in your bladder, it needs to be emptied by catheter. And because you may not feel any urge to push, the obstetrician may need to rotate the fetal head with forceps or manually.*

Since there is an increased chance of forceps delivery once an epidural has been given, you may want to refuse a replenishment and let the anesthetic wear off as you reach the very end of the first stage of labor. But if you have not felt the first-stage contractions at all and then suddenly have to cope with the long, hefty ones as you approach full dilation, you may find the experience completely overpowering.

Do not push just because you are fully dilated. Always breathe your way through contractions, which you can feel as waves of pressure, until the baby's head is well down on your perineum. If you push just because you think that you ought to be pushing, you are more likely to have deep transverse arrest of the baby's head, because with an epidural the natural tone of the pelvic floor muscles is lost. These muscles help the baby's head to rotate as it descends against them. If you have deep transverse arrest, you will need a forceps or vacuum extractor delivery.

An epidural multiplies the chance that your baby will get stuck in an occipito-posterior (see page 270) or transverse position.* Obstetricians often tackle this problem by setting up an oxytocin intravenous drip to make the uterus work harder, in the hope of avoiding the need for an assisted delivery later on. You can, however, do something about this yourself, and will reduce the risk of deep transverse arrest by more than half if you wait until the baby's head can be seen before starting to push. What you need most at this point is time, because, after an epidural and with a first labor, it may take two hours or longer from when you are fully dilated for this to happen.*

One side effect of having an epidural is that your temperature rises, which can make you feel very uncomfortable. Being overheated can be bad for the baby, too. Moreover, when a woman has a fever in labor, investigations are made to find out if she and the newborn baby are suffering from an infection, and the baby may be treated for infection "just in case." This means observation in the special care nursery, and the baby may be given intravenous antibiotics.

Epidurals may have long-term side effects for you, too. A small proportion of women have problems with backaches, migraines, neck aches, or numb areas of skin after an epidural.*

An epidural anesthetic passes into the baby within ten minutes. Studies are still being carried out on the possible effects of an epidural on the newborn.* Some suggest that the baby becomes nervous and jittery, while others show that the baby is very drowsy after delivery.* This may vary according to the drug and the dosage, how long the epidural is in place, and the condition of the fetus before the epidural is given. If you decide to have an epidural, bear in mind that some of the difficulty you might have in coping with the baby in the week or so after the birth could be connected with the effect of the anesthetic on the baby. It does not mean that you are an incompetent mother. You will soon be over this difficult period and everything will get much easier.

SPINAL BLOCK

This is used for Cesarean sections. Local anesthetic is given by injection into the cerebrospinal fluid in the lower spine, in more or less the same way as for an epidural. The effect is to numb you from the mid-chest down. Today, anesthetists use ultrathin needles to inject the anesthetic, with the result that post-spinal headaches (which used to be a major problem) are rare. This technique works well and has the major advantage of speed.

MOBILE OR "WALKING" EPIDURALS To achieve an epidural so that you retain some feeling in your legs and can move a little (also called a spinal/epidural), the drug bupivacaine is given in smaller doses than when full anesthesia is required, and this is combined with an opiate drug.

1. The first dose of anesthetic—half as much as usual—is injected into the subarachnoid space where cerebrospinal fluid circulates. A very fine spinal needle is used. This reduces the risk of your suffering a post-dural puncture headache.

2. Opioids and local anesthetics are injected into both the subarachnoid and epidural spaces. Again, when a drug cocktail that includes opioids is given, the bupivacaine can be cut by more than half.

3. Epidural injections are repeated when needed, or the drug is given by continuous infusion pump. Having "refills" reduces the drug dose by 35 percent compared with an epidural infusion.

Advantages of lower drug doses are that you can move around in bed, and possibly walk. But mobile epidurals can make you feel dizzy, your legs may feel rubbery, and you are unable to walk around, so you should have someone with you all the time and should not leave the labor room unaccompanied. There is less need to catheterize your bladder, and a mobile epidural reduces the risk of long-term backaches and possibly the need for assisted delivery. The problem is that there is still a high chance that you will have a forceps or vacuum delivery.*

WHAT WOMEN THINK ABOUT EPIDURALS

My own research into epidurals reveals that women are sharply divided in their opinions about them. In my study of women's experiences, many were very happy with their epidurals and said things like "It was a miracle!" and "It was pure magic." But, 18 percent of women very much regretted having had the epidural and said, in effect, "Never again!"*

Women praise epidurals when: it was their own decision, and theirs alone, to have one; they felt that they were among friends in the delivery room; the epidural provided them with effective pain relief; there was minimal other intervention; and they managed to push the baby out unaided. *Women are highly critical of epidurals when*: they felt that they could not make a free choice about having one; they did not feel that they were in an emotionally supportive environment; the epidural was not effective; delivery was by for-

"IF I HAD KNOWN WHAT I DO NOW ABOUT EPIDURALS I WOULDN'T HAVE AGREED TO IT, BUT IT WAS PRESENTED AS ENTIRELY RISK-FREE AND WITHOUT SIDE EFFECTS."

ceps; and there were side effects—they felt sick and dizzy, suffered headaches, or had long-term problems, such as pain or numbness, which they attributed to the epidural.

CAUDAL A caudal is like an epidural, except that it is injected into the epidural space around the sacrum and blocks only that area, rather than the larger area blocked by an epidural. A greater dose of anesthetic is necessary for a caudal than with an epidural, and a caudal is not of much use in the first stage of labor. It is usually given for short-term pain relief during a very difficult second stage of labor. It is uncommon in modern obstetric practice.

THE FUTURE OF DRUGS IN CHILDBIRTH

Hospitals should provide an environment and the kind of personal care in which each woman is free to accept or reject pain-relieving drugs as and when she wishes to do so. Whatever drugs are given, their effects and possible side effects on you and the baby should be fully explained, and your consent should always be obtained beforehand.

Unfortunately, drugs are often used in place of loving emotional support and encouragement and one-to-one care. Fear, anxiety, loneliness, and the feeling that you are part of a factory for producing babies all increase the experience of pain. Understanding what is happening inside you and what is being done to help you and your baby, being able to move freely, having nonpharmacological ways of handling pain, knowing what you can do to help yourself, feeling you are among friends, and having someone you love with you all make pain much easier to bear.

Pain-relieving drugs almost invariably have an effect on the progress of labor, and often prolong it or make an operative delivery more likely. This may be a price worth paying. It is up to you to decide. Nobody else should make the decision for you. Modern obstetric anesthesia, used only when necessary, is fairly safe for the baby, but little is really known about the effects, short- and long-term, on the child. One consultant anesthetist warns that "numerous questions about the effects of drugs given to the mother on mother–baby interaction and future child development require an answer,"* and stresses that long-term studies should be carried out to assess exactly what risks are being taken. For the present, this remains a largely unexplored field of research.

TOWARD THE MEDICAL CONTROL OF BIRTH

You have the right to decide what happens to your body before, during, and after childbirth. You are not bound, either by law or out of politeness, to agree to procedures and investigations to which you object. If things are done without your consent, it is a form of assault on your body.

It is worth remembering when you are in labor that your consent is implied when you are forewarned about an obstetric intervention and concur by remaining silent. Also, you are entitled to full information about anything that is done to you and your baby, and can reasonably expect to be able to ask questions and be given honest answers. You may also want time to think through the available alternatives, and should not be rushed into agreeing to any treatment that is proposed. If you do not ask questions, the professionals may assume that you do not want to know any more, and even that to offer further information might make you uncomfortable.

"I WAS MADE TO LIE FLAT ON MY BACK FOR HOURS. I FELT LIKE A LUMP OF MEAT, BEING POKED AND PRODDED AS IF MY BODY DIDN'T BELONG TO ME."

If birth is to be a fulfilling and satisfying experience, the important thing is to feel in control of what happens to you and your baby. Once you are secure in that knowledge, you can "let go" and allow your body to work freely. You are not fighting it or trying to rein in the power that is released from your uterus. Women are sometimes blamed for approaching birth with expectations that are "too high." But research into psychological outcomes of birth reveals that feeling cheated or let down has nothing to do with having had rosy expectations of birth that are destroyed by the grim reality of labor. In fact, women are more likely to be disappointed in their birth experiences when they did not expect much anyway. How you feel about the birth afterward has to do with human relationships. You are much more likely to have a positive birth experience if you are able to get the information you want, discuss everything fully, and share in all decisions that are made.*

YOUR RIGHT TO CHOOSE

In all medical procedures, it is a question of carefully balancing the relative risks of a policy of intervention on the one hand and one of "wait and see" on the other. To make an informed choice you may value the counsel of skilled professionals, but ultimately you make the decision. This applies to both *where* and *how* you have your baby. If you want natural childbirth, go all out to get it. Plan for it, prepare yourself for it, and do everything you can to create the right setting for it. But also be flexible, so that if something in your physical condition, or that of your baby, indicates that modern technology can be used to advantage, you will not miss out on its undoubted benefits, even if this means that the birth is less "natural."

A woman having a baby has responsibilities as well as rights. One of the most important of these is the responsibility to give the baby the best possible start in life. Some obstetricians believe that whenever a machine or a procedure is available that permits greater medical control of childbirth, it ought to be used. An equally valid view is that one should be selective in the use of technology, employing it where necessary, but bearing in mind that birth is also a psychological experience that affects the relationship among mother, father, and baby—perhaps for a long time afterward.

THE BEST ENVIRONMENT FOR BIRTH

The highest-quality childbirth and the best welcome for the baby must include emotional as well as medical aspects of birth. If you accept medical help, it does not follow that you relinquish concern about the psychological dimensions of the experience. Technology need not, and should not, be permitted to ruin a woman's experience of birth. When machines are used in place of warm and friendly human relations, they seem to take over. But when they take second place to emotional support and encouragement, and you feel free to reach your own decisions about how much aid to accept, they can be a useful adjunct to good care, especially when the risk to a baby is considered higher than usual.

Many couples can bear witness to ways in which sophisticated apparatus made them feel more secure in childbirth and helped rather than hindered. But for this to happen, the environment provided for birth has to be a very special one, and all those coming into contact with the expectant parents need to be able to give of themselves, not only lending their technical skills. For it is only in such a setting that there can be trust, honesty, and self-confidence.

THE GROWING USE OF TECHNOLOGY

Obstetricians are discovering new ways of controlling a process that in the past was left to nature. Many now say, "Why stand by watching and intervene only when something goes wrong?" and believe that, instead, labor should be regulated from start to finish. To do this effectively, they need to be able to monitor exactly what is happening in the uterus and to the fetus at every second, and to intervene at any point to ensure that cervical dilation, the strength of contractions, and the biochemical state of mother and fetus conform to a predetermined norm. This is called *active management of labor.**

There are many technologies on the market that obstetricians, eager to reduce the perinatal mortality rate, want to buy for their units. Some women hate this intrusion of machinery into what they feel should be a natural process, and question its benefits. Others find security in thinking that labor is controlled by the obstetrician and the machinery. They like knowing exactly when the birth day will be, and are relieved to know that labor will not last longer than 12 hours at most. There is no standard recipe that will suit all women.

COMMON PROCEDURES

The usual way to assess the progress of labor is by vaginal examination. The midwife is able to estimate the dilation of the cervix by inserting two gloved fingers through the vagina into the os, the mouth of the cervix. The examining fingers can also detect how soft the tissues of the cervix are, whether the baby is head down, how far the head has descended, and which part of the head is presenting.

The drawbacks to vaginal examinations are that they disturb your concentration, may be painful, can feel threatening, and introduce the risk of infection. However, some women like to be told that the cervix is dilating well and ask for an examination. Especially when you are in an undrugged state, an experienced midwife who has remained with

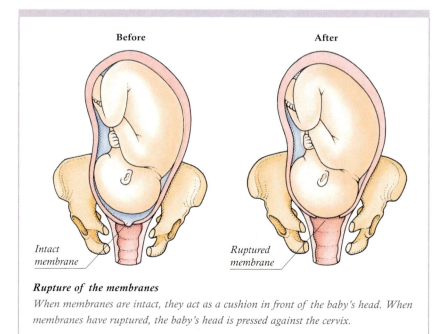

Before　　　　　**After**

Intact
membrane

Ruptured
membrane

Rupture of the membranes
When membranes are intact, they act as a cushion in front of the baby's head. When membranes have ruptured, the baby's head is pressed against the cervix.

you should be able to assess the progress of labor by observing the whole woman—this includes your facial expressions, movements, breathing, and any other sounds you are making—rather than relying on frequent vaginal examinations.*

When you arrive at the hospital, it may be assumed that you will have an amniotomy, be linked to a fetal monitor, and be hooked up to an intravenous drip. During the second stage, an episiotomy may be performed to hasten delivery. Some women experience many kinds of intervention during their labor, and unless you say that you do not want your labor controlled in this way, there is a chance that you will have at least one of them.

ARTIFICIAL RUPTURE OF THE MEMBRANES

Artificial rupture of the membranes (AROM or ARM), or amniotomy, has come to be accepted as a normal routine in many hospitals and is sometimes performed when you are admitted. If you don't want your membranes artificially ruptured, you can say so. It should not be done until you are in active labor (more than 4 cm dilated). The membranes surrounding the fetus are punctured with a small tool rather like a crochet hook, which is introduced through the open cervix.

When membranes are allowed to rupture spontaneously, they tend to do so toward the end of the first stage.* In 12 percent of women they remain intact until the birth. Some membranes rupture spontaneously when the midwife or doctor touches them during a vaginal examination.

"I WAS ASKED WHETHER I WANTED THE WATERS BROKEN AT FOUR CENTIMETERS, SO I CHOSE NOT TO HAVE THIS DONE. I ALSO STATED THAT I DIDN'T WANT AN EPISIOTOMY, NOR ANALGESICS IF I FELT THAT I WAS COPING. THESE DECISIONS WERE SUPPORTED BY THE MIDWIFE."

Since there are no nerve endings in the membranes, their rupture is not painful. All you feel is a gush of warm liquid. Be prepared for contractions to increase in intensity after this has happened. ARM can shorten labor by 30–45 minutes if the membranes have still not ruptured spontaneously by the end of the first stage, since the baby's head presses harder against the cervix once the cushion of fluid is gone. This produces a rush of oxytocin in your system, which triggers the start of strong contractions.

REASONS FOR AMNIOTOMY

Besides being a part of induction, rupturing the membranes also allows the obstetrician to assess the state of the amniotic fluid. When a fetus is in distress, it passes meconium, the first contents of the bowels, into the amniotic fluid, which is easily seen when the fluid is released. So amniotomy can sometimes be an important part of the assessment of the condition of the baby. Once the procedure has been done, an electrode may be inserted into the skin of your baby's scalp to provide a reliable record of the heartbeat (see pages 340–344). But with recent improvements in the technology of abdominal heart rate sensors, it is unusual to need to use a scalp electrode.

In some countries, obstetricians prefer to use an amnioscope in order to examine the amniotic fluid while still keeping the membrane intact. A cone-shaped instrument with a fiber-optic light positioned inside it is introduced through the vagina and cervix. Although it may be very uncomfortable, this technique is less invasive than ARM.

RISKS OF ROUTINE AMNIOTOMY

Inside the amniotic membrane, the baby is well protected against any kind of infection, and its head, body, and umbilical cord are all cushioned from compression. A routine amniotomy, on the other hand, carries some risks.

PRESSURE ON THE CORD Intact membranes protect the baby's head. The amniotic fluid equalizes pressure on the head, and amniotomy takes away the cushion of water in which the fetus lies, thus exposing its head to the direct effect of contractions. Rupture of the membranes also gives rise to the possibility of pressure on the cord, which may hinder the flow of blood through it. It is not rare for a baby to have the cord around its neck, and without the cushion provided by the amniotic fluid, these babies are particularly vulnerable to pressure on the cord. It has also been suggested that once the amniotic fluid is gone, the fetal surface of the placenta is compressed, which may reduce the flow of blood to and from the baby.*

INFECTION Amniotomy increases the possibility of an infection called chorioamniotitis that occurs in the membranes during labor.* This infection can extend into the uterine muscle and make contractions weak (metritis). The baby shows signs of infection, too, either during labor or after delivery.

Another risk factor is a bacterium called group B streptococcus (GBS) that about 30 percent of women carry in their normal genital and rectal flora. This infection is particularly severe in the newborn, causing pneumonia and meningitis. One prevention strategy is to test mothers for the bacteria around 35 to 36 weeks and give antibiotics intravenously during labor to those who test positive.

DECELERATION OF THE BABY'S HEARTBEAT Some studies have shown that after amniotomy there are more early decelerations of the baby's heartbeat. These occur at the start of a contraction, and the heart is back to normal by the end of the contraction. The slowing down is slight, by less than 40 beats a minute. Many obstetricians consider this quite normal.* Because babies who are born after amniotomy are generally in good condition, with high Apgar scores (see page 370), some doctors have concluded that the procedure does not subject the fetus to any special stress.

A TYPICAL HOSPITAL PARTOGRAM

This is a series of graphs used to record the main events of labor. It is used to isolate problems, as a record of progress, and is useful for any new staff who come on duty.

Fetal heart rate (FHR)

Charted in beats per minute, with 120 to 160 beats considered normal. (Any deceleration is shown as an arrow down to the lowest level.) The condition of the amniotic fluid (waters) is also recorded. I means "intact"; C means "clear."

Cervical dilatation / abdominal descent

The degree of dilation (X) is noted every 3 or 4 hours and a curve is drawn. If there is a two-hour delay compared with the norm, the doctor stimulates the labor with a pitocin drip. The descent of the baby's head through the pelvis (O) is also indicated.

Drugs

Any drugs given are noted on the partogram chart. In this case, Entonox (gas and oxygen) was given for pain relief and syntometrine to stimulate the delivery of the placenta.

Contractions

Frequency, strength (by shading), and length of contractions in seconds are shown.

Blood pressure and pulse

The mother's blood pressure and pulse are recorded. The upper level recorded is the systolic pressure, the lower one the diastolic.

Temperature

The mother's temperature is also taken and recorded on the partogram.

Mother's details

Facts about the mother are recorded including: her last period (LMP); the estimated date of delivery (EDD); when the membranes ruptured (two hours before birth).

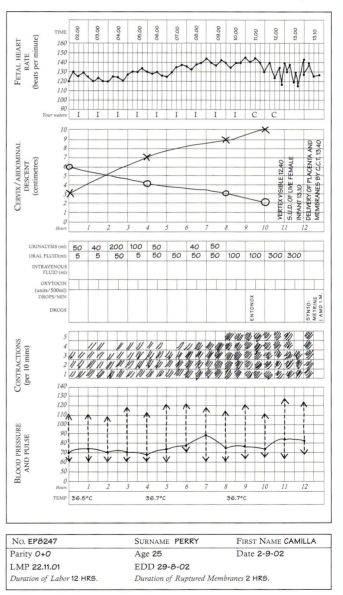

No. EP8247	SURNAME PERRY	FIRST NAME CAMILLA
Parity 0+0	Age 25	Date 2-9-02
LMP 22.11.01	EDD 29-8-02	
Duration of Labor 12 HRS.	*Duration of Ruptured Membranes* 2 HRS.	

HEAD MOLDING Some obstetricians are concerned about head molding and disalignment of the cranial bones, which may be increased after amniotomy. There is disagreement about this.

So amniotomy raises many questions that have yet to be answered. You can, if you wish, request that amniotomy be done only if the baby is showing signs of distress.

THE INTRAVENOUS DRIP

In almost all hospitals in the United States and many in Great Britain, an intravenous drip is set up for most women in labor. A fine catheter (hollow tube) is introduced into a vein in your arm or hand and fixed with adhesive tape so that fluids can be infused straight into your bloodstream. The argument for setting up a drip is that once a vein is open, emergency action can be taken rapidly and your strength can be kept up without your needing to eat or, sometimes, even drink anything. This means that if a Cesarean section turns out to be necessary (see pages 348–355) and a general anesthetic is used, your stomach is likely to be almost empty already and there is not much risk that you will regurgitate and inhale its contents. If need be, to lower the risk even further, you can have an antacid drink to reduce the acidity of your stomach contents.

"I AGREED TO HAVE A GLUCOSE DRIP BECAUSE I HAD BEEN IN LABOR FOR A LONG TIME AND WAS FEELING EXTREMELY TIRED. BUT I DIDN'T AGREE TO INTRAVENOUS PITOCIN."

Forcing women to go through labor without eating or drinking is bad policy.* It medicalizes the birth experience and is unnecessary. Labor is hard work. In the early phases, especially, you may get hungry and should be able to eat whatever you want. And you will certainly be thirsty and should feel free to drink.

Dextrose, a glucose solution, or "Ringer's lactate" solution containing electrolytes and water may be given through a drip to act as a "pick-me-up" in labor. Since it bypasses the stomach, you do not have to digest it. Dextrose may be useful if labor is long and you are becoming dehydrated, or if lactic acid builds up in the course of a difficult labor, causing acetone to appear in the urine—an indication that your body is short of glucose. But a dextrose drip can lead to hypoglycemia (low blood sugar) in your baby after birth.

If you have a drip set up, it is especially important to remember to empty your bladder regularly: every hour is not too frequent. You will be accumulating fluid and should urinate frequently to prevent urine from building up in your bladder.

Once a drip is in place, other substances can be introduced by the same route. If other drugs are given, make sure that you understand why. No extra medications should be given without your agreement. Oxytocin in its synthetic form, pitocin, is the most common drug. You can find more information about this in the section on induced labor on pages 334–339. Other medicines and opioids are also given via the drip. You need not consent to an intravenous drip unless you are confident that there are good reasons for it. It is another way in which women can be made physically uncomfortable in labor. The drip can be very helpful when needed, but it makes it difficult for you to move. In most hospitals where intravenous drips are administered as a matter of course, it is taken for granted that the woman in labor stays in bed.

EPISIOTOMY

An episiotomy is a surgical cut made to enlarge the birth opening. It is done with scissors, under local anesthetic, just before the baby is born. It can be midline (down from the bottom of the vagina toward the anus, at the place where small, "natural" tears often occur) or mediolateral (sloping out to the side, away from the anus, or down and then out again in the shape of a hockey stick). In Great Britain, the episiotomy is usually mediolateral, which can be more painful and cause more bleeding. Mediolateral incisions are done less often in North America, but midline episiotomies may make damage to the anal sphincter more likely.

Since the incision is made through both skin and muscle, careful repair of the wound must be made afterward. The local anesthetic given before the episiotomy is usually enough for the repair. If not, more can be given. This

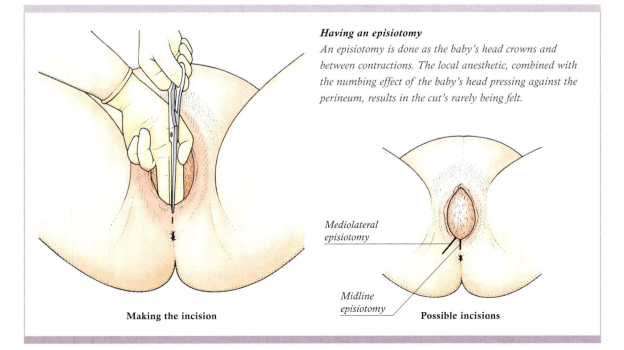

Having an episiotomy

An episiotomy is done as the baby's head crowns and between contractions. The local anesthetic, combined with the numbing effect of the baby's head pressing against the perineum, results in the cut's rarely being felt.

Mediolateral episiotomy

Midline episiotomy

Making the incision

Possible incisions

requires a few minutes to take effect, and the doctor or midwife should wait until the area is fully anesthetized before stitching the wound. The suturing is done with a curved needle, and it may take as long as an hour to sew up a mediolateral episiotomy or one that has been extended by tearing. Stitching a midline episiotomy is usually quicker, because there is a natural dividing line between muscles in the midline, which makes the repair much simpler to carry out. The stitches can be left in if they are the kind that dissolve, but you should have a look at the area in a mirror every couple of days to make sure that they have disappeared, since sometimes they do not drop out and become embedded in tissue. If you are sitting on thorns, the stitches should be snipped out by a midwife on or before the tenth day after the birth.

After an episiotomy, your perineum is likely to be very tender, swollen, and sore for days, or even weeks. Ask for a local anesthetic spray to apply to the area. This really helps.*

REASONS FOR EPISIOTOMY

Some obstetricians still believe that all first-time mothers should have an episiotomy to relieve strain on their tissues and get the baby delivered quickly. When there are signs of fetal distress, an episiotomy can speed delivery and make birth easier for the baby. You may be told that it is a good idea to have an episiotomy because "a straight, clean cut is better than a nasty, jagged tear," which is more difficult to sew up. Sometimes episiotomy is done in an attempt to prevent damage to tissues inside the vagina when there is evidence of "buttonhole" tearing (that is, a series of very tiny lacerations deep inside).

Routine episiotomy is still favored by many North American obstetricians and those on the European continent, but has practically disappeared in British hospitals. Episiotomy rates fell dramatically in the 1980s, not because of research that proved it was harmful, but because of women's outspoken criticism of the practice. In the 1970s, almost 100 percent of women had episiotomies in certain hospitals in Great Britain; now the proportion has dropped to below 14 percent. Research followed from women's protests. Moreover, as soon as a research project investigating episiotomy was begun in any hospital, the rate dropped by about a third, even before any results were obtained.*

PROBLEMS WITH EPISIOTOMY

Trials conducted in Dublin, Montreal,* and Argentina* revealed that women with an intact perineum, or only a superficial tear, experience less pain after childbirth than those who have undergone an episiotomy. Pain after an episiotomy is about the same as that from a second-degree tear (one that affects the underlying muscle). Women are also more likely to suffer severe tears into the anus with an episiotomy than when they have not had one.* Another trial, in England, as well as the Montreal trial, showed that there is no advantage to episiotomy over a first- or second-degree tear.*

Many women say that they feel terribly uncomfortable when making love for several months after an episiotomy, and they tend to resume intercourse later than women who have had a tear.

There are other problems with episiotomy: if done too early—before the perineum has thinned out—it can cause unnecessary bleeding; sometimes the cut is much larger than a tear would have been; and often the stitches get infected and antibiotics are necessary.*

With skilled guidance at delivery and a gentle birth (see pages 356–367), more and more women are now giving birth with no injury to the perineum—and this makes an enormous difference to how they feel in the days and weeks after the baby is born.

MANAGING THE THIRD STAGE

The third stage of labor is routinely managed by awaiting signs of separation and then using controlled cord traction to hurry the process along. Only after the placenta is expelled is medication given, usually pitocin by injection or intravenous drip. If there is no sign of separation after 30 minutes or so, the placenta may be trapped by the powerfully contracting uterus, and manual removal is considered.

If the placenta is left to separate naturally, it may take about half an hour or longer. Clamping of the cord immediately at delivery may make the chances of a retained placenta more likely. If the cord is not clamped

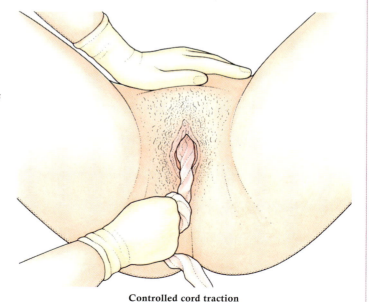

Cord traction

After the birth of your baby, your uterus continues to contract strongly to expel the placenta. You may be asked to push the placenta out, once it has peeled off the wall of the uterus, by pushing against the doctor's or midwife's hand placed against your lower abdomen, while he or she gently pulls on the cord with the other hand.

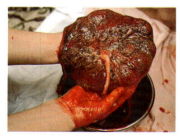

A healthy placenta

Controlled cord traction

until after it has stopped pulsating, there is much less chance of a retained placenta. This is because when the cord is clamped, blood cannot flow out of it, which would encourage the now defunct placenta to peel away from the uterine wall. A blood-packed placenta stays firm and full and is less likely to separate.

Your first physical contact with your baby produces a rush of emotion that is accompanied by the release of oxytocin. This natural oxytocin rush keeps the uterus firm and causes further contractions. Once the placenta has separated, the doctor or midwife gently places one flat hand over your lower tummy, just above the pubic bone, and you push against the hand, in order to deliver the placenta and membranes. It often helps to have a hand to push against like this. The doctor or midwife may use her other hand to gently pull on the cord. The alternative is to squat over a bowl or pail and to deliver the placenta with the help of gravity.

There is no reason for the cord to be clamped before the placenta has been delivered except for convenience, although sometimes the cord is so short that it is impossible for the mother to hold her baby unless it is cut first; or it is twisted in a succession of loops around the baby's neck and is cut so that the baby can slide out. If a woman is Rh negative with an Rh positive baby (see page 113), there is a case for delayed cord clamping. If the cord is clamped while still pulsating, fetal blood is retained in the placenta, blood vessels rupture as the uterus contracts, and the chances of Rh positive blood being pushed back into the mother's bloodstream are greatly increased.

INDUCED LABOR

When labor begins naturally, the uterus becomes sensitive to hormones present in your bloodstream at the end of pregnancy. When labor is induced, the doctor tries to obtain a similar result by flooding your system with hormones, until they reach a level much higher than that which occurs naturally. This is done by introducing synthetic hormones into your bloodstream through a continuous intravenous drip, or by inserting prostaglandin suppositories into your vagina. Both methods are usually combined with artificial rupture of the membranes.

INDUCTION PROCEDURES

Induction rates have greatly increased in the past few years in the U.S. You have the right to receive full details of exactly what is going to be done to you and why before being admitted to the hospital for induction, and you can choose to accept or refuse the treatment once you know all the facts. Ask for printed information so you can read up on induction of labor.

STRIPPING THE MEMBRANES Some doctors or midwives strip the membranes to stimulate labor. This is done by pushing the membranes away from the cervix by hand. It is rather uncomfortable, but may start things off. It is usually referred to as "stretch and sweep."

ARTIFICIAL RUPTURE OF THE MEMBRANES (see page 327) This may be performed as the only means of induction if your cervix is already starting to dilate. Most obstetricians believe that once the membranes are ruptured, the baby should be born within 24 hours, because there is some risk of infection if labor is long-drawn-out. So you need to be aware that if labor is started by ARM but is slow to get going, it may then be accelerated with hormones.

PROSTAGLANDIN INSERTS/GEL There are two forms of prostaglandin approved by the Food and Drug Administration (FDA) for labor induction: a gel (Prepidil), and a small plastic insert (Cervidil), which has a tail like a tampon so it is removable. While introducing these prostaglandins may not start labor, they help to ripen and efface a firm, thick cervix, making it more likely to dilate when pitocin is given. If they are inserted in the evening, labor may have started by the following morning. It may be unnecessary to have amniotomy (see page 327) and a pitocin drip. Prostaglandins have the advantage of allowing you freedom to move about in labor.

PITOCIN DRIP If induction involves being connected to a pitocin drip, ask for it to be placed in the arm or hand you use less. If the connecting tube is short, you will not be able to move your arm easily or change position without dislodging it. There is no reason for it to be short, and you can ask for it to be securely fixed so that you can still change position. Many women have discovered that they get a backache simply from lying in one position for too long, quite apart from the backache caused by contractions. A glucose solution may be passed through the drip first. The infusion can be slowed or stopped once contractions are effective and the cervix is 5 cm dilated. You can ask the obstetrician to do this. But the plastic cannula in your vein is usually kept in until after the end of the third stage, in case the drug is needed to control bleeding from the uterus by making it contract hard.

> **"I FOUND IT SO MUCH EASIER TO BE UPRIGHT AND MOVING THAT I GOT OUT OF THE BED AND WALKED AROUND ATTACHED TO THE INTRAVENOUS DRIP STAND."**

MISOPRISTOL This is a very powerful drug that makes labor especially painful and can cause uterine rupture, especially if a woman's uterus is already scarred from a Cesarean section. The U.S. manufacturers warn that Cytotec (the patent name) "may cause the uterus to rupture in pregnant women if it is used to induce labor." Clinical trials were stopped in the U.S.

after some women hemorrhaged, had to have hysterectomies, and even died. The Cochrane Database, in its 2002 review, states that the drug "cannot be recommended for routine use . . . further research is needed to establish safety." It adds, significantly, that "information on women's views is conspicuously lacking."

WHEN INDUCTION MAY HELP

Induction is useful when a baby must be born without delay. Many doctors believe that between 15 and 25 percent of labors benefit from either induction or acceleration. Some believe that these figures are too high, while a few contend that 60 percent or more of labors ought to be induced. Significant preeclampsia (see page 141), for example, including high blood pressure, albumin in the urine, sudden excessive weight gain, and edema (puffiness resulting from fluid retention), is a good reason for induction, since the baby may not continue to be well nourished in your uterus if the pregnancy is allowed to go on.

INDUCTION BEFORE THE EDD Some babies stop growing because the placenta, through which they receive nourishment and oxygen, is not working well at the end of pregnancy. This may occur even before there is any question of being "overdue," although the mother may be feeling fit and healthy. Such babies may flourish better outside the uterus and may be at risk if they remain inside.

INDUCTION AFTER THE EDD Between 10 and 12 percent of women go two weeks or more "overdue" (known as "post-dates"), but in only 1 percent is there evidence of postmaturity (the baby's skin is dry and peeling and the fingernails need cutting). In cases where no ultrasound was performed, the estimated date of delivery may be wrong. Alternatively, entirely normal biological variations in the length of pregnancy may be ignored. Growing a baby is not a factory process.

Having said this, there is an increasing tendency for obstetricians to advise induction of labor once women have gone beyond 8 or 10 days past their "proven" EDD. This is an area where obstetric opinion is deeply divided,* and you should certainly not feel pressured into being induced.

If you are 43 weeks pregnant, there is a chance that the placenta is not functioning so well because it is aging. However, you need to be sure that the baby really is overdue before induction. Fetal movement is an important natural sign of fetal well-being. Ultrasound can be used to check the flow of blood to the baby (Doppler scan) and the amount of amniotic fluid, and although these are not totally reliable tests, they may reassure you. Many women are sufficiently aware of their bodies and of their babies to feel instinctively that all is going well and so do not wish to be induced, and sensible obstetricians respect this self-awareness.

THE LENGTH OF INDUCED LABORS

Although you may have a rapid labor with induction, this cannot be guaranteed. Some obstetricians prefer labors not to last longer than ten, eight, or even five hours and deliver with forceps or by Cesarean section if labor is prolonged beyond that fixed point. When a policy of routine induction is introduced into a hospital, there is a large increase in the number of instrumental deliveries and Cesarean sections performed. Also, the proportion of babies with low Apgar scores (see page 370) goes up—evidence that a policy of routine induction is bad for babies as well as mothers.* Since there is so much variation in obstetric policy, it is a good idea when discussing the possibility of induction with the doctor to ask what his or her practice is. This may affect your decision about whether to agree to induction if it is not urgently necessary.

> **"I DECLINED THE OFFER OF INDUCTION AT FORTY-TWO WEEKS AND ASKED FOR SOME TESTS TO BE DONE INSTEAD. THE BABY WAS FINE, AND I WENT INTO LABOR THE NEXT DAY."**

Induction is an intervention that, while useful when necessary, is not without risk, and the relative risks of leaving the baby inside your uterus and of inducing labor have to be assessed.

UNRIPE CERVIX It has been stated that "the major factor governing the success of induction is the state of the cervix."* When the cervix feels soft—like your lips when you hold your mouth slack—it is ripe and ready for labor. Unfortunately, induction is often done before the cervix is ripe, and in consequence the uterus may not respond to hormones. If the membranes have been ruptured, the process may lead inexorably to Cesarean section. In cases where an induction is necessary and the cervix is unripe, prostaglandin inserts over a period of several days may be used before pitocin is administered.

PAIN If the uterus is triggered to work harder, labor is more violent than when it starts naturally. There are often two "peaks" to each contraction, and each may last one minute or longer. Women who have had babies before, and whose previous labors were not induced, say that induced contractions start more powerfully and that there is not much lead-up to each contraction, but instead a sudden "explosion." There is only a short interval between contractions; just time to let out one relaxing breath, and then you are into the next one! You need to go straight into the breathing patterns you will have learned for half-dilation (see pages 205–213).

INTERRUPTED BLOOD FLOW Extremely strong contractions are likely to interfere with the blood flow through the uterus. In one study it was discovered that fetal distress was significantly more common in women taking pitocin, that babies were more likely to have low Apgar scores (see page 370), and that far more of them than usual went to the nursery for special care.*

If labor is induced, the baby's heart is monitored continuously. If you experience a contraction that lasts longer than 90 seconds, let the midwife know immediately. Even with a small dose of pitocin, some women have a prolonged contraction in which the uterus clamps down on itself—and on the baby. There is no test by which the sensitivity of your uterus to oxytocin can be known beforehand, so it is best to start with a small dose and gradually build up until good contractions result. The aim should be to simulate normal labor.

MEASURING CONTRACTIONS

One of the potential risks of induction is that the contractions may be far too strong, so that you and your baby become stressed or even distressed by them. One way of measuring their strength is by using an intrauterine pressure transducer. When the strength is known, and if the contractions are being driven by an oxytocin (pitocin) infusion, it is possible to slow down the rate of the infusion. This technique is more "user friendly" because you do not have a tight belt fixed around your tummy for hours on end. If excessive contractions are caused by prostaglandins, there is no option of "turning down" the drug dose, and in this case the only course of action is to give a relaxant drug by injection.

> "IT FELT AS IF I WAS HAVING ONE NONSTOP CONTRACTION. THE DOCTOR EXPLAINED THAT MY UTERUS HAD GONE INTO SPASM, SO THEY WERE TURNING THE DRIP OFF."

INDUCTION AND EPIDURAL ANESTHESIA

In some hospitals you may be offered a "package deal" of induction and an epidural. (For more about epidurals, see pages 319–323.) Having an induction increases your chance of needing an epidural, so do not feel under pressure to have one.

As with any intravenous drip, if you are receiving a large quantity of fluid, it is important that you remember to empty your bladder regularly. If you cannot urinate (and you often cannot if you have had an epidural), the nurse will insert a catheter and draw off the urine for you.

ELECTIVE INDUCTION

Sometimes called induction for convenience, elective induction is induction with no medical indication. The practice reached its peak in the 1970s, and unfortunately there are still doctors who think it is the only way in which labor can be efficiently managed. Their reasoning is that it is important for women to be in labor when doctors and midwives are on duty, that hospital organization is easier when it is known how many women will be in labor each day, and that it is better if women are not in labor at night. Although there will still be women who go into labor spontaneously at inconvenient times, the belief is that the earlier they are induced, the less likely this is to happen.

In recent years there has been a shift in opinion. After considering the findings of research, the Food and Drug Administration withdrew approval for the use of pitocin for the elective induction of labor, asserting that it can expose both mother and baby to unnecessary danger. Fewer and fewer obstetricians now believe that induction without clear indication has any merit.

COPING WITH INDUCTION

Whatever your personal views about induction or acceleration of labor—and what that says about our increasingly technological style of labor and birth in the West—it is often a different matter if your doctor says that you should be induced.

Many women have enjoyed induced labors and coped with them well. But unfortunately many whose labors were induced say that they did not have any choice and that they were given inadequate information.

The important thing is to ask questions. Do not wait and hope that someone will explain things to you. Discuss it fully, learn about what might happen, and share in the decision-making rather than feeling it is all being decided for you. When you have the facts, take time to weigh them and choose what seems to be the best path, always leaving your mind open to new evidence that may later point to a different course of action. It is your baby and your body. Experts are there to help you, not to take over.

AUGMENTED LABOR

Labor is said to be augmented or accelerated when it has already started and then been speeded up by the use of an oxytocin (pitocin) drip. If a drip is used *before* the cervix has started to dilate progressively, even though you have felt contractions and have had a "false" labor or many Braxton Hicks contractions, your labor is being induced, not augmented. Labor may be augmented when there is uterine inertia or incoordination; that is, when the uterus is not working effectively (see page 285). If you are getting tired out with the stress of continued back pain, augmentation, perhaps surprisingly, may help you cope because it stimulates uterine action.

If it looks as if labor should be induced or augmented, there are a number of breathing skills you can use to help you deal with the challenge (see pages 205–213). Don't give up and hand yourself over to the doctors because have they have now "taken over." This is still your labor.

ACTIVE MANAGEMENT OF LABOR

This is a system of routinely controlling and hastening labor, and ensuring rapid and efficient uterine action. It is claimed that it cuts the Cesarean section rate. It was devised by obstetricians in the National Maternity Hospital in Dublin, Ireland, where 40 percent of women have their labors stimulated, and is increasingly popular with obstetricians all over the world.

"THE BIRTH WAS TURNED INTO A RACE AGAINST TIME, FOR NO REASON EXCEPT THAT THE OBSTETRICIAN BELIEVED THE BEST LABORS WERE THE FASTEST."

A woman is told that her labor will not be allowed to last longer than 12 hours, and if her cervix does not dilate by at least one centimeter every hour, the uterus will be stimulated artificially to work faster.

In Dublin, uterine stimulation is restricted to women giving birth for the first time. Its use is considered potentially dangerous for women who have already had babies—multigravidae.* In addition, an important part of labor management is one-to-one care from a personal midwife who usually stays with each woman until the baby is born.

Unfortunately, some obstetricians outside Dublin often use active management indiscriminately. They favor it for multigravidae as well as primigravidae (women having their first baby). And they neglect or forget that one-to-one care is part of the method, because it is administratively difficult. There is evidence, however, that it is not active management, but continuous one-to-one care, that reduces the need for Cesarean section.* Having a woman with you who has experience and who gives emotional support is the single most effective element in this method of labor management. The decision to have a birth partner with you is one of the best ways of keeping your labor normal and reducing the chances of a Cesarean.

ELECTRONIC FETAL MONITORING

An electronic fetal monitor (EFM) tracks the fetal heartbeat and records the pressure of the uterus. Either a transducer is placed over your abdomen near the baby's heart (external monitoring), or a spiral wire electrode is inserted through the open cervix and fastened to the baby's scalp (internal monitoring). A printout, usually in the form of a continuous graph on thermal paper, shows the baby's heart rate in relation to the work done by the uterus. The monitor is a compact box that amplifies the baby's heartbeat so that it is audible, and records the uterine contractions as peaks on a graph. It incorporates a flashing light that also registers the beating of the baby's heart and the contraction intensity, but this can be turned off. If anything goes wrong, the monitor sounds an alarm. This may indicate that there is something wrong with the machine rather than with the baby. Sometimes a nurse just kicks it and everything is all right again.

When EFM was invented in the 1970s, it was believed that it would make birth safer for babies, allowing fetal heart rates to be monitored constantly. But 12 prospective randomized controlled trials involving more than 55,000 babies in different countries have shown that it does not. Babies are just as safe when someone listens to the fetal heart after a contraction has finished and in the interval between contractions with a Pinard's stethoscope or a handheld Doppler machine. Babies who are intermittently monitored are no more likely to have low Apgar scores or go to the special care unit.* In fact, more babies suffer from cerebral palsy after EFM labors than when they are monitored intermittently. A study of EFM with babies who were being born preterm reveals a large and significant increase in cerebral palsy in the babies who were monitored, and no benefits.*

Research has shown that monitoring reduces the rate of neonatal seizures (fits). Some people concluded that this affirmed the value of continuous monitoring. Then it was revealed that this kind of neonatal seizure was not the type that produced long-term health problems, which occurred only in babies whose mothers received pitocin in labor.

The electronic fetal monitor shows when the next contraction is starting even before you feel it, so you can meet it with your breathing.

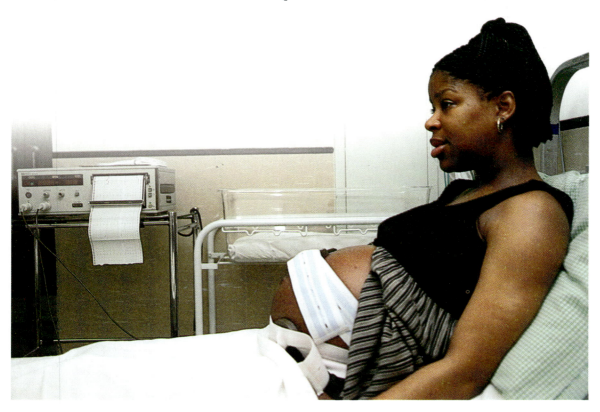

341

A major disadvantage of EFM is that it increases the Cesarean section rate by 160 percent, without any benefit to the baby.* This rate is reduced if fetal blood sampling is done before the decision to proceed to operative delivery, but there is still a 30 percent increase in the Cesarean section rate, again without any benefit to the baby.* Continuous monitoring also has a profound effect on the way that labor is conducted. With the monitoring setup, the woman is unable to move freely. She is more likely to be left alone at times during the labor, because the caregivers believe that the electronic equipment is doing the job of monitoring for them. She cannot use a birth pool or have transcutaneous electronic nerve stimulation for pain relief. For many women electronic monitoring makes the labor much more stressful than it need be.

ADMISSION MONITORING

Because of the unanswered questions about electronic monitoring, in many British hospitals it is used routinely only for 20 to 30 minutes when a woman is admitted to the hospital, and if all is well, no longer. Research shows that even this increases the risk of having a Cesarean.* So if you are healthy and pregnancy has gone well, you may want to say, "No, thank you."

THE EXTERNAL MONITOR

An external monitor has two straps that can be attached to your abdomen. One strap holds the tocodynamometer (the pressure gauge that records contractions). The other holds the ultrasound transducer that registers the baby's heartbeats.

THE INTERNAL MONITOR

The internal monitor, which is more accurate than the external monitor, is inserted through the vagina and cervix, and fixed to the skin of the baby's head. It is connected to a wire leading to the machine. An intrauterine pressure catheter is inserted into the uterus to record the pressure of contractions; or you may wear a single strap around your abdomen to hold the tocodynamometer. An internal monitor cannot be used until the membranes have ruptured and until the cervix is dilated at least 2 cm. It may increase the risk of infection.

ADVANTAGES OF MONITORING

The electronic monitor may be useful when labor is induced or augmented with a pitocin drip, since the length, power, and frequency of the contractions produced by the drip, and their effect on the baby, must be carefully observed lest they prove to be too stressful for the baby to cope with. Until recently, induction was often done "blind," and, as a result, enormous, turbulent contractions were produced that sometimes cut off the fetal blood supply. This is less likely today since, by monitoring these artificially aided births, it has been discovered that small amounts of pitocin are effective.

Another advantage of monitoring is that the monitor indicates when the next contraction is beginning, so that, however drowsy you are feeling, you can breathe out and relax and get ready to breathe over the contraction. Although you cannot get out of bed while you are wearing a monitor, you can make sure you are sitting comfortably in an upright position. This will help you when you use your breathing.

PROBLEMS OF MONITORING

Many women say that the abdominal strapping of the external monitor is very uncomfortable. Some even say that the pressure of the transducer on their tummies was the most painful thing about labor. Sometimes the internal electrode slips off the baby's head or, if an external monitor is used, the baby moves and its heartbeat is lost on the monitor. Some external monitors have transducers that track the position of the baby's heart so that they do not lose it in this way. As in the case of an intravenous drip, an external monitor requires you to remain more or less in one position lest the transducer slip off. This immobility results in discomfort for you and possible problems for the baby. So monitoring may sometimes produce the failing fetal heart rate that it then records. Do not allow the monitor to keep you from moving around within the range of the wires to which you are attached. The midwife can adjust the monitor when you move.

"I DIDN'T WANT A MONITOR THAT WOULD STOP ME FROM MOVING. SO THE MIDWIFE CHECKED REGULARLY WITH THE STETHOSCOPE INSTEAD."

Some women in labor are wired to the monitor only to find that nothing is being recorded at all because the machine is not operating. It is very irritating to be immobilized and connected to a machine when it cannot possibly be doing anything to help. Yet staff sometimes appear shocked at a woman's request for the transducer to be detached so that she can move around and get on with her labor unhindered. If this happens to you, you are entirely justified in insisting that the monitor be disconnected. However, when the monitor is working well, some women are reassured to know that every heartbeat of the baby is being recorded.

TELEMETRY

Monitoring by telemetry (radio waves) is an advance on the older method, allowing you to be up and around in labor, unattached to wires but continuously monitored at the same time. The equipment is not cumbersome and can be placed at some distance from you. Women prefer it, labors seem to go faster than with other methods of monitoring, and babies do better. Because you are able to stay upright, you may feel less pain, and the uterus can work more efficiently.

Even monitoring by telemetry can often be invasive, since internal monitoring methods are sometimes used. Any invasive technique (one that entails entering your body) introduces added risk of infection. This is a risk worth taking when there is reason to suspect that the baby is encountering difficulties, but not when everything seems to be straightforward.

A scalp electrode probably causes the baby some pain. It involves breaking the skin of the baby's scalp. It remains on the baby's head until after delivery, when it should be removed gently and deftly, not merely yanked. In 85 percent of newborn babies, a rash appears at the site of the electrode and in 20 percent a small abscess develops.* Sometimes the child is left with a permanent bald patch.

INTERPRETING THE DATA

Although it is estimated that the fetal monitor enables an obstetrician to save one life for every 1,000 babies monitored, the interpretation of data is of first importance. The machine itself can do nothing to make childbirth safer. It is only too easy to interpret normal variations in the fetal heart rate as pathological, sometimes because of the design of the machine, or to miss clinical signs that something is wrong because the monitor indicates that everything is normal. Obstetricians and midwives experienced in auscultating the fetal heart (listening with ultrasound or a Pinard's stethoscope) have a valuable skill that is neglected as more and more confidence is placed in electronic monitors.

Interpretation of electronic monitoring data sometimes causes more harm than good. Half of all babies show some irregularities of heartbeat during labor. Usually this is of no significance. We don't know how they manage it, but babies actually sleep during labor. They change from rapid eye movement (REM) or dreaming sleep to deep, quiet sleep for a period of up to 40 minutes, and then back again. As the sleep state varies, so the heart rate changes. In deep sleep the printout of the heart rate tends to be flat. Until deep sleep was understood, this trace made doctors anxious. But it has now been discovered that the baby only has to be roused a little for the heartbeat to pick up. One way of doing this is to touch the top of the baby's head. Mothers have their own ways of achieving the same result—changing position, for example—and this may reassure the doctors.

"THERE WAS SOME CONCERN ABOUT THE BABY'S HEART RATE BECAUSE IT WAS ABNORMALLY SLOW. THEN THEY FOUND THEY WERE PICKING UP MY HEARTBEAT, NOT THE BABY'S."

The baby's heart rate is usually between 120 and 160 beats per minute. A quicker rate than this is termed tachycardia, and a slower rate bradycardia. Incomplete understanding of the normal range of variation in the fetal heart rate during and between contractions leads to a great deal of intervention. Emergency Cesarean sections are often performed because of changes in the fetal heart rate that are judged to be signs of asphyxia. Yet more than 50 percent of babies delivered by Cesarean section turn out to be in good condition, so operating was unnecessary. What has actually occurred is a series of complex changes in the baby's heartbeat as a result of a normal catecholamine (stress hormone) surge. These alterations have then been misinterpreted as signs of fetal distress.

"I DIDN'T LIKE THEM PRICKING HER HEAD. BUT THE TEST SHOWED THAT SHE WAS FINE, SO I WAS ABLE TO GO AHEAD AND GIVE BIRTH MYSELF."

In Spain and Germany, when abnormal fetal heart patterns are recorded, obstetricians stop the uterus from contracting by introducing drugs into the mother's bloodstream. In all countries, electronic fetal monitoring has led to more forceps deliveries and Cesarean sections. The introduction of monitors in any hospital is always associated with a sharp increase in the rate of operative deliveries—although this tends to drop as staff become more aware of normal variations in the fetal heart rate.

The American College of Obstetricians and Gynecologists (ACOG), the Society of Obstetricians and Gynaecologists of Canada (SOGC), and now the British Royal College of Obstetricians and Gynaecologists (RCOG) support a policy of regular, frequent listening with an ultrasound stethoscope as equal or superior to electronic fetal heart monitoring in low-risk pregnancies. Despite this reversal of support for electronic fetal heart monitoring, most doctors and many midwives and nurses have not been well trained in auscultation, which also requires more staff time, and so continue to rely on EFM.

TESTING THE BABY'S BLOOD

If the fetal monitor suggests that the baby is under stress, the baby's blood should be tested in order to check the findings. If the baby is having difficulties, this shows up in the blood chemistry. But this testing is often not done. A biochemical test carried out in order to assess the pH level of the baby's blood cuts down the number of unnecessary Cesareans. One kind of electrode records the baby's heart rate and tests its blood.

It has usually been accepted that if a blood test reveals high levels of lactic acid, which builds up if the baby is short of oxygen in the second stage, the baby's brain will be damaged. But it is now known that if it does become short of oxygen, a healthy baby can switch to another kind of metabolism that allows it to draw on energy reserves that have built up over the previous weeks. In this way the baby can survive on less oxygen with no ill effects. Indeed, babies whose blood is acid at birth often have high Apgar scores (see page 370). Moreover, neurological studies on four-year-olds whose blood was acid at birth due to oxygen shortage show that this had no harmful effects.* But many obstetricians consider that pH levels remain the best method of assessing the fetus at present.

HELPING THE BABY OUT

If a mother needs extra assistance at the end of a delivery, the doctor may use forceps or a vacuum extractor to ease the baby out.

FORCEPS DELIVERY

Forceps look like metal salad servers and dovetail into each other so that they cannot press too far in on the baby's head. If the woman has not already had an epidural, an injection to numb the birth outlet is given first. The curved blades are inserted one at a time and cradled around the baby's head, one at each temple. Forceps are of different shapes for different situations: most draw the baby down the birth canal, though some are simply used to lift it out. If the head is occipito transverse or occipito posterior (see page 271), the obstetrician may first turn the head manually, or use curved Kiellands forceps to rotate it from transverse or posterior to anterior.

VACUUM EXTRACTION

A vacuum extractor works like a miniature vacuum cleaner designed to assist the mother's efforts by keeping the baby from slipping back up between pushes. A vacuum cup is attached to the head (this may take some time, and if you want to push during this time, push). There is evidence that vacuum extraction may be better than forceps for both mother and baby, but it is a skill that needs to be learned.* Newborn complications as a result of vacuum deliveries include bruising, scalp lacerations, and even bleeding into the brain. Vacuum delivery should be abandoned if delivery doesn't occur within a few contractions or the cup keeps slipping off.

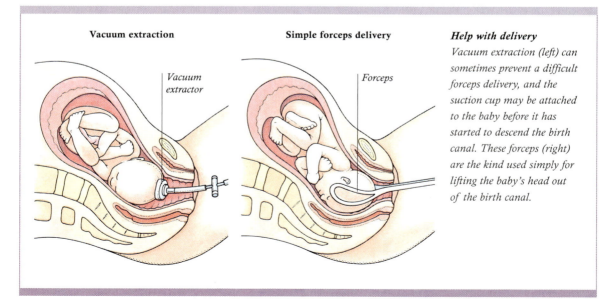

Vacuum extraction

Vacuum extractor

Simple forceps delivery

Forceps

Help with delivery

Vacuum extraction (left) can sometimes prevent a difficult forceps delivery, and the suction cup may be attached to the baby before it has started to descend the birth canal. These forceps (right) are the kind used simply for lifting the baby's head out of the birth canal.

REASONS FOR FORCEPS DELIVERY
OR VACUUM EXTRACTION

Forceps or vacuum extraction are used only during the second stage when delivery needs to be hastened because your blood pressure has risen dramatically, for example, or there are signs of fetal distress, or when the baby is in an unusual position, making its journey through the pelvic outlet difficult. Some women are advised, for medical or surgical reasons, not to push at all, and may need assistance.

The obstetrician has to use clinical judgment to decide whether your baby will pop out like a cork from a bottle given a firm, long pull, or whether it is so firmly wedged that it might harm both you and the baby to deliver vaginally. Sometimes a Cesarean section is performed after forceps or vacuum have failed. Forceps or vacuum extraction may also be used if you have had an epidural (see pages 319–323), because you may feel too numb to work with contractions.

A forceps delivery or vacuum extraction is frequently advised for a prolonged second stage. Different obstetricians have different ideas of what a prolonged second stage is. Some would say that it is any second stage longer than half an hour in which there are no signs of progress. Many set a definite time limit and instruct midwives to call them when it looks as if this stage is extending. Others believe that the important thing is to observe whether or not the baby is coming down the birth canal progressively, while checking its condition carefully and regularly.

Some women seem to be able to cope with long second stages without tiring, whereas others quickly become exhausted. If you have already had a long labor and then a slow second stage, it is difficult to retain enthusiasm and, unless given a great deal of encouragement, you may hope for someone to come and take the baby out of your body one way or another.

A woman may be encouraged to push or persuaded to hold her breath too long, when she does not feel any spontaneous urge to bear down. This is because the midwife knows that the delivery will be by forceps or vacuum unless the baby is born within the time decreed by the obstetrician. So she tries to avoid the intervention by encouraging the mother to push more strenuously in the hope that this will help the baby be born before the deadline.

AVOIDING A FORCEPS DELIVERY
OR VACUUM EXTRACTION

If you have been struggling to push the baby out and it is suggested that you need help because the second stage is taking too long, you are becoming too tired, or the fetal heart rate is slow, explore the effect of not pushing. You may not need to push at all for several contractions—a welcome rest for both you and the baby—and then there is an unmistakable and irresistible pushing sensation that is much more effective than pushing just because you are following instructions. It is a good idea to stand, squat, or kneel so that gravity can help the baby out.

CESAREAN SECTION

The most common reason for Cesarean section is the failure of labor to progress, due to malposition or cephalopelvic disproportion, when the baby's head appears to be too large to pass through the pelvis. But in retrospect, it is usually not too large. Some obstetricians prefer to deliver all breech babies, or all breech babies of first-time mothers, abdominally because they believe that it is safer for the baby. But the size of the baby in relation to the maternal pelvis and the way the baby is lying are factors to take into account. If fetal distress is picked up by an electronic monitor and the obstetrician becomes anxious about the state of the baby, he or she may decide to perform an emergency Cesarean section. A biochemical test of the baby's scalp blood should be done first to check whether the baby is finding birth hard going.

A Cesarean may also be performed for very low-weight babies, and in women suffering from active herpes or conditions such as kidney disease and severe hypertension. Research has been carried out on the outcomes of automatic Cesarean sections for multiple births and when women have diabetes, and it has been shown that this practice is unlikely to be of benefit.* Delivering all twins by Cesarean section does not save lives or produce babies in better condition. A study compared birth outcomes in two parts of Denmark, one where the rate of Cesarean section was about twice as high as the other, and found no differences in perinatal mortality or morbidity.*

THE CESAREAN EPIDEMIC

Cesarean rates vary. In Great Britain, they are about 20 percent of all births. In some cities in Latin America, a staggering 85 percent of babies are delivered abdominally, whereas in the Netherlands the overall rate is less than 10 percent. In South Africa the rate varies from 14 to 17 percent in state teaching hospitals to 33 percent in private hospitals. Private obstetricians there, as in other countries, are much more likely to opt for Cesarean sections than those in a national health service. South African obstetricians themselves report that they do Cesarean sections for convenience in 75 percent of cases.*

"IT WAS A SHOCK TO HAVE A CESAREAN SECTION—I'D LOOKED FORWARD TO A NATURAL BIRTH. I FELT CHEATED AND AS IF I WEREN'T A NORMAL WOMAN."

Hong Kong has the highest rate of all developed countries. There, one out of every two live births in private hospitals is a Cesarean, though the rate is far lower in public hospitals. There is a startling 64 percent difference in the Cesarean rate between public and private hospitals.* The Cesarean rate in the United States is approximately 24 percent and in some hospitals 50 percent or more. But there has not been a corresponding rise in the fetal survival rate. And Cesarean section imposes extra risk on women, as well as unnecessary pain and, often, postoperative infection. The World Health Organization recommends that Cesarean section rates should never be allowed to go higher than 10 to 12 percent.

In the past, an obstetrician would correct a breech baby's position by external version through the mother's abdominal wall (see page 241). This practice declined and it became the tendency to deliver by section rather than attempting to turn the baby first. As a result, doctors no longer knew *how* to perform external version. Now its value is being recognized anew, and doctors are starting to learn this technique again.

More and more women are now included in the category of "high risk." The age at which a woman is considered high risk went down from 40 to 35, then to 30. If you are over 35 and it seems likely that there may be problems with your labor, you may be advised to deliver by Cesarean section. Some obstetricians like to do a Cesarean just because a baby looks as if it is going to be big. This is not a good reason.* Throughout North America it is also the practice to do *repeat* Cesarean sections, even when the conditions that resulted in the first section are not present: "Once a Cesarean, always a Cesarean." Many repeat Cesareans are unnecessary. Only about one woman in four who had a Cesarean with one birth even tries for a VBAC (vaginal birth after Cesarean) with her next. Women often ask to have a Cesarean in order to avoid the pain of labor and because they can be conveniently scheduled. American doctors argue that the uterine scar might possibly break open during VBAC, but British obstetricians differ. They normally prefer a "trial" of labor but are ready to do a Cesarean if necessary. One professor of obstetrics says that problems of scar separation are "much less than the one percent that is often quoted," and that even if the scar is pulled open by strong contractions, "careful monitoring of the fetus and mother usually means that any harm to either is rare."*

> **"THEY SAID I HAD TO CHOOSE BETWEEN PITOCIN AND A CESAREAN. I FEEL SO ROBBED. EVERYTHING WAS TAKEN OUT OF MY HANDS. I DON'T FEEL LIKE SHE BELONGS TO ME."**

CHOOSING NOT TO PUSH

Some women are scared of having a baby vaginally and opt for a Cesarean because they think it will be less painful. A Cesarean is a major surgical operation. It takes at least six weeks to recover and it entails cutting through abdominal muscles that sag and bulge afterward.

Others choose a Cesarean because they are told they can keep a tight vagina and well-toned pelvic floor that way. Unfortunately, it does not work like this. Just being pregnant may put stress on those muscles, especially if the baby is big.* You can tone any muscles in your body by using them (see pages 120–124 for some exercises that help).

A Cesarean may have long-term effects, too. A study in the *British Journal of Obstetrics and Gynaecology** reveals that nearly half of all women who have a baby by Cesarean section do not go on to have other children—almost one in three because of infertility problems, and one in five because the Cesarean experience was so awful they could not face another birth by this method. Three times as many women are infertile following a Cesarean as those who have a spontaneous vaginal birth, and six times as many women suffer from the effects of emotional trauma.

Professor James Walker, one of the authors of the study, says, "When doctors and mothers assess the risks of Cesareans, they generally only think about what the risks are at that time and ignore the impact they might have five years down the line."* It's not that women ignore it. They are not told about it. Choosing to have a Cesarean section is not just a matter of how the birth will be. It can affect how you feel for many years afterward.

PLANNED CESAREAN

The decision to perform a Cesarean section is often made many days or weeks in advance. As one woman said, "I got out my diary and wrote 'BABY' in a square several months ahead." A Cesarean section will usually be planned if it is known that the baby is in a difficult position to be delivered vaginally. You may also be advised to have a Cesarean if there is evidence of cephalopelvic disproportion—although doctors can be certain that there is genuine CPD only when you are actually in labor.

> "I KNEW EXACTLY WHAT I WAS IN FOR, AND THAT'S WHAT I WANTED. IT WAS A STRUGGLE TO GET A CESAREAN AND I WAS RELIEVED WHEN IT WAS ALL ARRANGED AND SETTLED."

One circumstance in which the baby must be delivered abdominally is if the placenta is lying at the bottom of the uterus and over the os (the mouth of the cervix), in front of the baby's presenting part (placenta previa). You need to have a scan at 32–34 weeks to confirm that the placenta is still in this position, and surgery is arranged either for the 39th week or as soon as the baby's lungs are fully mature. This fact can be confirmed by going in for an amniocentesis. A mother with a low-lying or marginal placenta previa can often deliver vaginally, so long as the baby and any bleeding are carefully monitored.

A JUST-IN-CASE CESAREAN SECTION

During a long labor in which there is little progress, the obstetrician may decide to perform a Cesarean section for no other reason than that dilatation is slow. It is important that you share in the decision-making about this. It is up to you, and just one person who encourages you to go on can make all the difference.

EMERGENCY CESAREAN SECTION

Some reasons for a planned Cesarean section (such as cephalopelvic disproportion) may also apply to an emergency section, when the condition has not been obvious until labor. An emergency section may also be decided on during a long labor in which the baby is short of oxygen; if the placenta is failing to service the baby sufficiently or is becoming detached from the lining of the uterus, causing the mother to hemorrhage; or if there is a prolapsed umbilical cord.

ANESTHESIA FOR CESAREAN SECTION

Cesarean section in the past was always performed with the patient having first been given general anesthesia. Now epidural or spinal anesthesia is preferred. Although general anesthesia still has to be used when a very quick decision has to be made to do a Cesarean, those women who have epidural or spinal anesthesia are usually happy that they are awake, fully aware of what is going on and ready to welcome and hold the baby as soon as he or she is lifted out of the uterus.

GENERAL ANESTHESIA If general anesthesia is used, you are given as small a dose as possible for the baby's sake, and may be unconscious for only a few minutes. All the preparation for the operation is done while you are fully awake, and you are sometimes given pure oxygen to breathe during this time. It should be possible to arrange for the baby who is in good condition to be held by the father while you are still unconscious.

EPIDURAL ANESTHESIA You are given an epidural after being taken to the operating room, or an existing epidural will be increased. The dosage is higher for surgery than it would be if an epidural were being given just for pain relief. An anesthetist checks carefully to see that the anesthesia is sufficient for the operation, and is ready with general anesthesia if the epidural does not work effectively enough. With epidural anesthesia, you may have some postoperative nausea and vomiting, as is often the case with general anesthesia. An epidural is safer for you because there is no danger of inhaling your stomach contents, and safer for the baby, who does not receive a knockout dose of anesthesia. Another advantage of the epidural is that you can hold your baby and put it to the breast immediately after the operation.

SPINAL ANESTHESIA If you have had no anesthetic prior to the decision to do a Cesarean, a spinal anesthetic may be preferred to an epidural because it can be done more quickly and achieves good anesthesia more simply than an epidural. This is now by far the most common technique used for Cesareans in the U.S. and Great Britain.

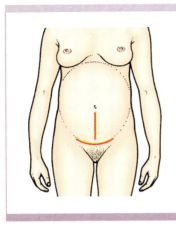

Cesarean incisions
The classic Cesarean incision is vertical. Although this is still used in emergencies, horizontal incision is now more common, because it reduces the risk of rupture in another pregnancy. The positioning of a vertical and a horizontal incision is shown left.

HORIZONTAL OR VERTICAL UTERINE INCISION

Incisions for Cesarean section are either horizontal or vertical. The classical incision is vertical, but this is rarely done now unless there is no time to spare or there are other problems such as large fibroids in the uterus. The main advantages of the horizontal incision are that it is made low down near the line of the pubic hair, in the area that would be covered by a bikini, and that a horizontal scar is less likely to break down than a vertical scar.

WHAT HAPPENS DURING A CESAREAN SECTION?

During a Cesarean, you should be given antibiotics, usually just after the delivery of the baby, because one very frequent problem is pelvic infection afterward.* A midwife will shave off your pubic hair (but not between the legs) and slip a catheter into your bladder so that it is kept empty. In the operating room, sterile drapes are put around your tummy. Because you are lying flat you will not see the surgery, but, if you wish, a screen can be erected at chest level to ensure that you see nothing. Your tummy is washed in antiseptic solution. If there is anything you want to know, ask.

You are given an epidural, spinal, or, rarely, a general anesthetic. When your whole tummy is numb, or you have become unconscious, small cuts are made through the layers in your lower abdominal wall until the lower uterine segment is revealed. Packs of surgical gauze are used to keep other organs out of the way. A horizontal slit is made through the uterus and the bag of waters bulges through it. The obstetrician pops the bag and sucks out the amniotic fluid—if you have had an epidural or spinal you hear the glug-glug-swoosh sound—and uses a forceps blade or a hand under the baby's presenting part to ease it out of the opening, at the same time pushing with one hand on the upper part of the uterus so that the baby is pressed out through the incision.

If you have had an epidural or spinal, it may be possible for you to watch the birth at this stage. Ask the doctor to lower the screen and prop up your head for a few moments. You see your baby emerging and, from your horizontal position, will not see anything gruesome. In fact, you will have eyes only for your baby. The baby is lifted out, suctioned with a mucus catheter, and, once it is breathing well, can be handed to you or your partner. The process from the beginning of surgery to the birth need take only about 4 minutes in an emergency, but can take up to 10 to 15 minutes.

As the baby is delivered, you may be given an injection of pitocin to make the placenta peel away from the wall of the uterus. It will then be lifted out through the abdominal opening that has been made. The obstetrician stitches the cut in the uterus, layer by layer, with absorbable sutures. Suction instruments are used to draw out blood and amniotic fluid, and then the obstetrician repairs the abdominal wall. This takes much longer than the birth—up to an hour—and entails repairing the skin with nonabsorbable sutures, staples, or metal clips, which are removed the next day.

HAVING YOUR PARTNER WITH YOU

Not all couples want to be together during surgery. You may worry that perhaps it will be too much for your partner to cope with, or he may expect the experience to be so distressing that he will be unable to give you any support. Those couples who do want to be together feel that the birth of a baby, by whatever route, is something they want to share, and that if the mother is not able to cuddle the newborn baby the father should be there to do so. A father who is present sits by your head, supporting you emotionally. There is no need to watch the operation, since the screen restricts his view.

AFTER A CESAREAN

When the operation is over, tell the staff that you want to hold your baby if he is not already beside you. An intravenous drip is left in for some hours so that you can be given plenty of fluids straight into your bloodstream in case this is necessary. If you were given general anesthesia, you may feel sick and weak for the first day or so. As soon as you feel that you can move around in bed a little, do so. Even small actions such as wiggling your toes and rotating your ankles are good for you and prevent pooling of blood in your legs.

"THE LAST THING I FELT LIKE DOING WAS GETTING OUT OF BED, BUT I MANAGED IT EVENTUALLY, AND ACTUALLY FELT BETTER— ONCE I WAS BACK IN BED AGAIN!"

Whatever anesthesia you have had during the Cesarean, nurses will help you to get up later the same day. Although it hurts, moving around is important in order to avoid thrombosis. To move off the bed, first work your way to the side of it, roll onto your side, and push yourself to a sitting position with your hands. As

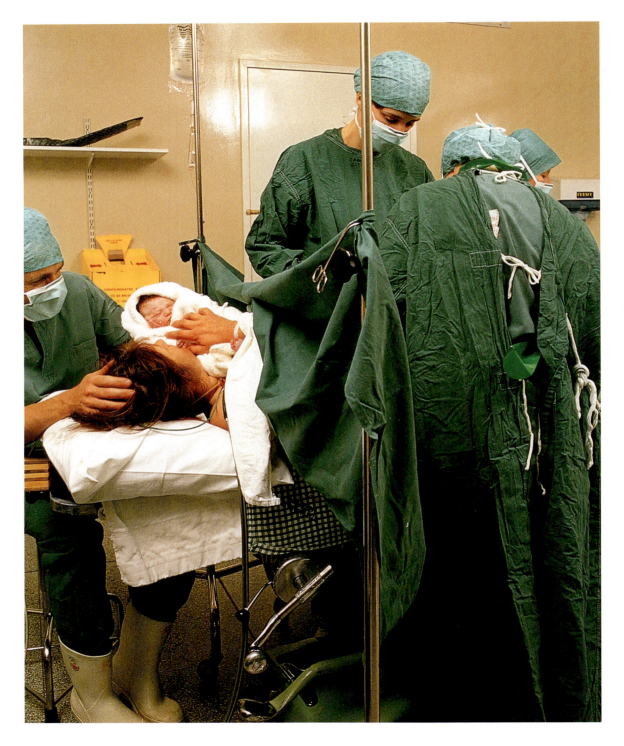

you get up you may have a lot of bleeding from the vagina. This also tends to happen after a vaginal delivery and is the blood that has pooled in your vagina. Stroll around the room in order to encourage good circulation and, as you do so, use the slow, complete breathing that you learned in your prenatal classes.

If you feel that you need drugs for pain relief, ask for them. Although you probably want to be awake to enjoy your baby, you cannot do this if you are in discomfort. The more your partner can be with you, even while you doze, the more you can relax, feeling that the baby is being looked after by someone who loves her.

A new approach to dealing with pain after a Cesarean section is to add a long-acting narcotic to the spinal anesthesia during the operation. This medication gives excellent pain relief for up to 24 hours after surgery. The paralysis wears off in a few hours and the mother can be out of bed with almost no postoperative pain for the first day. Much less medication enters the mother's blood than if she were taking intermittent doses by IV or mouth, so the baby is less likely to be affected by narcotics. An annoying side effect, however, is itching.

You will probably go home between 72 hours and five days after surgery, with instructions on self-care. Call the hospital or your doctor if you have problems or questions. Dressings will be removed three or four days later. Because the obstetrician has had to cut through muscle, your tummy will look very big and soggy. The stitches inside your body dissolve naturally, but the external stitches or staples will be removed before you go home. Do not worry about stitches bursting. With every layer stitched separately there is little chance of this.

After general anesthesia, fluid collects in the lungs and has to be coughed up. A midwife or physiotherapist will teach you the way to do this that causes least discomfort. The breathing techniques you learned in pregnancy can help, too.

It is natural to feel a flood of conflicting emotions after a Cesarean. Some women say that they are grateful to have the baby, but at the same time they feel "cheated." It is particularly upsetting if you have been looking forward to and preparing yourself for a normal delivery.

You may be able to hold your baby immediately and have precious moments together, even while work is going on down at the other end.

A Cesarean birth is a surgical operation, and you need time to recover from it, as from any abdominal surgery. For the first six weeks you should avoid any heavy lifting. If it is possible to arrange for extra help at home, especially if you already have a toddler who expects to be lifted, it is an enormous benefit if someone else does the more strenuous work.

GENTLE BIRTH

At birth, eyes open for the first time on a new world. Your baby's life outside your body begins. Yet the baby already has nine months' experience of life inside the uterus. The ancient Chinese dated life from conception rather than from delivery, and perhaps this corresponds more nearly to reality.

The baby started off as the chance collision of a ripe egg and a sperm. Forces that have their origin far back in time poured energy into the cells, nourishing and multiplying them to make an embryo budding on a stalk and drawing sustenance from your uterus. Gradually, as the days passed, a fully formed being developed, albeit in miniature, and there was already at the third month a fetus whose main task was one of growth and maturation. As week followed week, its senses became sharper so that it was increasingly aware of its surroundings, responding to your movements and to bright light, loud sounds, and music. This long-drawn-out period of preparation culminated in the dramatic journey into the brilliance and bustle of our own world.

WHAT IS IT LIKE TO BE BORN?

Birth is an intense experience not only for you: for the baby, too, it is the climax of a time of growing and waiting. The new human being is caught up in a rush of powerful uterine activity, which squeezes it out from the confines of the tight muscle enveloping it and the cradle of bone in which it has been rocked, into a separate existence.

Traveling from the depths of the uterus, under the arch of bone, and out through the soft, opening folds of the vagina, the baby passes through a barrage of different kinds of sensory stimulation. It is the original magical mystery tour, infinitely more astonishing than any tunnel traveled through in search of excitement in a fairground.

THE BABY'S EXPERIENCE OF BIRTH

Pressure builds up over the crown of the baby's head where it is directed through the dilating cervix, which is pulled up over the head like a turtleneck sweater. Simultaneously, pressure is also directed over the baby's buttocks as the uterus contracts down on them and propels the baby forward. The baby is fixed between the uterus gripping her bottom and the cervix being progressively drawn over her head. This pressure causes the baby to roll into a ball, with her head tucked in and knees bent up, and her arms folded over her chest. The upper part of the head, not yet hard bone all over, is molded so that the brow is pressed back.

As the baby is forced downward, the crown of the head confronts resistance from the pelvic floor muscles, which are springy and firm and are eased over her head little by little. The passage is narrow but yielding, and the baby's body is massaged vigorously with each new contraction as she gradually descends. Beneath the stretched abdominal skin and the thinned, translucent wall of the uterus, the baby has been

***Birth need not be violent** for a baby. Instead, there is welcome from loving arms and a gentle transition to life.*

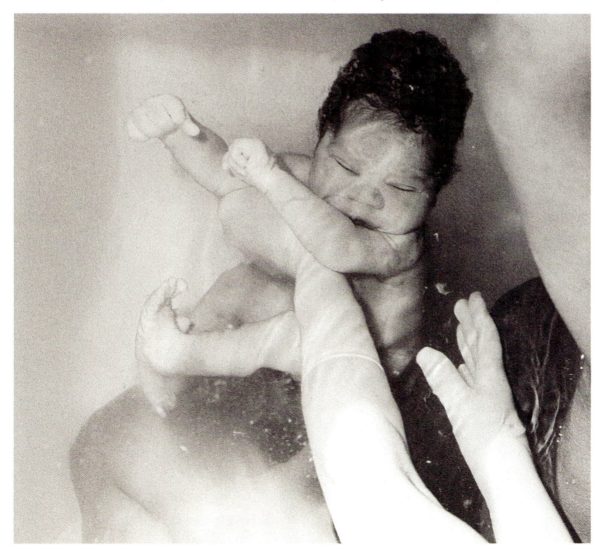

aware in the last weeks of pregnancy of glowing light whenever bright sun or artificial light shone on your body. It must be rather like firelight or the light cast by a red-shaded lamp. When the journey to birth begins, the baby is pressed deeper into the cavity of the pelvis, under arches of bone and a canopy of thick, supportive ligaments and muscles. Perhaps it is a sensation rather like traveling through a long, dark avenue of over-hanging trees.

The baby is not just a hunk of flesh or a life-sized doll but a human being fully equipped to feel pain and pleasure, a person coming to birth. The baby cannot remember or anticipate in the same way that we can, but nevertheless feels acutely and is a fully sentient being. The uterus holds and presses tightly in on the child not yet born, with steadily escalating power. By the end of the first stage it is embracing the baby tightly for one or two minutes each time. Each hug begins gently and grows tighter and tighter until at the height of the contractions the baby is gripped firmly for 20 to 30 seconds. Then the wave of pressure recedes again and the baby floats once more in her inner sea: she is in labor along with you.

NEWBORN REFLEXES IN LABOR

In some obstetric textbooks, the baby is described simply as "a passenger," and purely in mechanical terms as two ovoids, the head and the trunk, the long axes of which are at right angles to each other and which can take the curve of the pelvic axis independently. While this is accurate as a description of the mechanics of fetal descent, it omits any mention of what the baby might be doing during this process and how the reflexes with which he is born are already functioning during labor.

The baby changes position in response to the power unleashed in your body, and does this not only because of mechanical forces, but probably also because he is making active movements. Your baby is working with you toward birth, a partner in the struggle, not just a passenger, and can do this because of built-in reflexes (see page 372).

A newborn baby turns his head in the direction of a touch, moves his head up and down against a firm surface, curls his toes down when pressure is applied to the ball of the foot, lifts a foot up and puts it down at a higher level when pressure is applied over the top of the foot, and makes forward stepping movements when tilted forward with his feet against a firm surface. Two of these actions operate to help the baby onward in his journey. One is the reflex to move his head up and down against firm resistance, which means that he wriggles his way through the cervix and the fanned-out tissues of the vagina, with much the same action that we make when putting on a new sweater with a tight neck. The other is the reflex stepping movement when resistance is offered to the feet. When the baby feels the solid wall of the uterus as it tightens around him, he pushes away from it.

THE IMPACT OF THE OUTSIDE WORLD

In the second stage, the head has to take a nearly right-angled bend. The pressure builds up until it swivels the neck around so that the baby is facing downward and ready to slide out. You can imagine that this provides a very sharp stimulus to the baby, a message that says unmistakably, "Things are changing. Wake up! It's all systems go!" At last the crown of the head slides through the vagina and remains there. Perhaps you reach down with eager hands to stroke the damp, warm top of your baby's head. This is the first greeting.

The head slips out and suddenly the baby encounters space and air. The shoulders and chest slide forward, followed by the whole body. There is a gasp, and air rushes into the lungs, inflating them for the first time. The damp inner surfaces of the lungs, previously clinging together like wet plastic bags, open up with the first cry with which the baby meets life.

Air, space, the baby's own limbs moving in an unfamiliar medium, weight, strange sounds, lights, hands picking the baby up and turning her over—all at once a myriad of new sensations assail the newborn. Not only must the lungs fill with air and start to function rhythmically, but the circulation must find new pathways.

LABOR AS A STIMULUS

In his book *Birth Without Violence*,* Dr. Frederick Leboyer calls the mother "a monster" because of the pain he believes she cannot help but inflict on the baby as it passes through the throes of birth. But the process of being born can also be seen to involve stimulation and awakening for which the baby is ready and which prepares her for life. Looked at from this point of view, muscles hold and embrace the baby, triggering powerful sensations, then soften again in a rhythmic pattern. The space between contractions is like the trough between two waves. Inevitably the next wave comes and again the muscles tighten firmly around the child.

Although labor is undoubtedly traumatic for some babies, others look extraordinarily peaceful and contented after their journey. It may feel to you as if you are swimming in a stormy sea when you reach the end of the first stage of labor. You may be anxious that these massive squeezings of the great muscle of the uterus are causing your baby suffering. Yet in spite of the relentless onslaught of contractions as full dilation approaches, the baby who is pressed through the cervix and down the 9-inch (23-cm) birth canal responds more vigorously to life than do most babies who are merely lifted out through an abdominal incision.

The baby born vaginally has less mucus in her respiratory tract than one delivered by Cesarean section (especially an elective Cesarean) and is better prepared for the great new activity of breathing. The baby can also maintain her own body temperature better after a vaginal birth than after a Cesarean with little or no labor.

CATECHOLAMINES: THE AMAZING "STRESS" HORMONES

Stress is often talked about as if it were invariably harmful. But stress is part of active living. Labor is exciting, challenging—and stressful, for both you and the baby. As a result, hormones pour into your bloodstream and give you a "buzz." They are the same hormones that come with the triumph and satisfaction of at last climbing to the top of a mountain, or of drawing on all your reserves of strength and persistence in a race, the same hormones that flood through you when the curtain rises and you stand in front of an audience. There is striving, and the thrill of the unknown. It is like that, too, when labor begins. These hormones are produced by the baby as well as by you, and the baby produces them in vast quantities.

All hormones are chemical messengers. Catecholamines give the baby the message of life. A surge of the stress hormones—adrenaline and noradrenaline—courses through the baby's bloodstream before labor starts. They protect the baby from shortage of oxygen; shunt blood away from nonessential organs—the skin, for example—ensure a rich supply of blood to the heart, brain, and muscles; slow down the heart rate so that the heart does not have to work so hard or need so much oxygen; prepare the lungs for breathing by dilating the bronchioles; cause fat and glycogen to be broken down and available for quick energy; and in all these ways prepare the baby for the demands of life outside the uterus.

"MY LABOR WAS LONG AND HARD AND I FELT SORRY FOR THE BABY. BUT HE CAME OUT ALERT, PEACEFUL, AND SOON STARTED TO SEARCH FOR MY BREAST."

A scientist who researches the function of catecholamines at birth writes, "Nearly every newborn has an oxygen debt akin to that of a sprinter after a run."* This catecholamine surge is the reason why babies cope well with oxygen deprivation at birth. They handle it much better than adults, who develop heart rate irregularities after just a few minutes.

Catecholamine levels in the baby build up even in early labor, when the cervix is still only 2 or 3 cm dilated, and are about five times the concentration of those in a resting adult. These hormones surge still higher in the second stage of labor, and after the birth are double or triple the level of the early first stage, dropping to a resting level after about two hours.

Pressure on the head of the fetus causes increased secretion of catecholamines; babies who have not experienced labor and been delivered by elective Cesarean section have much lower levels. This is why whenever possible the mother should experience some labor. A baby who is removed through an incision is likely to have breathing difficulties because liquid in the lungs has not been absorbed during the process of birth, and because the lungs have not produced much surfactant—the substance like soap bubbles that prevents lung surfaces from sticking together. Both absorption of lung liquid and release of surfactant are dependent on catecholamines in the hours immediately before the baby is born. Some drugs used to treat hypertension in the mother also interfere with the action of catecholamines.

A newborn baby loses heat rapidly because of her high surface-to-volume ratio. If a baby gets cold after birth, catecholamines activate special heat-producing tissue called "brown fat." Another effect of catecholamines is to dilate the pupils of the baby's eyes and increase alertness. Mother and baby fix their gaze on each other. Each is for the other the most interesting person in the world. The baby is not only cuddly and warm, but also alert and responsive. In this way catecholamines are an element in the process of bonding between mother and baby.

BEING OVERSTRESSED

Catecholamine production is normal in childbirth. But if, as many women do these days, you begin to feel trapped and anxious—exposed under bright lights in an experimental lab—you get overstressed. Stress hormones in your bloodstream pass through the placenta to the baby. The result is high levels of cortisol not only in your bloodstream but in the baby's, too, and these can be a cause of fetal distress.*

WELCOMING YOUR BABY

Have you thought about how you want to welcome your baby into the world? This is not just a matter of safe or speedy delivery, of making sure that the baby has enough oxygen or is not traumatized by delivery, but also one of greeting the baby with gentleness.

Most babies cry at the shock of birth, and this first cry ensures that a rush of air enters the lungs. But if they go on crying there is something wrong. The crying of abandonment and distress is quite different from the healthy crying of the newborn. Yet people often take persistent crying for granted and even smile indulgently and say, "She's got a fine pair of lungs!"

The newborn baby continues to scream because of insensitivity to her needs and the lack of a sufficiently caring environment. If the setting for birth is changed and, above all, if the attitudes of those assisting are different, so that the baby is treated with respect, the child will become quiet, open her eyes, reach out her hands, and start to discover herself. But if this is to happen, the birth room must be calm and hushed, the lights dimmed, and those handling the baby must do so slowly, carefully, and lovingly. This is *gentle birth*.

A CARING ENVIRONMENT

Gentle birth need not start only as the baby is born. In the way that labor is conducted, and in the whole atmosphere of the birth room, an environment of peace and serenity can be created. As a mother you are in such a subtle and yet intense relationship with your baby that everything done to you during labor must affect the way in which you are able to respond to your newborn baby. If you are treated as if your body is merely the container from which a baby is removed, or as an irresponsible child who has to be given orders, you will find it very difficult to be in harmony with the forces that are bringing the baby to birth, with your own body in its work of creation, and also with the baby. The caring environment for the newborn starts with a caring environment for you, a respect for your rhythms, patience to wait and watch, and loving support.

DIMMING THE LIGHTS

It is irritating for you to labor under bright lights, just as it is for the baby to confront brilliant fluorescent light at delivery. For a gentle birth all unnecessary lighting is switched off so that the room is softly illuminated, with clear light only on the perineum. Instead of lying flat on your back or with your legs suspended in lithotomy stirrups, you need to be in a position you find comfortable and in which you can be an active birthgiver. Many women like to be sitting up, crouching, or kneeling so that they can catch the first glimpse of the baby's head and touch it even before it has started to emerge through the vagina. We have already seen (on page 252) that an upright position has many advantages for the mother in terms of mechanical function. If you are well raised, you are also in a splendid position for greeting your baby.

When the head crowns, some women put their hands down to caress the top of the baby's head. The head feels warm and firm, and as it eases forward you touch more and more warm, damp, silky hair. This very first contact between mother and child is beyond excitement; it is a moment of awe.

Then the head slides out and turns to align with the shoulders still inside, and you can see your baby's profile; with a rush the shoulders and whole body are born. As the baby slips out and starts to breathe, the lights can be dimmed further so that the baby can take her time to open her eyes in the half-light. Many decades ago, Maria Montessori, the educationalist, stressed that babies are assaulted by bright light. She said that they should be able to begin the gradual exploration of the world with their senses in a soft glow and shadows, similar to the uterine environment they have just left. Yet we have subjected newborns to harsh hospital lights and acted as if they were unable to see or hear.

REDUCING NOISE LEVELS

In nonviolent birth, there is no unnecessary conversation, and those attendants who speak do so in hushed voices. Dr. Frederick Leboyer believed that the mother should be quiet, too, and that excited voices can startle the baby. When he wrote his book, it was not known that

In a tranquil setting, *the midwife lifts the baby into the mother's arms, with her finger resting on the baby's chest to feel the heartbeat.*

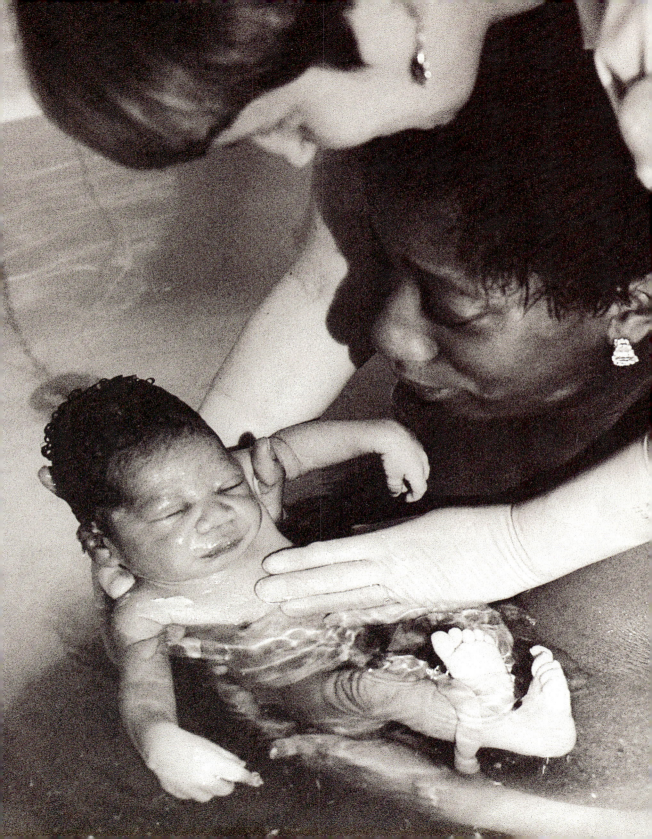

the intrauterine environment was full of sound, particularly the mother's heartbeat and voice and the voices of others. Dr. Michel Odent thinks that there is too much emphasis today on the father's presence in childbirth and that fathers sometimes get too emotional. Couples who value sharing birth together would not agree. I feel myself and know many women who also feel that it would not have been possible to go through labor and birth without the child's father there. In fact, couples often do cry out with astonishment and wonder when they see their baby leap into life. This is a spontaneous outpouring of emotion, of joy, an integral part of childbirth, which in itself is a life-enhancing experience for both parents. We do not carefully work out exactly what we are going to do when we are caught up in other sorts of peak experience; we do not weigh the different factors and come up with a formula. To do so would diminish the experience. Life is exultant and we are borne along with it. Birth is also an act of love, the culmination of the passion that first started the development of that baby.

PHYSICAL CONTACT

It is because birth is a peak experience that arms reach out to take and hold the baby and draw her close. It is not just that this small, wrinkled, vulnerable baby is yours and that therefore you decide to take her in your arms (although unfortunately this is just how it is for some women in a loveless, uncaring environment). If the right atmosphere exists, you are totally enveloped in a rush of intense feeling. This does not mean that the baby is neglected in an orgy of self-indulgent emotion. The baby is drawn into the warm circle of love between the parents and becomes part of it. This is what it means for not only a baby to be born but also a family. In nonviolent birth the baby is handled gently, without haste. There are no rough, quick movements. She is delivered onto your tummy or over your thigh. If you ask beforehand it is often possible to do this yourself.

Leboyer believed that the baby should be lovingly and gently massaged until she stops crying and gradually becomes calm. Only then does he think the baby is ready to go to the mother's arms. This was his own obstetric practice, but many women see this as yet one more way in which professionals, however caring, attempt to take over childbirth and to intrude on the mother's natural role.

Where gentle birth is practiced today, it is usually the mother who holds and caresses her baby. You do not have to learn how to massage your newborn. The way you explore and stroke her is spontaneous and right. But this is only possible if the baby is naked and in skin contact with you. Babies are often bundled up in wrappings in case they lose heat. It is true that new babies quickly become chilled unless they are in a warm atmosphere and are held close. Research has shown that even a low-birth-weight baby keeps warmer when in flesh-to-flesh contact with her mother and nestling against her breast than when wrapped and put in a crib. So ask a helper to slip your gown down over your shoulders or take it right off before the birth. A blanket can easily be thrown over you and your baby or a heater can be placed over you both. Mothers often feel chilled and shaky after giving birth and appreciate the warmth. Covering the baby's head also helps to avoid heat loss.

"I LIFTED HER OUT AND UP ONTO MY TUMMY AND HELD AND STROKED HER. IT SUDDENLY HIT ME THAT THIS INCREDIBLE LITTLE CREATURE HAD COME OUT OF MY BODY! SHE HAD BEEN A PART OF ME."

If your baby is handed to you bundled up in a cloth, unwrap the covers and cuddle her close. Do not be afraid to talk to your baby. She will respond to the sound of your voice and be especially sensitive to the higher-pitched tone of a woman's voice. The baby is also getting to know your unique scent. By the time she is a few days old she will already prefer a cloth that has been against your body to one that has been close to another mother.

DELAYING CLAMPING OF THE CORD

Ask your midwife or doctor not to clamp the cord until it stops pulsating. Immediate clamping may reduce the baby's red blood cells by over 50 percent. Midwives always used to wait, but now the birth is often so rushed that the cord is sometimes clamped and cut immediately while blood is still flowing back and forth between placenta and baby. Even though this blood is not well oxygenated—because the placenta begins to peel off the wall of the uterus as soon as the birth takes place—it is important that the correct balance between blood supply in baby and placenta be reached. The way to ensure that is to hold the baby at approximately the same level as the placenta and wait for the cord to become flaccid, indicating no further flow of blood in either direction. Occasionally, there are reasons for early cord clamping, such as an Rh negative mother who has produced antibodies against her baby (see pages 113–114), or a cord wrapped around the baby's neck. Otherwise there is no reason that the cord has to be cut until after the placenta is delivered.*

You can rest your fingers on the cord and feel the blood throbbing through it and wait for the moment when it stops completely. Cutting the cord between two clamps is a very simple procedure and something that a father may enjoy doing. If you would like him to do this, ask in advance.

Some obstetricians are concerned that blood could drain back into the placenta if the baby is placed above the placenta with the cord still un-clamped. This is not a sufficient reason for early clamping or not placing the baby against your body. The baby can be rested over your thigh at the level of the placenta, where you can hold him. Mucus usually drains out naturally, and there is therefore no need to use a mucus extractor, although the baby should be carefully observed and a mucus extractor used if the airways are blocked, followed by a few puffs of oxygen.

WAITING FOR THE ROOTING REFLEX

Your baby may emerge from your body already wanting to suck. But many babies need time to feel secure before they reach out to find the nipple. The rooting reflex is a sure sign that the baby is ready to be put to the breast. Wait until the baby shows interest rather than stuffing your breast into her mouth. Women often try to breast-feed before the baby is ready. They are anxious to put the baby to the breast immediately after delivery and try to rush things. Be patient. Let the baby rest against your bare breast, and in her own time she will start to explore with mouth, hands, and eyes. This time is precious for you both. It cannot be speeded up without interfering with spontaneous, natural rhythms. The baby begins to lick your nipple, and, with just a little help as you lift your breast into her searching mouth, latches on and begins to suck.

BATHING THE BABY

An important part of the Leboyer style of birth was the warm-water bath in which the baby is supported, and in his film illustrating gentle birth, the bath is given even before the mother holds her baby. Leboyer believed that the baby needs time to feel safe in the medium she has just left behind in the uterus—water—and that suspended in a bath the baby becomes peaceful and sometimes positively beatific, discovers herself, and starts to open her eyes and explore the world around her. It is true that some babies seem to enjoy the bath very much, but only if it is given slowly and calmly and if the water is deep enough for the baby to float. The ideal way to give a bath is in a container with a thermal lining and an air heater over it. Or you may prefer a water birth.

You may find that the hospital where you are having your baby does not allow a bath because of the risk of hypothermia (chilling). Unfortunately, cold air ventilation ducts have been incorporated into the design of many maternity units, and the baby in water or exposed to this air is likely to get chilled. Many hospital pediatricians are concerned that the baby can lose a great deal of body heat while wet through evaporation or in a bath that is too cool. They say that if a bath is given at all, it should be done speedily, which defeats its purpose. You obviously cannot add hot water to a bath when the baby is in it, and you know yourself how shivery you feel when you get out of a hot bath into a relatively cold atmosphere. It is much harder for a newborn baby, who cannot shiver yet and whose largest area of heat loss is her big head, to keep warm. The baby can maintain heat through brown fat that creates warmth, just as a bear or any cold-adapted hibernating animal does. A low-birth-weight baby does not have enough brown fat to do this. Muscular activity and crying also help the baby to keep warm. A baby in a cool room will hyperventilate, although one with respiratory depression cannot do this. Heat loss is also reduced when blood vessels near the surface of the skin tighten up. But babies who have received drugs from their mothers' bloodstreams, including narcotics, are not only sedated but also unable to prevent heat loss efficiently. So if you want the bath to be given, you should not have had narcotics in the last five hours, your baby should be full term, weigh more than 5 lb (2.5 kg), and not have breathing difficulties at delivery, and the room should be warm.

Parents are sometimes very doubtful about the advantages of the bath, preferring to be in skin contact with their baby and to let her suck at the breast indefinitely instead. If a baby is happy lying against her mother and is ready to go to the breast after a little while, it appears purely ritualistic to insist on putting her in a bath because of preconceived ideas about how babies *ought* to behave.

"SHE LOOKED AT ME VERY CRITICALLY AT FIRST AS IF TO SAY, 'DO YOU KNOW WHAT YOU ARE DOING?' THEN SHE RELAXED AND IT WAS LIKE WATCHING A FLOWER OPEN IN WATER."

Dr. Michel Odent* uses the bath in a different way. The baby goes first to the mother's arms and sucks if she is rooting. Only then is she immersed in a bath, and instead of the doctor bathing the baby, the father takes over this responsibility, but close enough to the mother so that she can see and touch, too. It can be moving to watch a father doing this first service for his newborn child.

A midwife described what happened in one case when a father bathed his baby in this way: "The baby, who had been resting quietly with its mother, now seemed to wake to its surroundings and gaze serenely around. It is this serenity that is so remarkable and such a joy to watch. The baby's body was totally immersed in the water, which kept it warm, and gave it total relaxation. After five to ten minutes, a midwife gently lifted the baby onto the warmed towel below the overhead heater. There was not one cry, and all handling was done with an awareness that the baby had never been handled before and that its skin was acutely sensitive. There were no sudden jerks or movements while the baby was being dressed. I now realize that the crying that accompanies these tasks is the result of sheer fright."*

AFTER THE BIRTH

Gentle birth does not end with the minutes after delivery. It is part of a continuum, a flow of interaction between you and your baby, beginning in pregnancy and going on following childbirth. It is a question not just of how the delivery is conducted or even whether you are able to hold your baby right away, but also of creating an environment in which throughout the 24 hours you have access to your baby, feel she is yours, and can act spontaneously. You need to know that everyone around you understands what you are feeling—and that you can have confidence in their emotional support as you and your partner learn to be parents.

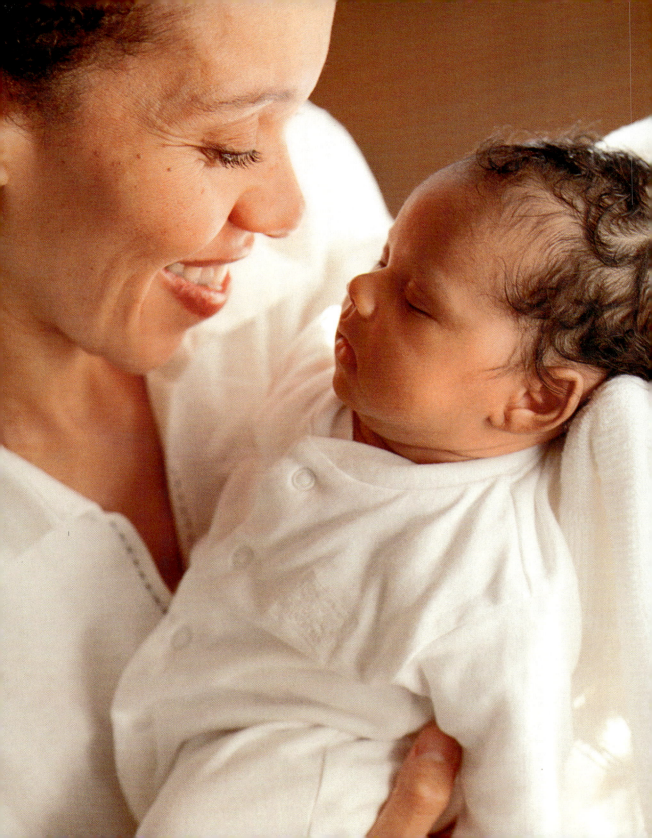

YOU & YOUR NEWBORN

370 | THE FIRST HOURS OF LIFE

380 | THE BABY WHO NEEDS SPECIAL CARE

386 | LOSING A BABY

394 | THE FIRST TEN DAYS

412 | THE CHALLENGE OF NEW PARENTHOOD

THE FIRST HOURS OF LIFE

The hours immediately following birth are for many
women some of the most intense of their lives. A peak
experience like that of giving birth does not suddenly
subside after you have spent half an hour holding
the baby or end when the lights are turned out.

After such a dramatic time, it is not surprising that some women cannot
sleep, and that many remain in a party spirit for hours or even days after.
Unfortunately, many hospitals treat the period after birth as a time for
quiet rest, once you are clean and tidy. If you are too excited to sleep, you
may be offered some sleeping pills or tranquilizers—feel confident about
refusing them. The staff may understand what you are experiencing, but
most hospitals do not make provision for this continuity of passionate
feeling after childbirth, which ensures that motherhood becomes part of
you as a person rather than something that you are straining to learn. The
overpowering emotions that fill you after childbirth propel you through
the period of knowing nothing about your newborn baby, who seems like
a tiny stranger, to the time when you realize that you know everything
about him. You have become centered in this tiny new existence as much
as you are in yourself.

THE APGAR SCALE

Immediately after birth your baby's vitality is tested. It is tested again after about
five minutes. Babies who get low marks the first time usually score nine or ten when
tested the second time; but a baby does not have to cry to be vigorous and healthy.

WHAT IS TESTED	0 POINTS	1 POINT	2 POINTS
Heart rate	Absent	Below 100 beats per minute	100 beats per minute or more
Breathing	Absent	Slow or irregular	Regular
Skin color	Blue	Body pink, extremities blue	Pink all over
Muscle tone	Limp	Some movements	Active movements
Reflex response	Absent	Grimace only	Cry

YOUR FIRST MEETING WITH YOUR NEWBORN

You look down at this new little person and feel the weight of the body as he begins to relax after the struggle to birth. The head is the biggest part, the hair silken and perhaps still wet and curled in damp fronds or streaked back as if after a swim. The ears are tiny and carved like convoluted shells, and the fingernails, too, are like the little pink shells you picked up from the sand when you were a child. If the baby is still crying, the mouth looks huge, a most efficient organ capable of reaching out to and grasping the breast for essential nourishment. And the cry itself, a high-pitched, almost animal wail, is well adapted to summon immediate attention, to drive you to find out what is wrong and how you can answer the baby's needs, and to be intensely anxious until you have stilled the crying. It is a biological mechanism of vital importance for survival. As you hold the baby, the hands start to scan the air, encountering space, meeting the face, perhaps brushing against your body or hand. The fingers move and undulate like sea anemones, embarking on the important task of finding out about this new world. If lights have been dimmed, the baby will open wide eyes and look straight at you some time during this process of unfolding. It has been discovered that newborn babies find the human face the most attractive thing to look at, far more so than fuzzy bunnies or painted ducks—and the moving, speaking human face is best of all.

THE EXPERIENCE OF BONDING

The environment into which the baby is born and the attitude of all those handling the baby are important not only for the baby's sake but for yours, too, and for the relationship between you. It is far more difficult for a mother to feel that her baby belongs to her and she to him—to bond—if she does not have time immediately following birth to begin to get to know her baby.* An important element in this is naked skin contact. The baby should not be wrapped up and turned into a solid little package that you are allowed to hold but not to explore. He should be delivered onto your body, and you should be able to put the baby to the breast as soon as he is ready to suck. Marshall Klaus and John Kennel, working at a hospital in Cleveland, recommended that mothers be able to hold their babies naked on the delivery bed and have undisturbed time to get to know them,

> "I KNEW I WASN'T WHAT PEOPLE CALL A 'BORN MOTHER' AND I'D NEVER PARTICULARLY LIKED KIDS, THOUGH I'M A TEACHER—PERHAPS BECAUSE I'M A TEACHER. BUT I FELL IN LOVE WITH MY BABY RIGHT AWAY."

and then be encouraged to look after them themselves, with help available if they needed it. They should have their babies with them and be responsible for them at least five hours a day, and be given ample emotional support from hospital staff. They found that when mothers and infants were allowed to remain together undisturbed for the first hour after birth, and then had extended contact

NEWBORN REFLEXES

Babies are born with reflexes to help them adjust to life
outside the uterus. Breathing, sucking, and swallowing
are the most important reflexes in a newborn baby.

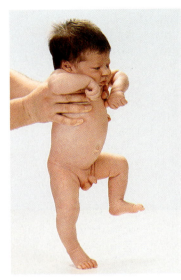 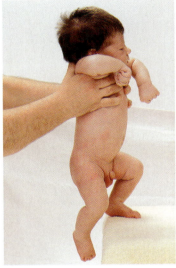 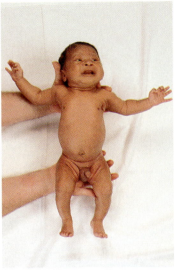

Step reflex
*Astonishingly, a newborn baby
makes movements that look like
"walking" if he is well supported
and firmly held.*

Stepping
*If you hold the baby under the
arms and let his feet touch a firm
surface, he will make "stepping"
movements.*

The startle reflex
*If the baby is handled abruptly or
roughly, the Moro or startle reflex
will be seen. The baby throws up
his arms and trembles.*

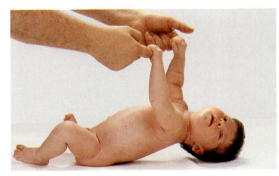 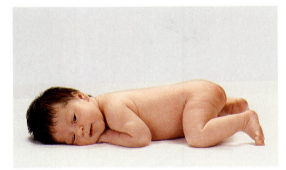

Hand gripping
*The baby will grip your finger tightly and has a
grasp reflex strong enough to support his weight.
Best not to test this yourself!*

About to crawl
*When you place a newborn baby on his tummy,
he will automatically assume a crawling position,
and may even creep.*

with their babies in the first 48 hours, the attachment between mother and baby was stronger than when minimal contact (for feedings only) was allowed.*

Still, in many hospitals, the hours after birth are used mainly for medically processing you and your baby. You must pass tests of fitness before being pronounced not "at risk" and discharged.

WHAT TESTS ARE CARRIED OUT?

As soon as the baby is born, the midwife, nurse, or doctor assesses the baby's condition and rates it at one and five minutes of age, according to the Apgar scale (see page 370). This is done by simple observation of the baby's breathing, skin color, muscle tone, heart rate, and reflexes. The important measurement is the one at five minutes, when a baby has had time to adjust to life and has received any help necessary, such as a whiff of oxygen. The highest score is ten and most babies get seven or higher. Once you have had a cuddle, a further check is made on the baby. Many women say they like this checkup to be done close beside them so that they can see what is happening and can discuss anything that they find worrying. If the baby stays by your side and never leaves you, this will happen as a matter of course.

The baby's weight is recorded. The depth of breathing is assessed and noted, whether the extremities are still blue, and whether he responds vigorously to stimuli and seems to be strong and healthy. Other things are looked for, too. These include the size of the head, the genitals, and—in a boy—whether both testes are descended. The anus is checked to ensure that it is normal. And the baby's heart is listened to (auscultated). The upper part of the mouth is examined to ensure that the palate is complete, and the legs are gently bent up and circled outward to make sure that there is no dislocation of the hips. Gentle feeling of the baby's tummy discloses whether the liver and spleen are the right size, and feeling around the top of the baby's head reveals the state of the skull bones. It is usual practice to give an injection or oral dose of vitamin K. This vitamin is necessary for formation of the enzyme thrombin, without which blood cannot clot.

Newborn eye prophylaxis is also required by law in most states to prevent "ophthalmia neonatorum" or newborn eye infection with gonorrhea or chlamydia picked up from the mother's genital tract. Prevention can be either drops of 1 percent silver nitrate or antibiotic ointment of erythromycin or tetracycline given as a single application soon after delivery.

RELATING TO YOUR BABY

The adjustment of mother and baby to each other is sometimes treated as of secondary importance to the process of medical screening. As a result, many new mothers lack confidence in handling and relating to their babies. Much of what is called "postnatal depression" is connected with a mother's inability to relate to her baby. It feels to her as if the baby belongs not to her, but to the hospital. It can be even more difficult for a man to

TESTING THE NEWBORN

These are some of the standard tests that are given routinely to
all new babies. You can ask that they be done right beside you
so that you can discuss the results.

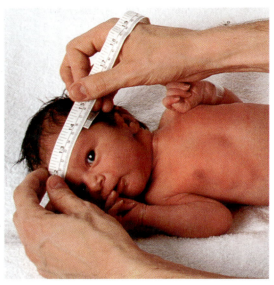

. . . the diameter of the head is measured . . .

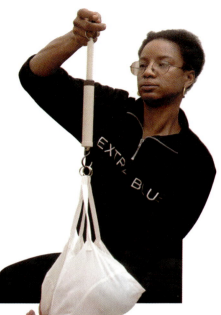

. . . the weight recorded . . .

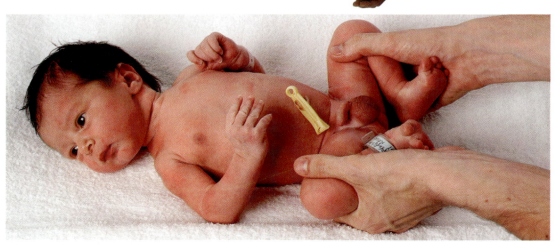

. . . jaw and hips tested for dislocation . . .

feel that his baby belongs to him. In one Stockholm hospital, men were shown how to handle, change, bathe, and weigh their babies and were helped to understand the emotional and physical stresses of pregnancy and birth on their partners. This was done on two separate occasions while the women were in the postpartum ward. These fathers became more involved in baby care later on, and it seemed that they were more understanding than another group of fathers who had not been given the chance to become involved with their babies in this way. Research shows that *both* parents need an unhurried and peaceful time with their baby in the hour following birth.

HOW YOUR BABY MAY LOOK

Your new baby may have a low, sloping forehead; a receding chin; hair in sideburns (low on the brow, in the nape of the neck, and sometimes down the back as well); an odd, bumpy head that has been molded like a ripe grapefruit in its passage down the birth canal; a squashed boxer's nose; and blotchy skin. Yet to most new parents, their baby looks beautiful! You respond in a loving, protective way to the wonder of this new human being.

"I NEVER THOUGHT I COULD CREATE SOMETHING SO BEAUTIFUL. HE IS PERFECT, AND I JUST LIE AND STARE AT HIM IN WONDER. AND WHEN HE OPENS HIS EYES AND LOOKS AT ME, I AM BOWLED OVER."

Even if you are unaware of feeling anything remarkable at the time, you will probably look back at those moments as being special, as you piece together the fragments of the birth experience. This reflection and thinking back is especially important after a difficult labor. It comes spontaneously to most women if they allow themselves time, and do not try to forget about what happened to them.

HOW THE BABY HAS HAD TO ADJUST

Enormous changes occur as the baby adjusts to the challenges of an extra-uterine existence. One of the most dramatic things, although unseen, is the change from fetal to newborn circulation, with the blood flowing along different pathways. When the baby is inside you all the blood flows in and out through the umbilical cord and bypasses the lungs, which do not need to function (see page 76). Since the placenta is doing much of the work that will later be performed by the baby's liver and kidneys, little blood needs to be carried to these organs in the intrauterine state.

At birth, the first great gasp of air causes pressure changes in the whole circulatory system so that the baby's blood enters the lungs, liver, and kidneys. The increased pressure in these organs brings about the collapse of the umbilical blood vessels and of the bypasses around the lungs, liver, and kidneys. Once these pressure changes have taken place, the system is all set to work for a lifetime, and the blood vessels that are no longer used waste away.

WHY YOUR BABY MAY SEEM STRANGE

Many things you notice about your baby may worry you. It helps to realize that the baby may look very different once she has uncrumpled after a few days.

LANUGO The dark hair that may cover large parts of the newborn's body, especially if it is preterm, is called lanugo and drops out over the next week or so. The hair on the head is often a different shade from that which will grow later. One of my babies was born with almost black hair and in a few months was a flaxen blonde.

VERNIX The creamy substance that may coat the baby's skin, sometimes thickly, is vernix. It is produced by skin cells as they drop off into the amniotic fluid and forms a protective coating. Vernix is gradually absorbed. It is not necessary to wipe it off, except on the head, where it tends to stick to the hair, and in the folds and creases under the arms, in the neck, and in the groin.

CAPUT Some babies are born with a peculiar bump like a large blister on their heads, often just off center. This is where the head was pressing down through the cervix. The swelling does not affect the baby's brain, and will gradually go away.

MOLDING Usually the brow is sloped back and rather low in a newborn baby, but some babies who were in a posterior position have high-domed heads like figures in an Egyptian hieroglyph, but this is temporary. A baby who was presenting by the face is usually very swollen, bruised, and puffy but, again, this gradually goes away.

MONGOLIAN SPOTS Some babies have patches of slate-blue skin on their tummies or backs. These are called "Mongolian spots." They are completely harmless. They occur most often in families of African, Asian, Mediterranean, or Native American and Canadian origin.

SEXUAL CHARACTERISTICS A newborn baby's genitals can look very large, especially if the baby is preterm. Sometimes there is milk in the breasts of both girl and boy babies. It is harmless and disappears without treatment. This is a result of the withdrawal of estrogen received from the mother's bloodstream and the action of prolactin released by the baby's

Meeting a new brother or sister, encountering the amazing reality of a newborn person, is a very important event in a child's life.

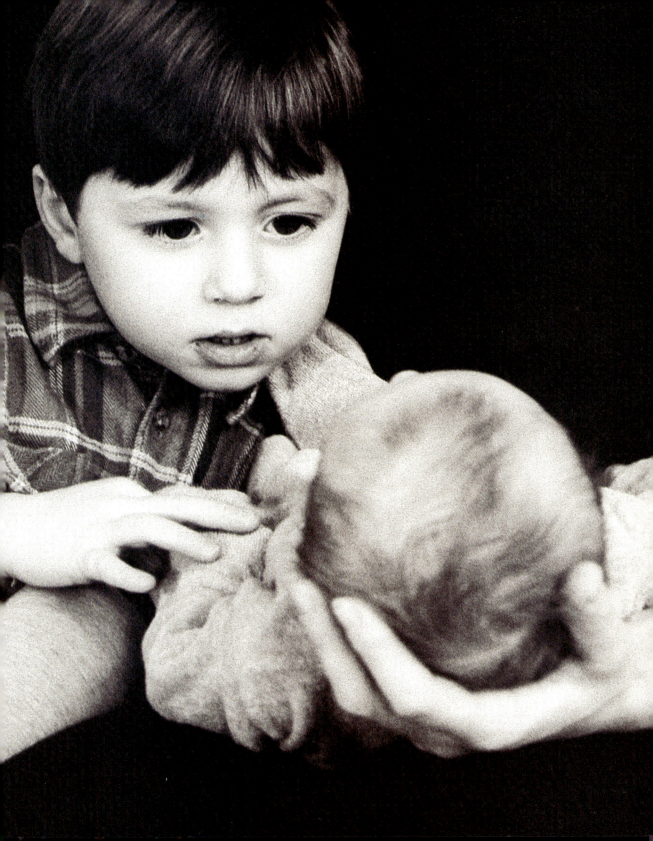

pituitary. Some baby girls even experience pseudo-menstruation as the result of the withdrawal of maternal estrogen. It is nothing to worry about, and stops within a few days.

BONDING—A GRADUAL PROCESS

Some of the reactions that you have to your newborn baby are instinctive. You respond to the sight of the baby's plumpness, the rounded head, the large forehead, the smell of the skin, the bright gaze of her eyes (which look as if they say "So that is who you are!"), your baby's cry, her exploring hands and mouth, her vigorous movement, and the extraordinary compactness of her neat little body. But even instinctive behavior needs the right setting if it is to be triggered and to unfold into appropriate nurturing. Then you can go on to learn from the baby how to respond to her signals.

"I TURNED MY HEAD AWAY AND SAID, 'YOU HOLD HER.' I COULD SEE THEY WERE WORRIED THAT I WASN'T BONDING. BUT LATER SHE STARTED TO CRY AND REACH OUT AND I FELT A SURGE OF LOVE FOR HER."

Bonding is often talked about as if it were instant glue that sticks a mother and baby together the minute after birth, and some women who do not have their babies with them after birth worry that they have failed a test in motherhood and that this will have lasting effects. In fact, bonding is a gradually unfolding process that starts then and develops each hour you and your baby are together. During all this time, you are both learning about each other, and further physical changes in you are set off by stimuli provided by the baby. The most obvious of these is the milk ejection reflex, which is stimulated by the baby's crying and searching for the nipple, the touch of her mouth against the breast, and her sucking.

One measure of the quality of hospital care is the way in which caregivers support the family—not just the mother, father, and baby, but also other children. Older brothers and sisters should be allowed to have close contact with the baby, too, and be made welcome. In practice, some hospitals still restrict sibling visits.*

THE IMPORTANCE OF THE TIME AFTER BIRTH

Wherever you are having a baby, even if you are "high risk" and need obstetric help, provision should be made for a quiet, intimate time together after birth. This can be done in a big teaching hospital just as it can in a small birth center, *and it is part of the job of the hospital to create that environment for each mother, each father, and each baby*.

The minutes, hours, and days after birth are a time for emotional "work" that may be no less significant in the lives of the newborn baby and of both parents than the physical work of labor. The hospital should provide an environment that supports these unfolding emotional processes. New parents do not need to be shown how to develop a relationship with their babies. They do need, however, to feel among friends, to be handed the baby at birth, and to be left in peace and privacy together.

THE QUESTION OF CIRCUMCISION

Circumcision is an unnecessary operation. It can be dangerous, too. It may result in excessive bleeding or infection. Sometimes the penis is damaged irreparably. Some babies have to be rushed to an intensive care unit because of complications. Occasionally a baby dies.

Newborn babies feel pain. In fact, they may feel it more acutely than adults. An adult knows that the pain caused by an operation will end. A baby cannot know this. Amputation of the foreskin, even if it is done with local anesthetic, is an intensely painful and traumatic procedure. It is true that some babies do not cry during circumcision. They are too deeply shocked to do so. Instead, they withdraw. Whether a baby cries inconsolably or is overwhelmed by shock, he has a raw and painful scar afterward. He is often so distressed that there are feeding problems, and a woman who longed to breast-feed may be unable to do so. Sometimes a mother observes that her baby's personality seems to have changed. Perhaps it is not only the pain. Trust has been destroyed. The rhythms of love and intimacy between a mother and her newborn have been disrupted.

"WE WERE UNDER PRESSURE FROM OUR PARENTS TO CIRCUMCISE HIM. WE DID RESEARCH AND DECIDED THAT WE COULD NOT DO THIS TO OUR CHILD."

Although few doctors still defend circumcision as medically necessary, they are often slow to criticize it because they believe that babies cannot feel much, and they are concerned that to challenge circumcision may appear to be anti-Semitic. Men who were circumcised themselves may believe that it never did them any harm. Some parents want a son to be circumcised so that he can be the same as "everyone else"—an argument that is also used to support the practice of female clitoridectomy and infibulation in Egypt and Somalia.

The foreskin protects the tip of the penis. You do not need to retract it or work it loose. Trying to do so may tear delicate structures and hurt the baby. By the time a boy reaches adolescence it will be more flexible.

If you are Jewish or Muslim, you may want to welcome your baby into your faith in a ceremony of blessing and thanksgiving that does not entail mutilation. Do not expect grandparents to find this an easy adjustment. You may need to acknowledge the pain that your decision causes them. But ultimately it is a choice that *you* make.

THE BABY WHO NEEDS SPECIAL CARE

About 6 percent of all babies weigh 5 lb (2.27 kg) or less (the internationally agreed definition of a low-birth-weight baby). Such babies can be divided into two categories—preterm and small-for-dates—and they generally require special care.

Half or more of low-birth-weight babies are born too soon—preterm babies. Maternal illness, smoking, poor nutrition, a high-stress lifestyle, and poverty are all associated with preterm delivery, but sometimes none of these factors is present.

Small-for-dates babies are born at the right time but have not flourished in the uterus in the last months of pregnancy. Sometimes this happens because of malnutrition in the mother, because of her smoking, preeclampsia, or high blood pressure, because the placenta has not been working well (placental insufficiency), or because she was carrying twins or more. These undernourished babies often have difficulty during labor, are short of oxygen, and have problems with breathing after birth. They may suffer from hypoglycemia (low blood sugar) or have convulsions. Some small-for-dates babies, however, are small right through pregnancy because of intrauterine infection, or for genetic, chromosomal, or other reasons.

THE BABY WITH POOR TEMPERATURE CONTROL

Low-birth-weight babies may have problems during labor and are more likely to have poor temperature control, because there is very little fat under the skin. They may be jaundiced, difficult to feed, and susceptible to infection. Their skin is usually red because the blood vessels are visible through the thin layer of fat. They are kept in a nursery that is warmer than the wards and may be cared for in incubators. A thermostat may be strapped to a baby's tummy so that the temperature can be regulated. Sometimes a baby is placed under a plastic heat shield and wears a hat. Tiny babies who are kept warm grow faster.*

THE BABY WITH BREATHING DIFFICULTIES

Preterm and low-birth-weight babies may have interrupted breathing (apnea) in the early days after the birth. This is why a very tiny baby is kept on a mattress that sets off an alarm should breathing stop. All that is usually needed to start the baby's breathing is a little stimulation of the baby by touch. One in every ten preterm babies has insufficient surfactant in its lungs. Surfactant reduces the surface tension in the lungs, allowing them to expand and stopping them from deflating entirely with each breath out; it normally develops before the baby is born.

A baby usually inflates its lungs with the first breath after birth, when they pop open like parachutes. With the first breath out, half the air is retained, so that breathing after this is much easier. The baby without enough surfactant has to work hard to breathe and may become exhausted in the struggle to get enough

Phototherapy
A jaundiced baby can be treated beside his mother's bed or at home using a blanket that is equipped with fiber-optic bands.

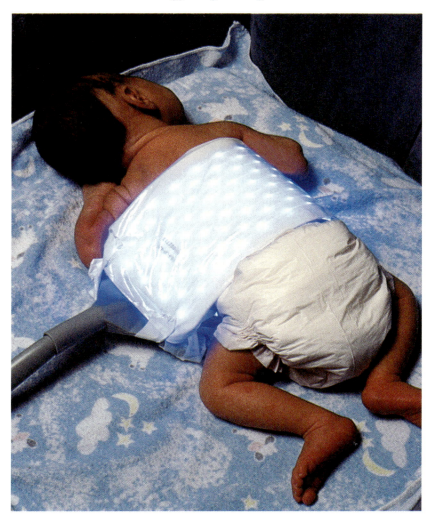

air. She breathes very quickly, the chest collapses with each breath out, and she looks blue and grunts as she breathes. This is called respiratory distress or hyaline membrane disease. It is important in these cases to give the baby oxygen to help with breathing.

Other babies who may suffer from respiratory distress are those born to diabetic mothers (even though they are usually large babies), those who have not had sufficient oxygen during labor, those who have been delivered by Cesarean section, and those who develop pneumonia as a result of infection.

If the pediatrician decides to give the baby oxygen, blood oxygen is measured by means of a monitor held against the baby's skin. A small catheter can also be inserted through the cord stump into an artery so that blood samples can be taken when necessary to test the amount of oxygen in the baby's blood.

Oxygen can be administered with continuous positive pressure so that the baby's lungs are kept open. A tiny catheter is inserted through the nostrils, or a face mask or headbox is used.

THE BABY WITH LOW BLOOD SUGAR

A baby may have low blood sugar (hypoglycemia) if he has a low birth weight or is preterm, if the mother received large amounts of intravenous dextrose during labor, if she is diabetic, or if she had a difficult delivery. The hypoglycemic baby may have breathing difficulties and be jittery, or lie limp and apathetic. Hypoglycemia can be dangerous for a baby if left untreated, and for this reason a small baby may be tested for it in the first 48 hours or so after birth.

Treatment involves giving the baby ample nourishment, so the pediatrician may decide to set up an intravenous glucose drip. Because of the risk of hypoglycemia, a very tiny baby may be given additional feedings, even though there are no symptoms of low blood sugar.

For babies who are of 30 weeks' gestation or more, cup feeding works well. They lap the milk from a cup with their tongues, like kittens. When they are over 34 weeks' gestation, they can often sip it. The transition to breast-feeding is often easier than after tube feeding, perhaps because the baby has already had a satisfying oral experience and has learned to work to get milk.*

NEONATAL JAUNDICE

If your baby looks beautifully suntanned, as if just back from a cruise in the Bahamas, this is jaundice. A newborn baby has a surplus of red blood cells that are broken down after birth. During this process, a yellowish substance called bilirubin is produced, which has to be excreted by the baby's liver. Sometimes the liver is unable to cope rapidly with the large amount of bilirubin, so it builds up in the blood, giving the skin a yellowish tinge. Bilirubin levels peak between the third and fifth day and then drop.

PHYSIOLOGICAL JAUNDICE About half of all babies develop jaundice. It is usually harmless and is then called physiological jaundice. It is most likely to develop after the second day of life and to disappear after a week. In preterm babies, jaundice tends to be most marked on about the fifth or sixth day of life and to go on longer—often for ten days or more.

A jaundiced baby needs sunlight and frequent feeding. If you have the chance, put your baby beside a window and, if it is warm enough, uncover the baby so that light can reach her limbs and trunk. Jaundiced babies tend to get very sleepy. They need to be roused for feedings—about every two hours.

If the bilirubin level is high, the pediatrician may decide to use phototherapy to bring the level down. This light treatment produces a photochemical breakdown of bilirubin into substances that are passed out in the urine. The baby is blindfolded so that the light cannot harm her eyes. This can be distressing for a mother, who may feel out of touch with her baby when she cannot make eye contact. When you lift your baby away from the light for a feeding, take off the eye covering.

"THEY GAVE MY BABY PHOTOTHERAPY TREATMENT RIGHT BESIDE MY BED, INSTEAD OF IN THE NURSERY. THAT MEANT SO MUCH TO ME."

Another form of phototherapy is a blanket filled with fiber-optic wands that emit light. The blanket is wrapped around the baby and glows. This type of phototherapy, as well as standard phototherapy, can be used in the home.

PATHOLOGIC JAUNDICE Pediatricians always watch the jaundiced baby carefully because, although neonatal jaundice is common, the baby may be jaundiced as a result of other problems, the most common being a blood group incompatibility with the mother. This is called pathologic jaundice and can damage the baby's nervous system and brain cells. Sometimes jaundice is associated with infection or with a metabolic condition such as low blood sugar, or is the result of drugs taken by the mother in pregnancy.

FEEDING THE BABY IN SPECIAL CARE

Very small babies do best if they are fed soon after birth.* The best food is the mother's breast milk, but it will take a few days to be produced in quantity. The baby can be put to the breast if strong enough to suck, to derive benefit from the protein and antibodies in the colostrum that is already there.

A baby who cannot suck is usually fed through a small, soft catheter, a nasogastric tube, which is passed through a nostril down into the stomach. Feedings should be small and frequent—about every half hour. You can help with the feedings once you can express your own breast milk. Breast milk offers protection against necrotizing encolitis, a disease in which the baby's intestines become damaged; formula-fed preterm babies are at risk of developing this illness, which can be fatal. If you have any difficulties, contact one of the organizations listed on pages 427–428.

RELATING TO THE BABY IN SPECIAL CARE

It is distressing for parents to see their baby in intensive care, attached to tubes and wires, isolated in an incubator. Your baby may look like an odd, misshapen doll, or a little animal. On the other hand, you may feel passionately that the baby belongs to you and want to grab him away from all the machines and other contraptions to hold him close. The obvious skills of those working with sophisticated technology can make parents feel clumsy and awkward, so that they lack confidence to handle their baby. Yet it is important to do this. All babies need touching and talking to and, if they are well enough to be taken in your arms, they like being cuddled. If your baby is in an incubator, you can stroke him through the portholes. Tender, loving care may be just as important for the health of your baby as modern medical technology.

Mothers and fathers are encouraged to spend time in the special care nursery. They can touch their baby through portholes in the incubator.

Many hospitals now have rooms where mothers of babies in special care can stay to be close to them, help look after

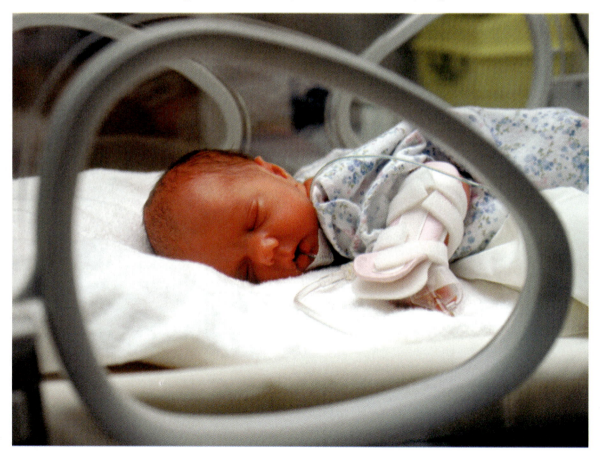

them, and breast-feed. It is easier to build close links if the mother stays in the special care unit rather than merely visiting. When a woman can start to look after her baby herself, she begins to feel that her baby belongs to her. One model intensive care unit has rooms where babies are cared for by their mothers, with a glass wall at the side of the babies' cubicles so that nurses can keep a constant eye on them. A nurse in this unit said: "One thing the nurses must not do is to take away the mother's responsibility for her baby. We always try to make a mother feel that it is her baby, even when it is very small and sick."

THE BABY WITH A DISABILITY

The moment when someone tells you, or when you yourself recognize, that your baby is not "normal" is engraved on your mind forever. This happens to 3 in every 100 women. The most common disabilities are cerebral palsy, which can affect both brain and body, and Down's syndrome, which has a genetic cause. For many disabilities no cause is known. It used to be thought that cerebral palsy was always caused by lack of oxygen during labor and birth, but it is now known that it is much more likely (90 percent chance) to be a result of oxygen deprivation during pregnancy. There is no way a mother could have known about this or taken steps to avoid it.

"WE COULDN'T BELIEVE IT. WE HOPED THAT THEY'D SAY, 'THERE HAS BEEN A MISTAKE. THE BABY IS GOING TO BE FINE.'"

Your first reaction to being told that an abnormality is suspected may be simple denial. It cannot possibly be, or if there is something wrong they will discover that it is minor. As tests are done and information trickles in, you may start to feel cheated. You see other mothers with their perfect babies and ask, "Why me?" Having a baby with a disability sets you apart from other mothers and may make you feel not only different but stigmatized. There may be an overwhelming sense of guilt: "What did I do wrong?" Although you are assured that nothing you did or did not do brought about this outcome, you probably continue to blame yourself even when your rational mind acknowledges that bad things happen in life that you cannot possibly control. Other people's attitudes are often difficult to cope with, whether it be their careful avoidance of the topic, their pity, or ways in which they try to be positive and reassuring. Feelings of shame and resentment jostle with anger. You want to blame someone, but there is no one to blame and, of course, you feel realistic anxiety about the future. One of the most painful things about having a child who is different is the isolation that often results. So contact an organization that enables you to meet parents who have children with the same disability, to learn more, share experiences, and develop coping strategies. Some addresses are on pages 427–428.

LOSING A BABY

Many women have an interrupted pregnancy, although the distress caused by even an early miscarriage is often underestimated. Stillbirth, however, is now rare. But still today, for a small number of women, birth is also a death.

Women who make the painful decision to have a termination, because of fetal disability or for any other reason, grieve deeply, too. This is so even though they know that they have made the best choice and have behaved sensibly. A termination should never be dismissed as a simple expedient to get rid of an unwanted pregnancy. Yet it is still largely a taboo subject, and women often have to go through the experience alone, without any help, socially isolated and deprived of the emotional support they need.

Most people find it easier to sympathize with a woman whose baby dies at birth. Yet often they do not know how to help and they withdraw from her grief in embarrassment. After all the woman's preparations and her happy expectations, she goes through a labor that culminates in the delivery of a stillborn baby, or of a frail or disabled baby who dies a week or so after birth. Her arms are empty and she is left alone. The more medical advances reduce perinatal mortality, the more isolated is the woman whose baby dies.

MISCARRIAGE

A miscarriage usually comes as a terrible shock, and yet one in every five pregnancies probably ends in miscarriage or "spontaneous abortion." In three out of four cases this occurs before the tenth week and sometimes even before you realize you are pregnant.

THREATENED MISCARRIAGE

In the first three months of pregnancy, you may notice a heavy feeling around your pelvis and in the pit of your tummy and have periodlike twinges and aches.

Sometimes you have bleeding that is really a suppressed period. This happens when there is insufficient pregnancy hormone to stop your period, even though it is scanty. Such bleeding is not a miscarriage, and the blood comes from the endometrium (uterine lining), not from the placenta or the baby. Sometimes this also occurs at the time when each period would have been due, and through the early months of pregnancy each would-be period is marked by slight bleeding. Some doctors advise injections of progesterone to stop this bleeding. Bleeding in pregnancy is not the baby's blood but yours, and comes from the maternal side of the placenta where it is not adhering to the uterus, or from around the cervix. It used to be thought that the best thing was to go to bed and stay there until the bleeding stopped. There is, however, no evidence that this helps at all.* So do whatever makes you feel more comfortable.

INEVITABLE ABORTION

An "inevitable abortion" is a miscarriage that occurs because the baby is no longer alive and, whatever you do, the bleeding is bound to continue. If the fetal heartbeat cannot be detected by ultrasound (see pages 229–232), the abortion is inevitable and you might just as well be up and about and let it run its course. If ultrasound picks up the baby's heartbeat, there is only a 10 percent chance that you will miscarry, even though you may go on bleeding for a while.

CAUSES OF EARLY MISCARRIAGE

The cause of early miscarriage is often not known. Embryos with abnormalities that would not allow them to survive after birth are usually miscarried, and a very large proportion of miscarriages are nature's way of getting rid of imperfect babies. Sometimes there has been no development beyond the very early stages of segmentation, and what is termed a "blighted ovum" is passed. It is estimated that one in six miscarriages result from fertilized eggs that do not develop properly.

"I'D BEEN IN TWO MINDS ABOUT BEING PREGNANT, BUT I WAS SURPRISED BY THE SADNESS AND SENSE OF FAILURE I FELT WHEN I REALIZED THAT I HAD LOST THE BABY."

After it had been noted that more women than usual miscarry in early pregnancy during flu epidemics, it was discovered that a high fever can result in miscarriage. There is more about this on page 111. Sometimes uterine fibroids (common in older mothers) or an oddly formed uterus result in there not being enough space for the pregnancy to develop.

CLEANING OUT THE UTERUS Some doctors take it for granted that a woman who has had a miscarriage should go to the hospital for a D & C (dilatation and curettage) to scrape out surgically any remaining contents of the uterus, in order to avoid infection. This can be a traumatic experience. Research shows that surgery is no better than waiting, if the amount left in the uterus is small.*

There may be a hormonal factor in some miscarriages, since one third of women who have repeated miscarriages have also found it difficult to get pregnant. (Insulin-dependent diabetic women with poor glucose control have up to three times more miscarriages than other women.) Occasionally, recurrent miscarriage is a sign of an autoimmune condition known as antiphospholipid syndrome (APS). The mother produces antibodies that cause blood clots in the placenta. Low doses of aspirin given throughout pregnancy help these women, and injections of the anticoagulant heparin raise the chances of a live birth from 10 percent to 70 percent.

LATE MISCARRIAGE

Miscarriage after the 12th week of pregnancy is approximately three times less common than in early pregnancy. It is more likely as you grow older (over 35), if you had difficulty in conceiving (if it has taken longer than six months), and if you have had two or more previous miscarriages. If you have had only one miscarriage before, there is no reason why the next pregnancy should not be straightforward. After three miscarriages there is a 50/50 chance of miscarrying again, so talk to your doctor before you become pregnant again, and plan your time to include extra rest from the first days after possible conception.

INFECTION Twenty percent of late miscarriages are due to infections such as listeriosis. Antibiotic treatment is effective.

"INCOMPETENT" CERVIX Late miscarriage is sometimes the result of a weak cervix that starts to dilate long before it should. The bag of waters is wedged between the baby and the cervix and ruptures as the cervix starts to dilate, so the first sign may be the breaking of the waters. This type of miscarriage is particularly likely if a woman has already miscarried repeatedly in mid-pregnancy. A weak cervix may be the result of a previous abortion if it was done after the 12th week, or of a previous difficult labor, or of certain treatments for abnormal pap tests that can shorten and weaken it. More information about this can be found on page 115.

PLACENTAL INSUFFICIENCY Miscarriage after the 20th week may occur because the placenta has failed to function in servicing the baby. (After 24 weeks the loss of the baby is termed a stillbirth.) If there is evidence of poor placental function and inadequate growth of the baby in the uterus, bed rest will allow a better flow of blood through the placenta to the baby. One way you can improve the efficiency of the placenta is by making sure that you have a good diet during pregnancy. If you have had a miscarriage, start a high-standard diet before you become pregnant again (see pages 96–101). If you have had a series of miscarriages, keep any large blood clots from the latest one for the doctor to see and have tested in a laboratory.

GUILT ABOUT A MISCARRIAGE

Every woman who has had a miscarriage wonders if anything she did or failed to do caused it. A miscarriage can happen at any time, so most women will be able to think of some event that might have triggered it. You had an argument with someone in the office, your mother-in-law came to stay, you slipped in the street, had just had intercourse, or were overtired from a party the night before. Whatever your guilty suspicions, none of these things has been shown to cause miscarriage. However, it can be difficult to convince yourself that you are in no way responsible.

GRIEVING FOR THE LOST BABY

Miscarriage, however early it occurs, is for most women the loss of a baby. If it was to be your first child, it is also the loss of yourself as a mother, and with repeated miscarriages you experience this loss over and over again. It may also be the loss of your partner as a father and of your parents as new grandparents. It may be a child's loss of an expected sibling. But women are often ashamed of this and fear that they are being "overemotional" or "silly."

> **"I MISCARRIED LATE IN PREGNANCY, SO I STARTED TO LACTATE. IT FELT AS IF MY BREASTS WERE WEEPING MILK FOR MY LOST BABY AND IT WAS ALL BEING WASTED."**

Talk with your partner about your feelings. Even if you have not yet felt fetal movements, the loss of your baby is sometimes emotionally shattering. If you have had miscarriage after miscarriage or are slow to conceive, you may experience every single period as the loss of a baby.

Your partner, however, may not have accepted the reality of the pregnancy by the time you miscarry, so it can be difficult for him to understand why you need to mourn. You may find you can talk more easily with another woman who has been through a miscarriage herself.

After it is all over, the longing to start another pregnancy can interfere with relaxed and spontaneous sex. If you feel that you are getting anxious and that this is hurting your sexual relationship, try taking a vacation from each other and coming together again at the time when you expect to be ovulating (see pages 68–70).

STILLBIRTH

"I'm so sorry. Your baby has died." Almost every expectant mother has thought at some time that someone might say these words to her. For some women it is a fear that haunts them as they punish themselves for negative feelings they have about the baby and about becoming a mother, or for daring to expect too much of the birth and the baby. Sometimes, but not as often as in the past (in about 8 out of every 1,000 births), it really happens and the baby dies before, during, or shortly after birth.

THE EXPERIENCE OF LOSS

Despite everything that anyone can do, you are suddenly confronted with the experience of loss. This is a loss not only of the baby, but of all the expectations of yourselves as parents and the new images of the self and the family that have been built up through pregnancy.

Nothing can take away the suffering that accompanies stillbirth. This is so even when the care that is given to you is loving and sympathetic, although such emotional support can help you deal gradually with the experience and eventually come to terms with it. Unfortunately, some members of the hospital staff cannot cope with their own feelings of guilt and distress when a baby dies, and you may be left alone in your room, avoided as much as possible because they do not want to "upset" you by referring to what has happened. When they talk to you, they may urge you to put it behind you, say that you will forget when you have another baby, or tell you to think of your partner. The more such advice is given, the longer it takes to live through and come to terms with the experience.

You will be offered bereavement counseling, and although you may not feel like it at the time, it helps to have someone to talk to who is not a friend or relation. The task of grieving is a personal and intimate one. It consists of slowly and painfully integrating the experience into the total pattern of your life and finding a place for it in which it has meaning. (Sometimes you may feel that you will never succeed in doing it.) Once you have done this, you will be able to stand back from it a little. This process cannot be hurried, and if an attempt is made to force the pace, grieving will be delayed and you may be overpowered by grief at a later stage of your life.

STILLBIRTH IN TRADITIONAL SOCIETIES

A hundred years ago, everyone expected a certain proportion of babies to die. A woman bore ten and reared six if she was lucky. In many traditional societies even today, babies are not named or spoken of publicly for the first few weeks in case they do not survive.

In these societies, death is incorporated into the web of life and there are supportive rituals to deal with it, whereas we are ill-prepared in Western society for facing death. We struggle individually to find our own way and are often left with the feeling that we are the only people who have ever faced such emotional upheavals. Death is a shocking intrusion into the normality of our existence.

FACING UP TO THE LOSS

If professional helpers know that something is going wrong with your birth, you have a right to expect them to give you clear information, discuss the difficulties openly and honestly, and stand by you as you try to cope emotionally with what is happening. Women who have been through this ordeal say that it helped to be told the truth and to be fully involved rather than shielded from the event by the mystique of medical practice. If your baby dies while still inside the uterus, you know that you are carrying a dead baby. It feels then as if your uterus, a place of life, has become a grave. The obstetrician may advise that it is safer to wait to go into labor naturally, which often happens within a couple of weeks, but may offer you induction if you wish. Many women feel an urgent need to "get it over with." Others feel that they want to spend the last remaining days possible with the baby inside them.

When something so distressing happens, there is no easy "solution," no one course of action that can wipe out the anguish. Sometimes a man asks what he can say or do to help his partner and to make the suffering less, or other family members or friends want to help but do not know how. People are so different in their responses to loss that the most helpers can do is to make themselves available, reach out and be ready to receive whatever the bereaved person wants to tell them, without holding back for fear of intruding or feeling embarrassment at her grief. The most valuable thing they can offer is a *waiting silence*.

MOURNING FOR THE BABY

This may sound simple, but it can be very difficult, because grieving is a matter not just of tears and sadness, but numb shock and guilt and anger, all of which are felt at different phases of the experience. It is not easy to acknowledge destructive guilt, and even harder to cope with anger that involves hostility toward people, including doctors and midwives who did all they could to help.

> **"I NEEDED TO BE HELD AND HUGGED,** BUT IT WAS HARD FOR MY HUSBAND TO DO THIS BECAUSE HE WAS TRYING TO BE STRONG AND HIDE HIS EMOTIONS."

The time immediately following the death of a baby may be a time of frozen half-awareness of what has happened, and frequently it is not until at least three weeks afterward that you begin to live through these other phases of grieving.

It is sometimes difficult for a mother to mourn her stillborn baby because she never really knew this person for whom she is grieving. It can be still more difficult if you have not seen the dead baby. This is why most grief counselors and pediatricians think it is a good idea for a mother to touch her stillborn child, and encourage her to do so. You can ask to hold your baby and to be left alone to say good-bye. Take as long as you need.

THE BABY'S BURIAL

You and your partner may wish to discuss together arrangements for the baby's burial. Some women feel afterward that perhaps the baby was a figment of their imagination and never actually existed at all. It was removed from them like a tooth that was causing trouble. You may think of your baby's body being handled with indifference and lie awake wondering what might have happened to it. This is why it often helps to involve yourself in the arrangements.

THE EFFECT ON YOUR RELATIONSHIPS

Being depressed affects all our relationships with other people, including those we love and need the most. Although the death of a baby may draw you and your partner closer together, it introduces stresses that may be too severe for you to cope with. You both may need help from other people. Your partner has to grieve, too, and yet may feel that it is "unmanly" to show any emotional weakness and that he must be strong to support you. The result may be that he simulates a matter-of-fact acceptance of the inevitable and leaves you feeling isolated because he seems not to understand.

"I DIDN'T WANT TO FORCE HIM TO TALK ABOUT IT, AND HE FELT THE SAME WAY ABOUT ME. SO WE GOT ON WITH OUR LIVES AND AFTER A WHILE FOUND WE HAD DRIFTED APART."

If the baby lived for a time and went to the special care nursery, your partner probably had a chance to go there and see and touch the baby while you stayed on the maternity ward. So you rely on his descriptions to build up a complete picture. Yet a man who is himself depressed and grieving may find it difficult to talk without showing his own distress and may resist it, giving the impression that he is holding back on vital information.

Losing a baby almost invariably causes a deterioration in the couple's sexual relationship. It is difficult to feel sexually excited when you are depressed. Even when you are beginning to "function" again, feelings of pleasure can be followed by a rush of grief. When you start to enjoy life, or to feel sexually aroused, you may both feel at times that you are betraying your dead child.*

If you want to be in touch with other people who have undergone this experience and are willing to share experiences and support, contact one of the organizations listed on pages 427–428.

THE NEXT PREGNANCY

If you have had a termination or have lost a previous baby as a result of miscarriage or stillbirth, or if your baby died after birth, the previous experience tends to cast its shadow forward. This tends to happen even if you really did not want that particular pregnancy to continue.

A woman who has lost a baby through accident—who has had miscarriages, for example, or a crib death—may feel angry that the emotions of one who has had a termination should be discussed in the same context as her own ordeal, and may even feel that the woman who got rid of a baby deserves whatever happens to her. Yet the experience of loss may be equally haunting and the sense of guilt even greater.

We tend to compare and contrast the progress of the present pregnancy with past pregnancies. If a previous pregnancy had an unhappy outcome, it colors our view of the whole experience, and it is natural to be acutely conscious of risks and dangers.

A woman who feels guilty about aborting a previous baby or who feels responsible for a miscarriage may transfer this guilt to the present pregnancy and be anxious that she is going to have a terrible labor, bear an abnormal baby, or lose the baby as a kind of retribution or punishment. This is not a rational or even a conscious thinking-through of the risks but a primitive expectation that automatic punishment comes from the gods.

"IT WAS AS IF I WERE BETRAYING MY DEAD BABY WHEN I BECAME PREGNANT AGAIN. I COULDN'T HELP FEELING GUILTY."

If you try to forget what happened or to push it to the back of your mind, you will be unprepared for the emotions that may assail you in stressful situations—when you have a vaginal examination, for example, or when you go into the hospital. When labor starts, you may find that you cannot help thinking back to the loss of the other baby.

You may tell yourself to be sensible and not dwell on negative thoughts. This is rarely successful. You are right to acknowledge your feelings and justified in getting those who care for you to take them seriously. But do not postpone this process until the end of pregnancy, certainly not until you go into labor. Try to find the kind of preparation for birth that includes frank and open acceptance of any previous unhappy experience.

In a pregnancy following the loss of a baby, women often experience painful, disturbing dreams about bearing a damaged child or losing the baby and feel that in some awful way this is their own fault. The dreams may be clearly about birth and babies or may be heavily disguised. The baby is often represented in such dreams as a doll or small animal, or one's own tooth or limb, and death as the irretrievable loss of something that is treasured.

You may feel that you are carrying a baby of the same sex as the previous one or even that you are pregnant with the child you lost before. Some people even say, "Have another baby and you'll forget about it." But of course you cannot substitute one baby for another, or replace a lost baby by getting pregnant again. It is vital for both you and the baby you are bearing that you acknowledge that this baby is its own unique self.

THE FIRST TEN DAYS

For much of the time, you may feel ecstatic and on a permanent high after the birth, but the chances are you will experience a range of other emotions, too. However perfect and welcome your baby is, this is a new beginning, and it entails leaving behind some aspects of yourself.

EMOTIONS AFTER BIRTH

Many women need time to part with the fantasy baby they carried inside them before they can come to terms with the real one. The real baby is often astonishingly different from the one they imagined they were bearing. The death of a fantasy that has been cherished can be painful. It is especially threatening if the baby is preterm and needs special care, or suffers from a disability. But even a healthy, mature baby may be so unlike what you expected that you cannot come to terms with the reality.

CHANGES IN MOOD

All the intense feelings you have during the hours and days after having given birth have biological survival value for the baby. Without them you would be just a caretaker. Sometimes your emotions are mind-altering and, had you not just had a baby, would be thought pathological. But during the first week after birth they are perfectly normal and experienced by many more women than ever openly admit to them.

It is not just a matter of depression. In fact, you may feel on a permanent high. But it is likely that at some time during the first five days after the birth you will experience an abrupt drop in mood and a sudden feeling of depression. Your stitches are uncomfortable, the first days at home are like a thick fog, you start to worry about the baby or whether you will be a good mother, or you simply feel flat because the party is over and it is now "the morning after the night before." Then again, you may experience violent mood swings and feel you are on an emotional roller coaster in the days immediately after the birth. Our society often has a very romanticized stereotype of the new mother in a frothy pink negligée with a cherubic baby in her arms. The violent mood swings that you may experience can come as a shock because they are so different from the way you think you *should* feel.

A mother gives her newborn his first taste of one of the great pleasures of the first year of life.

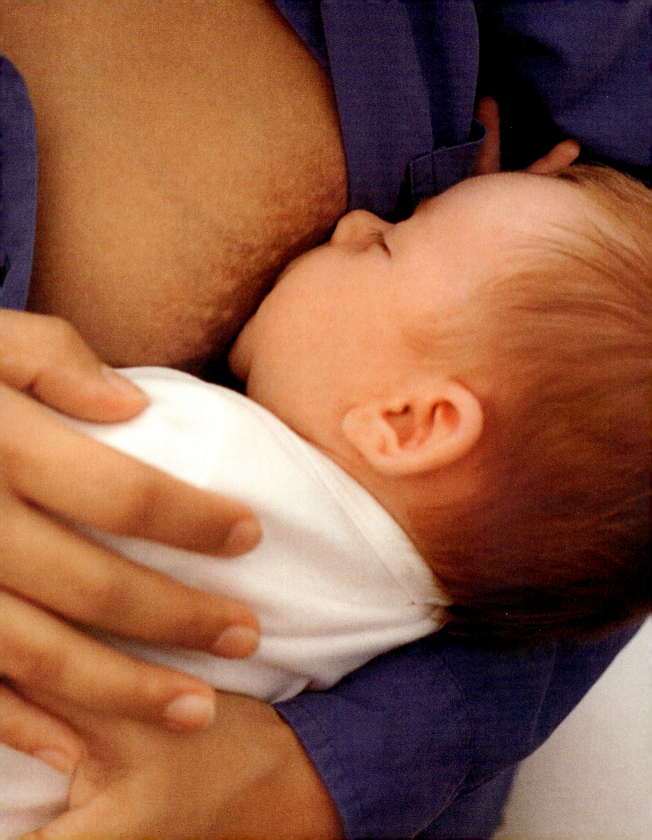

THE NEED TO BE SPONTANEOUS

You do not become a different person once you have a baby, but all the colors of your personality become more vivid. You want to cry and then a short while later laugh helplessly at something that is not really very funny. This is why any indignation you may feel about something or someone in the hospital—and, above all, longing for your baby if he is in a nursery—seems to have a physical impact, knotting your stomach, drying your throat, burning you up.

Some women who have their babies in a hospital are emotionally unsettled until they get home. They have a great need to be *in their own place*. On the other hand, if you are sent home within 24 or 48 hours of the birth, you may not feel ready. You may not have successfully breast-fed your baby; you may have painful stitches; there may be no one there to help you. You may feel frightened and helpless at the prospect of taking on all that responsibility so soon after the birth. There is nothing abnormal about feeling like this.

"I WAS DEPRESSED BUT TOLD NO ONE, SINCE NO ONE ASKED AND I FELT TOO TERRIBLE ABOUT IT TO BRING IT UP. SURELY I OUGHT TO BE HAPPY."

If all is going well with you and the baby, and you have help at home, it works well to leave the hospital as soon as possible. If you are discharged from the hospital sooner than 48 hours after delivery, or if you or your baby have certain complications, it is sometimes possible to arrange a home visit by a postpartum nurse.

COMPLICATED EMOTIONS

Your partner may be experiencing violent emotions at this time and be torn between laughter and tears. Our society tends to stress that men should be strong and offer broad shoulders for a new mother to lean on, but some men are so deeply touched by the experience of birth that they undergo much the same emotional turmoil as the new mother. A father may suffer as he goes back home after the birth, because he is surrendering you and his newborn baby to the care of strangers. In spite of rejoicing and excitement, there may be an undercurrent of grief. The intimate bond linking him to the woman who has borne his child is cut by enforced separation. When he returns to the hospital it is as a visitor.

YOUR CHANGED BODY

After you have had a baby you encounter your body in a dramatically changed state. Whereas before you enjoyed your smooth body heavy with fruit, the curve of your abdomen like an enormous melon still awaiting the harvest of birth, after birth you may feel astonishingly alone, bereft, and empty. If you are in the hospital without people you love near you, in the care of people who treat you as just another "mom" or, worse still, as an involuting uterus, a sutured perineum, and a couple of lactating breasts, you need time to come to terms with your changed body and to rediscover yourself as a person.

For many women, the euphoria of having given birth and of having produced a real baby, which comes as a delightful surprise at first, gives way to this confrontation with the body. Changes in the breasts associated with breast-feeding can be an ordeal for some women. Many set their sights on the birth, seeing this as the challenge, and are ill-prepared for the new challenges that follow. One mother who felt a revulsion at her much-changed body exclaimed: "But it was all supposed to be *over!*"

YOUR PERINEUM

You are likely to feel swollen, tender, and bruised. A packet of frozen peas or ice chips wrapped in a washcloth placed over the sore area gives relief. Your perineum probably stings when you pass urine, so keep a small pitcher of boiled saltwater in the bathroom and pour some over as you empty your bladder or bowels. Pour some of this water over after you have finished, too, and dry with a hair dryer on a low setting or gently pat with soft toilet paper. If you had a slight tear, it will heal naturally. If you had stitches, they should be absorbed in about a week. It helps if you press a piece of cut-up sanitary pad over the sore area as you empty your bladder or bowels. Avoid constipation by eating laxative foods like prunes, figs, and puréed fruit of any kind, and drink plenty of water. If you are finding it difficult to pass urine, tell your doctor or midwife. It is important not to let your bladder become distended with urine. Sometimes a catheter helps for a day or two.

WEIGHT LOSS

Immediately following delivery you probably feel beautifully slim and lightweight. You have lost the combined weight of the baby, the placenta, the amniotic fluid, and membranes. But when you first put your hand down on your tummy, you become aware of folds of skin, like a soft and soggy cream puff. When you first catch sight of yourself naked in a full-length mirror you may be horrified at the amount of weight you have put on: thickened waist, heavy thighs, and (if you are breast-feeding) ballooning breasts—which you and your partner may enjoy if you were small and flat before, but which can be too much of a good thing if you were top-heavy anyway.

WATER LOSS During the week after childbirth most women sweat out and pass as urine the excess fluid they no longer need, and any puffiness you may have noticed in your legs and ankles will disappear. So will the plumped-out facial features and any fluid retained in your fingers. You may be pleasantly surprised by the difference this makes to your shape.

RESTORING MUSCLE TONE If you use your abdominal muscles your tummy will flatten after a few weeks. Some exercises for the early postpartum period are illustrated on pages 416–419. Brisk walking is good for abdominal muscles. If the weather is suitable, put the baby in a carrier against your body and walk, in the country if possible. At first your pelvic floor muscles may feel as if they are sagging like a heavy hammock, but their tone will be gradually restored over the next three months and, if you use them regularly, without straining them, rehabilitation will be complete.

BREASTS AND BREAST-FEEDING

The sooner you put your baby to the breast, the sooner her stomach will be lined with colostrum, a substance that forms a protective "paint" and a barrier to invading bacteria. Colostrum also provides the baby with antibodies to diseases to which you yourself are resistant. Ready in your breasts at the end of pregnancy, it is the earliest form of milk, rich in protein, and an ideal first concentrated food for your baby. Do not wash your nipples before breastfeeding. Babies are attracted to the breast partly by their sense of smell, and prefer an unwashed to a washed breast.*

THE MILK EJECTION REFLEX

When your baby sucks, the action stimulates an area in your brain (the hypothalamus) that activates the pituitary gland at the base of your brain to release oxytocin into your bloodstream. Oxytocin flows into the blood vessels in your breasts and causes cells around the milk glands deep inside them to contract. This has the effect of squeezing milk out through the tiny holes in your nipples.

Oxytocin also makes your uterus contract, so you have the odd feeling of milk being pushed down into your baby's mouth at the same time as your uterus is squeezing tight. After about a week you can no longer feel uterine contractions when you breast-feed. You will probably feel the warm, tingling glow of the milk ejection reflex immediately preceding the flow of milk. This occurs as the oxytocin-carrying blood rushes into the breasts and you feel them getting warmer. Infrared photographs of lactating breasts show that they really do grow hotter in response to the baby's cry.

THE FIRST FEEDINGS Notice what happens when you put the baby to the breast. He should have the nipple deep in his mouth and as much of the areola as will make a good mouthful. Cuddle the baby close and wait. Drop your shoulders: if they feel stiff, *pull* them down and then let them go. Sometimes it may take a few minutes for the sensation to come and then suddenly it is there! Deep inside both breasts, not just the one the baby is sucking, there is a prickling, buzzing feeling as if champagne were flowing through your veins, while a wave of heat flows toward your nipples. You

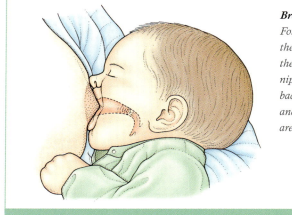

Breast-feeding
For breast-feeding to go well, the baby needs to suck at the breast, not just the nipple. The nipple is drawn back into the baby's mouth, and the jaws press on the areola to pump the milk.

see the baby's jaws beginning to work, and the strong, steady movement of the bone at the top of the baby's jawbone, just by his ear, as he begins to swallow as well as suck.

The milk ejection reflex can occur spontaneously when you just think about feeding the baby or hear his crying. If he is not in your arms, press the palm of a hand firmly against your breast and the milk flow—a slow but steady dripping from the nipple—will stop.

THE DIFFERENCE BETWEEN SUCKING AND FEEDING

Having milk in your breasts is just the beginning. Obviously the important thing is to *release* it so that it flows into your baby. For nutritional purposes it is not enough to have a baby sucking at your breasts, although he will enjoy this anyway. He needs to swallow in a steady rhythm, and until this happens he is not feeding.

Hospitals are more relaxed than they used to be about the time babies spend at the breast, but if you are in one where feeding time is still restricted, you should count the time from the moment the baby is actually feeding, not from when he is just sucking.

Even before the reflex occurs the baby gets some milk, because it collects in the ducts just behind the nipple. This is called "foremilk" and is thirst-quenching. It usually keeps the baby happy until the rush of milk comes with the reflex. But if you give a baby foremilk only, because he is not sucking long enough to stimulate the reflex, your milk supply will dwindle or never build up.

If you feel embarrassed or self-conscious or experience strong emotions of anxiety, fear, or anger, the milk ejection reflex will probably be slower in coming and sometimes may not occur at all. This is why the setting for breast-feeding in the first days after birth is so important and why emotional support from your partner or someone else who understands how you feel is helpful. Even though you may think you have emptied a breast, a fresh reflex can occur when you put the baby back to it again. A breast is not like a jar of milk but produces a constant supply, provided that the baby gives the right stimulus.

BLISSFUL BREAST-FEEDINGS

If you can, keep your baby with you all 24 hours of the day, and feed whenever the baby wants. Some babies, especially in the first four to six weeks of life, enjoy sucking more or less continuously at certain times of the day. Look at your baby's little clenched fist: her stomach is just about the same size. Feeding her frequently is important, but so is the length of the feeding, because milk becomes progressively richer as your baby feeds. Although the milk starts to get creamy as soon as she begins to suck vigorously, keep her at the breast until her eyes close and she begins to feel heavy. Then you can be sure she is taking enough.

The shape of the baby's face is perfectly adapted to sucking at the breast: a snub nose, receding chin, and a mouth that opens wide and latches on.

Most babies find breast-feeding so blissful they don't want it to end. You can unplug the

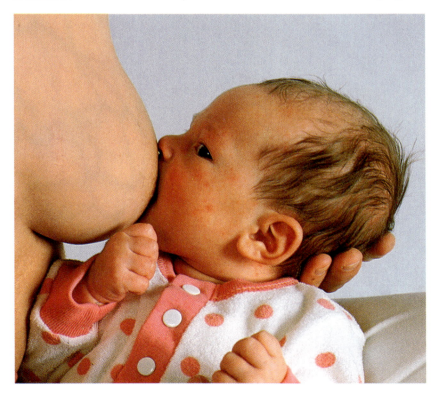

baby's mouth gently by depressing the breast with a finger, or slip a finger just inside the baby's mouth to break the vacuum—but don't just pull the nipple out. If she eagerly grasps the nipple again, breast-feed a bit longer.

BABIES LIKE SUCKING FOR COMFORT

You may feel very "drained" when nursing is long and drawn out: if you are tired and the baby is constantly demanding to be fed, it is easy to think that you cannot be providing enough milk. Although this is sometimes the case, many babies want to go on feeding nonstop because they like it so much, not because they are starving. So after about ten minutes' sucking, it is sensible to put the baby down or hand her over to a friend or your partner for a cuddle. Relax a bit; offer some more breast milk on whichever side feels more generously supplied; then take another break, and so on.

EACH BABY HAS A DIFFERENT FEEDING PATTERN

Breast-fed babies do not suck continuously through a feeding. They enjoy bursts of sucking, stop for a while, then start again. If you think about meals you enjoy, you will realize that you do not chomp away nonstop, either. Nor do you want an equal quantity of food at each meal. Babies are the same.

Think of each feeding as divided into different courses. Some will be seven- or eight-course banquets, but others will be only two courses. You will gradually be able to work out when the baby likes the banquets, and then you may be able to cater to them by arranging your day to fit this pattern. Anticipating and preparing for feeding sessions of this kind makes them much easier to cope with, and you are less likely to feel exhausted by them.

IS BREAST MILK ENOUGH?

You may wonder if and when your baby needs food other than breast milk, especially if you secretly feel that he is not getting enough milk from you, or he cries a lot. But introducing extras can make the problem worse.

WATER Some hospitals still give water or sugar water. The baby needs milk, not water. If your baby is producing six or more wet diapers in the course of 24 hours and frequent bowel movements and is having no other fluid, and if the urine is pale amber or colorless, then this shows that he is getting enough milk from you. You will probably find that *you* are thirstier than usual. Drink as much as you like, although there is no point in having more than you want, since it will not produce more milk. Giving a newborn baby any fluid other than breast milk is harmful.

SUPPLEMENTARY BOTTLES If you think your baby is not getting enough milk and you start to give bottle feedings, the amount of milk you are producing will diminish, since demand stimulates supply.

SOLID FOODS When you introduce solid foods, your milk supply is reduced. This is one reason that introducing solid foods early is counter-productive. It replaces food the baby needs, human milk, with food he does not need until he is about six months old. A baby's appetite cannot cope with human milk *plus* a range of other foods that are on the market. Manufacturers who promote the early introduction of so-called "baby foods" at three to four months are often responsible for breast-feeding difficulties. It is no coincidence that when the baby is three to four months old, mothers who have started mixed feeding begin to discover that they are failing to produce enough milk.

TEST WEIGHING Weighing the baby before and after a feeding (test weighing) is a pointless exercise unless done over a 24-hour period, since the baby takes different quantities of milk at different times. Even then, it tends to increase your anxiety and make you feel inadequate. A much better guide to your baby's well-being is good muscle tone and alert responses.

MORE FREQUENT BREAST-FEEDING When you want to increase the quantity of milk you are making, put the baby to the breast more often. If the baby has not gained weight, or has lost weight, breast-feed every time he stirs over a 24-hour period. If the baby is very sleepy, rouse him every two and a half hours if you can, except at night. Unwrap him, talk to him, and "woo" him with the breast. I call this my "Twenty-Four-Hour Peak Production Plan." It works in the first weeks after birth and is also useful at about six weeks.

BREAST-FEEDING DIFFICULTIES

The early days of breast-feeding are often beset with minor and more challenging difficulties that may make you feel you are not cut out for breast-feeding. Take heart—they are only temporary problems.

ENGORGED BREASTS Many new mothers are engorged on the third or fourth day after birth, when the milk really floods in. The longer you go between feedings the more likely you are to be painfully engorged. A cold compress, such as a cloth with ice inside, resting against your breast will ease the pain, and the baby's frequent sucking will help you through this difficult transitional phase. The hospital will have a breast pump that you can use if it is important to draw off some milk and you find it difficult to express by hand, but make sure to draw off only enough for comfort.

SORE NIPPLES Nipple soreness, especially when the baby is a vigorous sucker, is common in the first few weeks after birth and does not mean that you will fail at breast-feeding. Studies show that those mothers who go on to enjoy breast-feeding include many women who have had initial trouble with sores and cracks, and that the only difference between these and others who give up is that they persevere. The easiest way to prevent sore nipples is to make sure your baby is well positioned when she feeds. Check that she is well latched on the breast and has a good mouthful.

Go topless whenever you can. Avoid using soap on your nipples or using plastic-backed breast pads against them; and let them dry off after a feeding, exposed to warm air. Don't use cotton balls to protect them, because the cotton tends to disintegrate and stick to your skin.

CRACKED NIPPLES Sometimes a crack appears at the point where the nipple joins the areola. This is almost invariably because the baby has not fixed well on the surrounding tissue and has not obtained a really good mouthful. If a baby drags on the nipple stem and does not draw the nipple into the back of the mouth, not only will you have problems with sores and cracks, but the baby will not be able to take enough milk after the first spurts at the beginning of a feeding. A soft, flexible nipple shield made of silicone, with a wide brim like a Mexican sombrero, can sometimes help to relieve the soreness

"MY LAST BABY TOOK TO BREAST-FEEDING LIKE A DUCK TO WATER. BUT MY LITTLE BOY WAS QUITE DIFFICULT—HE HAD TO BE TAUGHT HOW TO LATCH ON."

that is caused by cracks and make nursing tolerable until the nipple has had time in which to heal. Avoid using plastic-lined breast pads, since if there is any leaking, your nipples will be sitting in dampness.

SORE ABDOMEN After a Cesarean section, breast-feeding may be difficult because it is almost impossible to settle with the baby in a position where she is not pressing on the wound. Try placing a pillow on the wound and lie on your side, or sit up and prop the baby's legs under the arm on the same side as the breast you are using.

BREAST TENDERNESS If you develop a red area on a breast, feeding more frequently can help. Ensure that the baby is well latched on. Exercise your arms to increase the circulation to your breasts (see page 419). If an infection develops with red patches on your breast and you run a temperature, this is mastitis. Cold compresses and oral antibiotics prescribed by the doctor will quickly treat it. Continue breast-feeding the baby, since this makes it far less likely that you will develop an abscess. An episode of mastitis shows that you have plenty of milk. Women who have mastitis are more likely to breast-feed successfully.*

EXCITABLE BABIES Some babies nurse with great bluster and excitement, spluttering and coughing and really making a meal out of it. In the first weeks they suddenly draw back as they start to choke, pulling on the nipple at the same time. Or they may let go for a second and then grab on again, but because they have jerked their heads back they now have only the nipple stem in their mouths so that they are dragging on the place where the stem joins the areola. This kind of baby needs a calm environment to feed in. Reposition him securely and talk to him soothingly.

UNSETTLED BABIES Babies do not need "burping" unless they are obviously uncomfortable. In the past, mothers spent hours trying to achieve a burp. At last the baby gave a belch and then fell asleep, exhausted (often to wake again after half an hour or so). Yes, a baby who has taken a feeding very fast may act as if bubbles are trapped in his gastrointestinal tract. Resting him, tummy down, over a warm towel or a very well covered hot-water bottle on your lap and slowly rubbing his back can help. Holding him upright over your shoulder, or sitting him up and gently rocking him up and down to produce rhythmic pressure and release on his tummy, often works. But the important thing is to prevent it. A baby who gets ravenously hungry tends to gulp feedings, so offer the breast before he is desperate. Some babies feed most calmly if they are still drowsy or if they are rocked gently while they feed. It may help if you are in a semiconscious state, too, instead of trying to get the feeding over and done with as fast as possible.

A baby who does not suck vigorously, or for long, gets low-solute milk, because the milk gets creamier throughout the feeding. A relaxed atmosphere in which a baby can go on happily sucking after immediate hunger is satisfied ensures he gets the high-calorie milk and helps settle his stomach.

GIVING BREAST MILK IN A BOTTLE

If your partner wants to give the baby some feedings, you could express some breast milk after each feeding and store it in the refrigerator in a sterile plastic container. (This is perfectly safe for two or three days.) If you want to keep the milk longer, freeze it. Express milk after each feeding. If it shoots out of one breast when you put the baby to the other, collect this milk, too. If you find it hard to express milk by hand, buy a small breast pump.

A woman who meets obstacles to breast-feeding—who discovers, perhaps, that her partner does not like her nursing in front of other men, or who sees disgust on people's faces when she is breast-feeding in a public place—is coming up against a social system in which breasts are considered exclusively as playthings for sexually aroused men, and in which the life-giving milk for her baby is treated like an unclean physical discharge.

Breast-feeding is an intimate personal experience and a way of loving. Once it is going well, many women find it brings sensual feelings of closeness to and pleasure in their babies. When women fail to breast-feed, it sometimes has less to do with failing to get the techniques right and more to do with the fact that breast-feeding can be a lonely struggle in a culture that disapproves of its being visible.

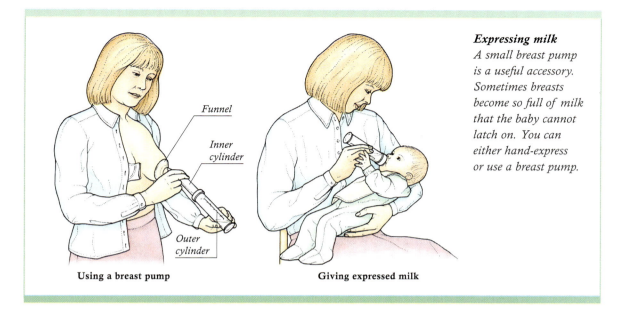

Funnel

Inner cylinder

Outer cylinder

Using a breast pump

Giving expressed milk

Expressing milk
A small breast pump is a useful accessory. Sometimes breasts become so full of milk that the baby cannot latch on. You can either hand-express or use a breast pump.

It helps to get together with other women who are breast-feeding to discuss your experiences, including any problems and the strategies you have worked out to deal with them. Organizations that can put you in touch with other breast-feeding mothers are listed on pages 427–428.

BOTTLE-FEEDING

If you decide to bottle-feed, avoid lactation suppressants. Bromocriptine, the generic name of the drug that was once used widely to suppress breast milk, is not safe. Some women had strokes or seizures. If you bottle-feed, the formula you choose should be as much like your own milk as possible.

No manufacturer has yet been able to invent anything better than an *approximation* of human milk, because your own milk adapts to your baby's individual needs. Substitute milks are a great improvement over unmodified cow's milk, however, and those that are "humanized" have the proportions of fats, sugars, and trace elements changed to be more like the real thing.

DIFFERENT KINDS OF FORMULA

If there are allergies in your or your partner's family, breast-feeding is the easiest way to protect your baby against eczema, asthma, and other allergies, although it is no guarantee that a child will never develop such conditions. Some babies are allergic to the protein in cow's milk. With this in mind, formula companies promote milk containing hydrolyzed protein, although it does not always solve the problem, and there are reports of babies becoming ill from it. Another alternative is to use soy milk, but this may not be a good idea. Babies fed on soy milk receive the equivalent of up to five contraceptive pills a day, because soy milk contains 100 times more estrogen than breast milk. Such an estrogen overdose may have toxic effects in the long term.

Human milk also contains long-chain fatty acids that help brain development.* For this reason, some formula companies are now adding long-chain lipids derived from egg yolk or bioengineered yeasts. But some babies are allergic to these lipids.

MAKING UP BOTTLES

You need to be scrupulously hygienic when preparing formula. It is vital that your kitchen and all utensils be clean and that you sterilize both bottles and nipples carefully, and follow the instructions on the can. You can make up enough feedings for 24 hours, put caps on the bottles, and store them in the refrigerator. It is then easy to feed your baby whenever she shows signs of hunger, just as if you were breast-feeding.

Never leave warm formula out for more than a few minutes—harmful bacteria may multiply. After the feeding, always throw away any leftover milk, clean out the bottle immediately, and sterilize it. Keep nipples in sterilized, covered containers. When you go out, do not take warm milk with you. Take it cold, straight from the refrigerator, and reheat it in an electric bottle warmer. It is tempting to tuck the bottle under the baby's covers to keep it snug and ready as soon as the baby wants it. But if you do this you are running the risk of harboring bacteria that cause gastrointestinal illness.

Although it seems nicer for a baby to have warm milk, this is not strictly necessary. If the baby is impatient for a feeding and you are in a hurry, it is all right to give a cold bottle. Powdered formula must be thoroughly mixed. Some brands dissolve more easily than others. Even the tiniest lumps can block the hole in the nipple and, if your baby splutters or vomits, can be inhaled and cause trouble with breathing. When making up dried milk, measure it very carefully, and never be tempted to put in an extra scoop to make it richer, since this overloads the baby with minerals that her system can absorb only with difficulty.

The baby who is fed on formula may go longer between feedings, since the milk takes longer to digest. Avoid trying to make the baby finish the bottle just because there is milk in it. In hot weather give drinks of water, too, and introduce sips of fruit juice for vitamin C at any time from six weeks. Formulas contain extra vitamins, so do not give vitamin supplements to your baby unless you are advised to do so by your doctor, and take care that you do not exceed the prescribed dose.

When giving milk in a bottle, hold the baby close. Never feed a baby who is lying in a crib or leave a baby with a propped-up bottle.

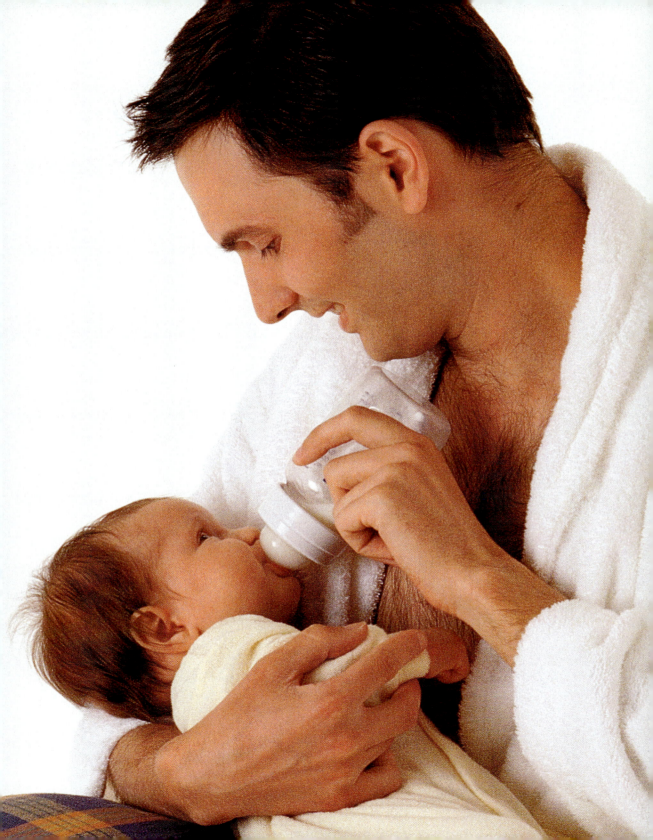

FEEDING FOR PLEASURE

When bottle-feeding, remember to hold the baby close, cheek against your breast, just as if you were breast-feeding. Although it may produce a less comfortable cushion for the baby's head, a man can also do this. The baby may sometimes like to lie nestled against your partner's bare skin, and fathers who give a feeding like this in the middle of the night say how much they enjoy it. Never feed a baby while he is lying in a crib or stroller, or even worse, prop up a baby to feed on his own in a crib, however rushed you are. It can be dangerous.

SLEEP AND CRYING

After being awake and alert, eyes wide open, for an hour or so after birth, the baby often sinks into a deep sleep for about 24 hours, waking only to suck, and dropping off to sleep again while still at the breast. This period is often followed by another lasting about 24 hours in which the baby is sucking almost continuously. This is a normal pattern. Frequent sucking stimulates your milk supply. Some babies suck in short bursts, get drowsy, then suck again. Others sleep for two to three hours between prolonged sucking sessions. Some babies start a pattern of evening fussing when they are one or two weeks old, which may continue for three months or longer. Although this is tiring for you, it is completely normal. It may be a sign that the baby is overstimulated and needs to discharge tension.

SLEEP PATTERNS OF NEWBORN BABIES

When your baby is asleep you will sometimes notice that the eyelids flicker and the eyeballs move behind them. This is rapid eye movement (REM) sleep similar to that which adults have—the dreaming time. REM sleep is essential for mental well-being and to prevent exhaustion.* These little eye movements also stimulate the flow of blood to the brain. Even if the baby seems to be stirring and is making little jerking movements or fussing noises, it is not a time to wake her. This kind of sleep is probably just as important for babies as it is for adults.

THE MEANING OF YOUR BABY'S CRY

Another innate biological mechanism is your baby's cry on waking, which alerts you to care for her. Your baby may also cry whenever you undress her and hate being without clothes. This is nerve-racking, especially if you are about to bathe her. But remember that the baby was held firmly inside your uterus, hugged by its tightly enclosing walls. If your baby startles and cries when you change a diaper or start taking off her clothes, keep your movements slow and firm. With one hand, hold the baby's arms over her chest, as they would have been folded inside the uterus at the end of pregnancy, and speak soothingly.

You will soon discover that the baby has different cries to express different needs such as hunger, discomfort, or simply boredom and loneliness. But in the first weeks the cry nearly always means hunger, and the right thing to do is to let the baby suck. At this age a wet or dirty diaper does not concern most babies.

PRACTICAL CARE

There is a great gap between studying something in a book and doing it in practice. Experiment and see what works best for you and your baby.

BATHING YOUR BABY

It does not matter how you bathe your baby, so long as he is head-above-water, keeps warm, and has a chance to enjoy it. Many babies abhor being bathed in the first weeks of life, and make you feel that you must be a tyrant for ever doing this to them. And because your baby cries, you are convinced that you must be incompetent and hopeless as a mother. The single most important thing to remember is to talk calmly to your baby while you are undressing, bathing, and dressing him.

"I MADE SURE THE ROOM WAS VERY WARM SO I COULD BATHE HIM SLOWLY AND LET HIM DISCOVER THE WATER. I COULD SEE HIM BEGINNING TO MOVE FREELY AND ENJOY IT."

If you do not want a hot bath yourself, try taking the baby with you into your own bath. Start by placing him facing you on your knee so you can smile at him and begin a conversation. Then you will discover that you can work out little games together. As he relaxes and becomes more confident, your baby will find out what fun it is to splash. Have ready the biggest bath towel you can find and make the patting dry fun, too.

DIAPERS

The main choice is between cloth diapers and disposables. Many women who choose cloth diapers find that, with extra organization, washing them becomes routine and they do not mind the extra laundry. Although cloth diapers may be expensive initially, you can often get them secondhand, and they work out more cheaply in the long run if you have a washing machine. Even so, you would be wise to buy a packet of disposables before the baby is born. You are bound to resort to them occasionally when you go out for the day. Babies often soil or wet their diapers before, during, and after a feeding. Since many like to suck every two or three hours or more, you may need as many as 24 diapers to see you through 24 hours. You can save some washing by buying disposable diaper liners and plastic pants. A diaper service may solve all the problems.

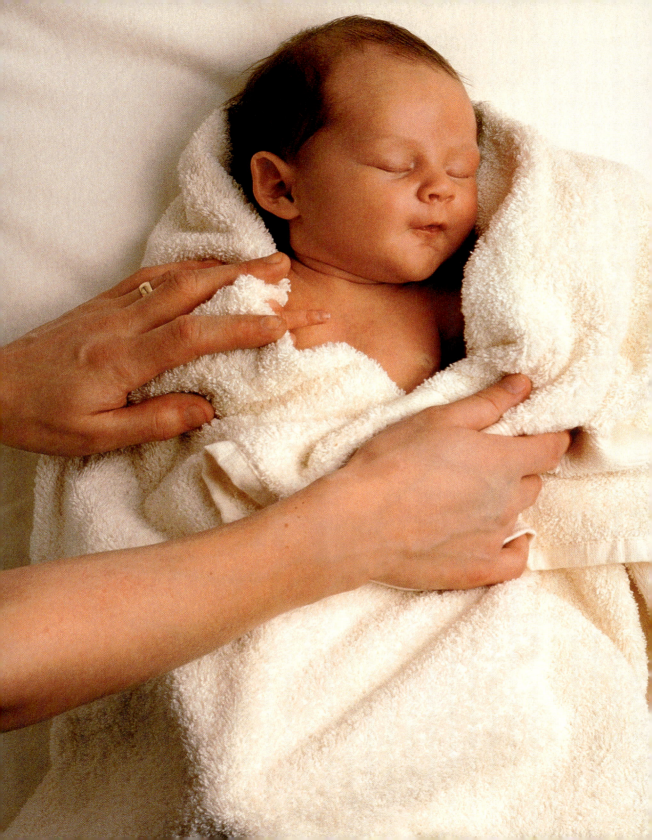

On the other hand, disposable diapers save time and work. There will be no pails of dirty diapers soaking, no frantic hunt for clean ones on days when you have not been able to catch up with yourself, and no waiting for diapers to dry. Mothers tend to change their babies more often when it is simply a matter of taking another diaper out of a packet, rather than estimating how many clean ones are left, and that must be more comfortable for their babies. But disposables end up being more expensive, and none are completely biodegradable.

MOTHERS WITH DISABILITIES

If you have a disability that makes caring for your baby difficult, you will want special equipment to help you. A woman in a wheelchair, for example, welcomes a crib and a bath on a stand the height of which can be adjusted, and with space underneath so that she can get up close to the baby. If you have back pain, you will want equipment that reduces the need to bend and lift. (For organizations, see pages 427–428.)

DRESSING YOUR BABY

Newborn babies lose heat rapidly, so they need to be warm and cozy. Several fine layers are usually warmer than one thick one. Choose clothes that do not have to be pulled over the head, since most babies hate narrow neck holes. In cold weather the baby's head should be covered outdoors.

Avoid strings and ribbons near the mouth and hands, and lacy knitted jackets and shawls in which the baby will catch fingers and toes. You are bound to be given bootees and mittens; these can be wriggled off or lost, and they can become dirty and germ-ridden. Stretchy one-piece suits are better for keeping feet covered. Babies should be able to get at their hands and explore with them.

A baby carrier is not strictly clothing but is important for your mobility. The sling you use to begin with should be one of those in which the baby is held in front of you and the head is supported.

Most babies love to be bathed when handled gently and reassuringly, although they might not take to it the first few times.

And the most useful item of clothing in cold weather is something for you, not the baby. It is a big, wraparound overcoat or cape. You can tuck the baby underneath it in a sling against your body, with just her face peeping out. Your body heat will provide warmth, and the outer garment will hold the warmth around the baby.

THE CHALLENGE OF NEW PARENTHOOD

The first days at home with a new baby can be filled with unexpected worry and even a sense of panic as you try to cope with the needs of this demanding person. However, you will soon learn to interpret the different cries of your baby and understand what he is trying to tell you.

POSTPARTUM CHECKUP

Your postpartum checkup takes place between five and seven weeks after the birth. It is important to ensure that you have complete physical rehabilitation after childbirth. You have an internal examination to see if your pelvic floor muscles are well toned and that the uterus and bladder are correctly positioned, and to check the state of any scar tissue. If you have been finding that sexual intercourse is difficult and uncomfortable, or you are feeling depressed and unhappy, tell the doctor at this visit. If you are dissatisfied with any aspect of the care you received or seek further explanation of things that happened to you in labor, take the opportunity to discuss these things, too.

TIREDNESS

Tiredness is inevitable because you are unlikely to get much sleep in the first four months. A survey by a parenting magazine found that women get on average only four hours of sleep a night.*

In some ways, a new baby seems like an alien from outer space. Babies do not care about the time or observe any social rules. They fuss and cry, wet and dirty themselves, spit up, and want to be held close and reassured, or walked around, regardless of adult agendas. In the first weeks, they need to be fed every two to three hours. It is not wise to put a baby out of earshot. You should be alert to respond, if only with a sleepy cuddle. In this way you show your love for your baby and lay the basis for happiness and self-confidence. A child needs love as much as food.

If you can, organize your day flexibly so that you can rest when the baby sleeps. Your impulse may be to catch up with work or housework when the baby is not in your arms, but this is unwise. Sleep deprivation is a well-known form of torture. It is disorienting, and, if it goes on long enough, can drive anyone to the edge of despair. Discuss this with your partner and devise a strategy to deal with it. Unplug the phone when you need to, have a notice ready to stick on the door, "NEW PARENTS RESTING," when you are both at home, and take turns on baby duty, even though this may mean that your partner brings the baby to you and fixes her to the breast while you are still half asleep. See what help you can get with housework, laundry, and cooking. Recognize that this transition to parenthood is exciting, but very stressful.

UNHAPPINESS AFTER BIRTH

"It's going around and around in my head. I can't forget it. People say that I should put it behind me because I have a lovely baby. But I can't forget it—it's like I have to live it over and over again."

Any woman who feels birth was taken out of her hands and that she was simply the body on the bed is likely to feel abused by the professionals who attended her, and even by her partner who stood by and let it happen. For a woman who has been treated like a baby-producing machine rather than a person, birth can seem like rape.

You need time to fall in love with your baby, being together in a relaxed, peaceful atmosphere.

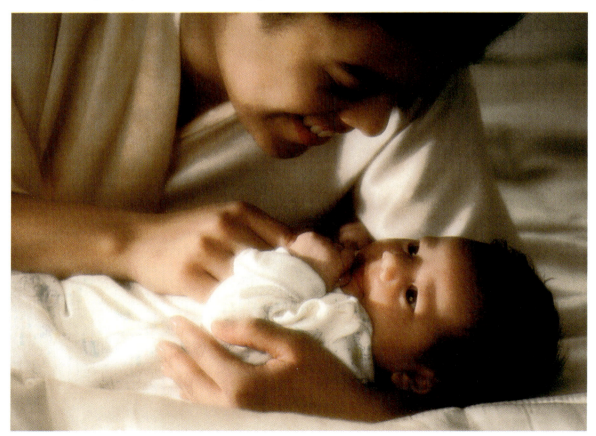

413

Though she may seem grateful and positive immediately after the birth, glad that it is all over, or numb with shock and smiling automatically, distress may overwhelm her weeks, or even months, later. She may have flashbacks, nightmares, and panic attacks, and feel different from other women and isolated from them. She lives every day as if on red alert.

This is often defined as post-traumatic stress disorder (PTSD). It is similar to the distress experienced by anyone who has been trapped and helpless in a frightening situation or who has witnessed terrible things that they were unable to do anything about. In World War I, it was called "shell shock."

You can be shell-shocked after birth, too, and if you feel like this, you are not being weak, self-centered, or ungrateful, though some people will imply that you are. Women suffer this unhappiness because they are disempowered in childbirth. Post-traumatic stress after birth is iatrogenic— a medically produced disorder.

It is different from either "the baby blues" or postpartum depression, although you may be misdiagnosed with these conditions. Drugs for depression are not the right treatment and can make you feel worse. There is no quick-fix pill. You are reacting in a normal way to violence and dehumanization.

To get help, talk to your doctor or midwife and ask if you can be referred to a counselor or psychotherapist, preferably a woman who has herself had children. Or contact a support group to talk to another woman who will listen in a nonjudgmental way and help you find the power within yourself to cope. (See page 427.)

INCONTINENCE

Up to 30 percent of women wet their pants occasionally—when they cough, or laugh, run, climb stairs, lift something heavy, or exert themselves physically—after having a baby. For some this continues and becomes a permanent problem. Yet many do not seek help. This is partly because it is an embarrassing subject, partly because they think it is the inevitable consequence of childbirth. They may also believe it is their own fault because they have not done pelvic floor exercises regularly. Sometimes, even when a woman does tell her doctor or midwife about it, she is told, "Give it time. It's early days yet. It'll get better."

If you are incontinent, ask your doctor to refer you to a urologist who specializes in women. These specialists have nurses trained to work intensively with patients once testing indentifies the cause of the incontinence.

Pelvic floor exercises are important, but specialists have equipment that enables you to locate the exact muscles you need to strengthen, and measure your achievement, so that you really understand what you are doing and can test your progress.

Fecal incontinence (and gas) can also occur, although more rarely. This is often even more difficult to discuss with your midwife or doctor. Do mention it, though: the sooner you get help, the better it will be in the long term.

SEX AFTER CHILDBIRTH

For many women the full flood of passion is slow to return after childbirth. This is not surprising, considering that so much has happened in your body and to your emotions. You may need time to find yourself again. If the birth was unpleasant or traumatic, you may need additional time, too, to like yourself again and regain trust in your body.

If you have had stitches, you will not feel relaxed about sex until the wound has healed completely. You may feel at first as if you will never want to make love again. If you do not have stitches you may not be able to wait to make love. So there is a great difference to making love after giving birth, depending on the state of your perineum. The initial healing of the tear or episiotomy wound often takes two weeks or more, and even then you may be very conscious of a knot of scar tissue at the lower end of your vagina.

"I WAS SORE, AND A BIT SCARED. THE BABY HAD AN UNCANNY KNACK FOR KNOWING WHEN WE WERE MAKING LOVE, AND WANTING A FEEDING."

REDISCOVERING TOUCH AND SENSATION

Make sure that your partner knows which areas are likely to feel sore, and help him to discover what feels good and where. Do not attempt to have intercourse at first, and certainly do not try to prove anything to yourselves. Choose a quiet time when you need not be rushed, perhaps after a feeding when the baby is most likely to settle and sleep soundly. Squeeze a little lubricant jelly onto your partner's fingers and, taking his hands in yours, guide him, showing him where you like to be touched. Many couples need two or three exploratory sessions like this before they feel sufficiently confident to have complete intercourse. If you rush it, you may have unexpected discomfort and will tense up in anticipation of pain next time, and because your pelvic floor muscles have contracted will have more pain.

When you feel that you are ready for intercourse, adopt a position in which your partner's weight is not going to pull and drag on the lower part of your vagina or on your breasts. For example, if you lie or sit with your legs over the side of a low bed, feet on the floor, your partner will be able to penetrate you gently without pressing against or pulling on any tender areas. You will probably feel extraordinarily full. Release your throat, and this will help release muscles around your vagina. Do not aim for simultaneous orgasm. It is usually very much more comfortable and pleasurable for you in the weeks immediately after birth if your partner comes to orgasm first and then stays inside until you have an orgasm, too.

POSTPARTUM EXERCISES

Many of the exercises for pregnancy are also good for
getting your figure back after birth. Postpartum exercises
should be progressive. Do only the gentlest exercises for the
first day or two. Then move on to the more strenuous ones.
Never do an exercise that hurts.

PELVIC ROCK

Lie on your back on the floor, knees bent, soles of feet flat, and your
baby lying between your legs and along your tummy. Breathe out
and push against the floor with your feet. Allow your pelvis
to roll and your lower back to press against the floor. Then
release your feet and rock your pelvis so that the pressure
of your lower back is lifted away from the floor. Notice
the movement all along your spine
to your head, and how your back
flattens as your chin rolls up from
your chest and arches as it rolls
down onto your chest.

THE LEG SLIDE

Lie on your back, knees bent, feet flat
on the floor. Place one hand under the
small of your back. Release your
chest, press against the floor with
your feet, and notice how your
back also presses against
your hand.

Keeping up this pressure against
your hand, slowly allow both feet
to slide forward so that you extend
your legs and feel the pull of your
abdominal muscles. Let your
toes come up off the floor.
Continue to breathe.

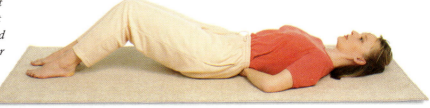

UNFOLDING

Sit on the floor, knees bent and together, soles flat, with your hands crossed on your chest. Relax your chest and let your back drop slowly backward with your legs sliding forward. Feel how vertebrae in your lower back press on the floor one after the other like a string of pearls unfolding.

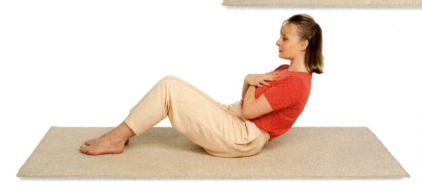

Fold yourself together by moving your knees and then lean back and unfold again, continuing this folding and unfolding movement rhythmically.

SIDEWAYS CURL-UP

Lie on your back on the floor, knees bent, with your right hand tucked behind your head. Breathe in, breathe out, let your chest become soft, lift your head and shoulders, and lift your right knee.

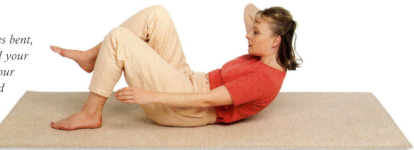

Continue to lift your knee until it touches the elbow. Stay in the position for a few seconds, breathing gently. Then slowly return to the starting position. Continue the movement on your left side, then repeat the right side again, and so on.

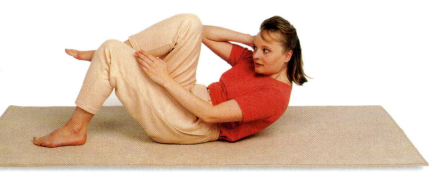

THE HAMMOCK

Lie on your back on the floor, knees bent, feet flat, holding your baby sitting on your tummy. Soften your chest and press your feet and head against the floor, allowing your bottom to lift up off it. Rock your baby by swinging from side to side in this position. Then relax your body and let your bottom drop back to the floor.

ROCKING THE BABY

Lie on your back, knees bent, feet up off the floor so that your lower legs are parallel with it, and your baby is resting on your lower legs, face down and supported under the arms. Tuck your chin in and, slowly lifting your head and shoulders, rock forward and back, alternately lifting and lowering to and from the floor.

COMPLETE ROCK

Lie on your back, knees bent, feet lifted off the floor, your hands behind your knees. Rock backward and forward, keeping your back rounded and a steady distance between your nose and your knees.

You may find that you rock completely until you sit upright, but do not force it.

ROLL UP

Lie on your back, knees bent, your hands holding your lower legs, elbows forward. Let your head and knees roll toward each other, then apart, then together again and continue this rocking movement. You may find that you roll right up until you are sitting. Do not force this. You can also do this movement with your hands behind your head.

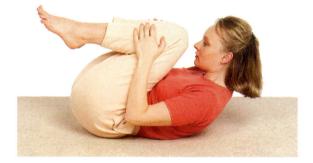

UP, UP, AND AWAY

Lie on your back, knees bent, feet flat on the floor, your baby lying on your chest and your hands supporting her under the arms. Gently lift the baby up above your face, noticing the pressure of your lower back against the floor as you do so. Hold the baby in this position for a few seconds. Then slowly lower her onto your chest and rock her gently.

ADJUSTING TO YOUR CHANGED BODY

You and your partner will learn a lot more about each other after the birth and, as a result, sex will sometimes be funny, sometimes tender, and occasionally passionate. Even if you do not feel that you are making a wild success of your sex life in the first few months after birth, lovemaking helps both you and your baby by releasing oxytocin into your bloodstream. This helps the uterus to contract so that it returns to its previous size and shape, and also encourages the flow of breast milk. When you have an orgasm, milk may actually shoot out of your nipples.

"I DIDN'T WANT HIM TO TOUCH MY BREASTS, BECAUSE I FELT THAT THEY BELONGED TO THE BABY. BUT I FOUND THAT WHEN I WAS AROUSED MY MILK SHOT OUT. THAT BROKE THE TENSION AND WE BEGAN TO GIGGLE."

The shape of your body has changed after giving birth to a first baby. The labia, like the outside petals of a flower, are now softer and fleshier, and if you did not have an episiotomy you may find the entrance to the vagina also more yielding. If your uterus is still involuting, you will also feel after-contractions following lovemaking. This is a good sign. If they are uncomfortable, use a hot-water bottle against your lower tummy or against your back. Even if you thoroughly enjoyed lovemaking, you may feel slightly sore afterward, once the sexual intensity has faded. Again, this is quite normal. A cold witch-hazel compress held against the area may feel soothing and help to bring relief.

PAINFUL INTERCOURSE

For some women, intercourse is acutely painful after childbirth, and no amount of trying to relax does away with the pain they experience. This is called "dyspareunia." It can occur when stitches have been inserted too tightly and the surrounding flesh has become puffy and swollen (edematous) and is perhaps infected. Many zealous junior doctors pull stitches so tightly that there is no space for the inevitable swelling that follows tissue injury. Ask your doctor or midwife to look at the sore area as soon as possible. Sometimes it is just a question of snipping a few stitches, sometimes a matter of taking antibiotics. Occasionally, a small operation may be needed. If you have pain up near your cervix, it may be that the transverse cervical ligaments have been torn, and it will take time for them to repair themselves. Make sure that your doctor knows that you are having this sort of pain.

Many women worry that they have become "frigid" after childbirth. Often a lack of interest in sex is directly caused by tiredness. Try to rest regularly with your feet up and, if it is possible, sleep at some time during the day when your baby sleeps. Even the most active baby sleeps sometimes, and you could try to discover your baby's pattern and then take advantage of it yourself. This is more difficult if you also have a toddler, but many toddlers enjoy a cuddle in bed or on the sofa.

Although you may not feel like making love for some time after childbirth, it is sensible to have explored sensations and had intercourse before your postpartum checkup. Most women with new babies are so busy that it is not easy to fit in another appointment in order to discuss sexual difficulties, and they may hope that if they take no notice then the problems will disappear gradually of their own accord. Make a note of where and when you feel pain during intercourse, and let the doctor know that you are experiencing dyspareunia and that you want help.

Sex after childbirth takes you on a new journey with your partner. It involves discovery, change, for many women a fresh awareness of the depth of their own sexual feelings, and for both of you a new kind of closeness and tenderness as parents of the baby who has been born of your love.

CONTRACEPTION

There is no easy answer to contraception, and what pleases one couple may be completely unsuitable for another. Many couples consider the matter in advance, so that they can have intercourse safely whenever they feel ready. It is not worth being worried about another pregnancy when you are only just beginning to enjoy the results of the last!

BREAST-FEEDING

If you are breast-feeding, your periods may not come back until you wean the baby or introduce solid food. Ovulation, and the possibility of conception, can occur a couple of weeks or so *before* you have this first period. Breast-feeding reduces fertility but is not an effective contraceptive unless you are suckling the baby intermittently right through the 24 hours and giving no other food or fluid. A fully breast-feeding woman may not have a period for a year. In many traditional cultures, lactating women rarely conceive. Since children are breast-fed for three years or longer, this is an effective method of family planning. But bear in mind that in these societies, intercourse is often prohibited during lactation, too.

WITHDRAWAL

Hoping that your partner will withdraw before ejaculation is not a reliable method, though it is common throughout the world. In spite of working well for some couples, it demands great self-control on the man's part and may lead to dissatisfaction for you both. You should also be aware that sperm can flow from the penis *before* ejaculation, and if you have intercourse again within a short time, live sperm may already be present in your partner's urethra and be introduced into your vagina before ejaculation. Sperm do not have to be deposited inside your vagina for you to get pregnant. Even a drop or two of semen leaking against the labia may contain a million sperm or more.

NATURAL FAMILY PLANNING

Natural methods entail identifying ovulation, the phase of the menstrual cycle at which you are most fertile, and abstaining from intercourse during that time. It is impossible to calculate ovulation accurately using a calendar alone. The only methods of birth control officially approved by the Roman Catholic Church are the rhythm method and the symptothermal method. With both, you keep an accurate record of your menstrual cycle and also a daily chart of body temperature, using a special thermometer. By doing this, you identify when ovulation occurs and avoid intercourse at that time. With the symptothermal method you also observe changes in the cervical mucus, which gets thinner during your fertile period. There are drawbacks, however: in the first year or so after childbirth, a woman may not have a regular menstrual cycle. Natural methods require instruction from someone who is really skilled in using them, and a firm commitment from both partners.

CONDOMS

The big disadvantage of using condoms after childbirth is that your vagina may not be well lubricated and may be tender following an episiotomy. The latex sticks and drags, interfering with pleasure. Use some artificial water-based lubrication—preferably a spermicidal cream or jelly. Avoid Vaseline because it causes rubber to disintegrate.

THE DIAPHRAGM

If you used a diaphragm before you became pregnant, you will probably need a larger size now. It must be fitted by a doctor or midwife, and they will not be able to do it accurately until about six weeks after childbirth. It should be left in place for at least six hours after intercourse. Do not, however, leave it for longer than eight hours if you have had a bladder infection during pregnancy or following the birth, since the pressure of the rubber rim on your bladder could cause irritation and infection. Sometimes ligaments running across the cervix are slack after childbirth, so that the diaphragm cannot be wedged up under the pubic bone and slips.

"AFTER THE BABY CAME WE USED A CONDOM OR A DIAPHRAGM, DEPENDING ON HOW WE WERE FEELING. I DIDN'T WANT TO INTRODUCE CHEMICALS INTO MY BODY WHILE I WAS BREAST-FEEDING."

THE INTRAUTERINE DEVICE (IUD)

It is usually easier for an IUD to be inserted and retained without cramping once you have had a baby. Pelvic infection within three weeks to three months after insertion is common, but after that is unlikely if you have only one partner. Infection should be treated with antibiotics, which pass through into your milk, though the only effect may be that the baby's stools become loose.

Rarely an IUD perforates the uterus. This is most likely to happen if it is inserted a short time after delivery, when the uterine wall is thin and soft. There are three models of IUD currently available in the U.S. All are T-shaped, and two of them release the hormone progesterone that decreases menstrual loss. There is no consensus on whether the hormone-containing IUDs can be used while breast-feeding.

ORAL CONTRACEPTIVES

The pill is the most reliable method of contraception. But if you have high blood pressure that continues after the birth, or diabetes, you should probably not take the pill. If you are suffering from severe postpartum depression, it may also be wiser to avoid the pill. If you developed varicose veins during pregnancy, watch for pain in your legs that could be a sign of a blood clot. If you have had a blood clot in a vein (thrombophlebitis), you should not take the pill.

THE COMBINED ESTROGEN-PROGESTOGEN PILL is definitely out if you are breast-feeding, because it affects your metabolism and indirectly the baby's. It may alter both the quantity and the quality of milk, and there could be long-term effects on your child.

THE PROGESTOGEN-ONLY PILL OR "MINIPILL" is often prescribed to women who are breast-feeding. Though your milk supply may be diminished for a few days after you start taking it, feeding the baby on demand brings the supply up to normal again.

THE VAGINAL RING AND THE SKIN PATCH

Two new delivery systems for combined estrogen-progesterone contraception are the vaginal ring (NuvaRing) and the contraceptive skin patch (Ortho Evra). They are very similar to oral contraceptives except you don't need to take them every day. They are not for use while breast-feeding.

GAINING CONFIDENCE AS PARENTS

Many women in our society have no experience of babies, and some have never held a newborn baby in their arms. They are anxious that they will not know when the baby is hungry, that they will drop or drown him in the bathtub, that they will never be able to stop his crying, or that the baby who is not crying has ceased breathing. New mothers are often too ashamed to talk about such feelings. Talk with other mothers and you will find that you are not alone with anxieties such as these. Talk about good feelings, too—when the baby falls asleep and lies in your arms in perfect contentment, the soft, downy head resting against your skin, when he opens his eyes wide

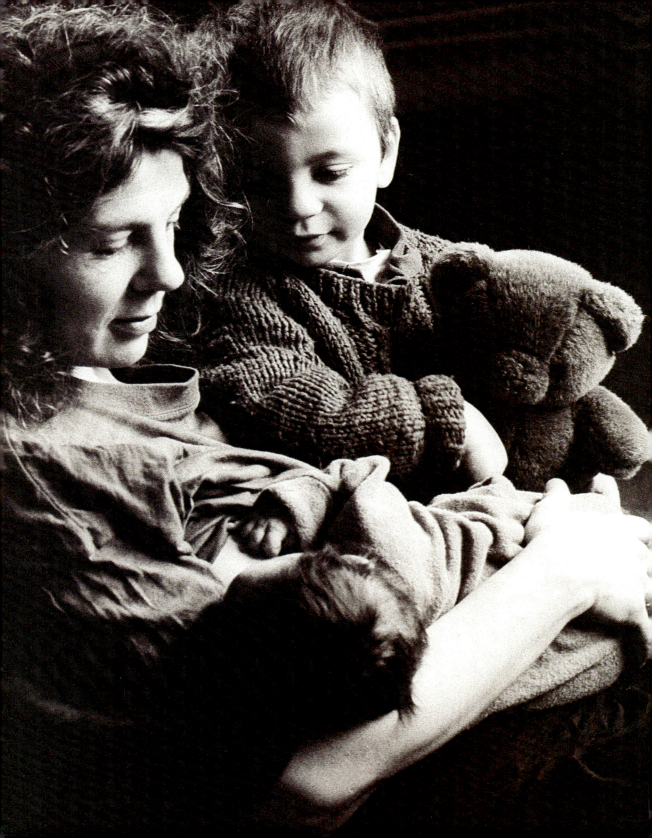

and gazes at you with excited attention, or when you watch and feel him contentedly sucking at your breast.

You are not just a caretaker of the baby but a partner in a unique and evolving relationship. In your new roles, you and your baby learn more about each other every day, synchronizing with each other like dancers. You respond to facial expression, eye movement, muscle tension—even breathing—spontaneously. When you act on these impulses you are invariably doing the right thing. When you are self-conscious, you miss steps in the dance and confidence drains away.

The developing relationship between a mother and her baby is a process that needs time to unfold and blossom, patterned, just as a hyacinth bulb or a crocus is patterned, by the laws of its own inner energy. Yet this is only part of the dance. The baby's father has his own special kind of interaction with his child, as well as with you. When a man is fully involved with his baby, enjoying her, responding to her needs, and by his getting to know her as intimately as you do, the pattern becomes even more intricate and exciting.

SHARING IN PARENTHOOD

Babies have astonishingly strong personalities. They are quite different from one another, even in the early weeks of life, so take time to get to know the person who is your child.

To be a parent is all about learning. A child with a younger sibling has new opportunities for development, too.

Being a parent is not just an endless series of repetitive tasks or a heavy responsibility, though all parents see it like that at times. It is a journey of discovery—discovery of the baby's personality, of who you are, who your partner is, and who you are becoming together.

USEFUL READING

Balaskas, J.
Easy Exercises for Pregnancy.
Hungry Minds, Inc., 1997.

Balaskas, J.
Natural Baby.
Creative Publishing International, 2001.

Balaskas, J.
New Active Birth.
Harvard Common Press, 1992.

Balaskas, J., and Gordon, Y.
Water Birth.
Unwin Hyman, 1992.

Bryan, E.
Twins, Triplets and More.
St. Martin's Press, 1992.

Chamberlain, G. (Ed.)
Pain and Its Relief in Childbirth.
Churchill Livingstone, 1997.

Clement, S.
The Cesarean Experience.
Pandora, 1991.

Enkin, M., Keirse, M., Renfrew, M.,
and Neilson, J. (Eds.)
*A Guide to Effective Care in Pregnancy
and Childbirth.*
Oxford University Press, 2000.

Gordon, Y.
Birth and Beyond.
Random House, 2002.

Graham, I. D.
*Episiotomy, Challenging Obstetric
Interventions.*
Blackwell Science, 1997.

Kitzinger, S.
Becoming a Grandmother.
Fireside, 1997.

Kitzinger, S.
Birth over Thirty-Five.
Penguin, 1995.

Kitzinger, S.
*Birth Your Way: Choosing Birth at
Home or in a Birth Center.*
DK Publishing, 2002.

Kitzinger, S.
Breastfeeding Your Baby.
Knopf, 1989.

Kitzinger, S.
Rediscovering Birth.
Pocket Star, 2001

Kitzinger, S.
The Year After Childbirth.
Fireside, 1996.

Kitzinger, S., and Bailey, V.
Pregnancy Day by Day.
Knopf, 2001.

Lawrence Beech, B. (Ed.)
Water Birth Unplugged.
Butterworth-Heinemann, 1997.

Lothrop, H.
Help, Comfort and Hope.
Perseus, 1997.
(For anyone who has lost a baby.)

Maxwell-Hudson, C.
Aromatherapy Massage.
DK Publishing, 1999.

National Childbirth Trust.
*The National Childbirth Trust Book
of Pregnancy, Birth & Parenthood.*
Oxford University Press, 1992.

Odent, M.
The Farmer and the Obstetrician.
Free Association Books, 2002.

*Pregnancy and Childbirth,
Module of the Cochrane Library: Issue 3.*
Update Software, 1998.
(An excellent source of all research
results based on randomized
controlled trials.)

Smale, M.
*The National Childbirth Trust Book
of Breastfeeding.*
Vermilion, 1999.

Thiro, R. (Ed.)
Baby and You.
Blue Island, 2002.

Thomas, P.
Every Birth Is Different.
Trafalgar Square, 1998.

Thorn, G.
Having Your Baby.
Perseus, 1997.

Wagner, M.
Pursuing the Birth Machine.
ACE Graphics, 1994.
(P.O. Box 173, Sevenoaks, Kent,
TN14 7EZ, UK)

USEFUL ADDRESSES

American Academy of Husband-Coached Childbirth (AAHCC) (Bradley Method)
P.O. Box 5224
Sherman Oaks, CA 91413-5224
http://www.bradleybirth.com

American College of Nurse Midwives (ACNM)
818 Connecticut Ave. NW
Suite 900
Washington, DC 20006
(202) 728-9860; fax (202) 728-9897
http://www.midwife.org

American College of Obstetricians and Gynecologists (ACOG)
P.O. Box 96920
Washington, DC 20090-6920
(202) 638-5577
http://www.acog.org

Bereavement Services RTS
1910 South Ave.
La Crosse, WI 54601
(608) 775-4747

Birth and Life Bookstore Cascade Health Care Products
141 Commercial St. NE
Salem, OR 97301
(503) 371-4445

The Compassionate Friends (Perinatal bereavement)
P.O. Box 3696
Oak Brook, IL 60522-3696
(877) 969-0010
http://www.compassionatefriends.org

Depression After Delivery (DAD)
91 E. Somerset St.
Raritan, NJ 08869
(800) 944-4PPD
http://www.depressionafterdelivery.com

The Dr. Edward Bach Center (Bach flower remedies)
Mount Vernon, Sotwell
Nr. Wallingford, Oxon
UK
011 44 1491 834 678

Doulas of North America (DONA)
1100 23rd Ave. E
Seattle, WA 98112
(206) 324-5540
http://www.dona.org

Global Maternal/Child Health Association, Inc. (Water birth information)
P.O. Box 1400
Wilsonville, OR 97070-1400
(503) 673-0026
http://www.waterbirth.org

Hygeia Foundation, Inc. (Perinatal loss)
P.O. Box 3943
New Haven, CT 06525-3943
(800) 893-9198
http://www.hygeia.org

International Childbirth Education Association (ICEA)
P.O. Box 20048
Minneapolis, MN 55420-0048
(952) 854-8660; fax (952) 854-8772
(800) 624-4934 for book orders
http://www.icea.org

International Lactation Consultant Association
1500 Sunday Drive
Suite 102
Raleigh, NC 27607
(919) 861-5577; fax (919) 787-4916
http://www.ilca.org

La Leche League International (Breast-feeding support and information network)
1400 N. Meachum Rd.
Schaumburg, IL 60173-4808
(847) 519-7730
http://www.lalecheleague.org

Lamaze International
2025 M St.
Suite 800
Washington, DC 20036-3309
(800) 368-4404
http://www.lamaze.org

March of Dimes
1275 Mamaroneck Ave.
White Plains, NY 10605
(888) MODIMES
http://www.marchofdimes.com

Mothers of Supertwins (For mothers of triplets, quadruplets, etc.)
P.O. Box 951
Brentwood, NY 11717-0951
(631) 859-1110
http://www.mostonline.org

National Association of Childbearing Centers
3132 Gottschall Rd.
Perkiomenville, PA 18074
(215) 234-8068; fax (215) 234-8829
http://www.birthcenters.org

National Organization of Circumcision Information Resource Centers
731 Sir Francis Drake Blvd.
San Anselmo, CA 94960
(415) 488-9883; fax (415) 488-9660
http://www.nocirc.org

National Organization of Mothers of Twins Clubs, Inc.
NOMOTC Executive Office
P.O. Box 438
Thompsons Station, TN 37179-0438
(877) 540-2200
http://nomotc.org

National Women's Health Network
514 10th St. NW
Washington, DC 20004
(202) 347-1140
http://www.womenshealthnetwork.org

Nurses for Newborns
(Crisis intervention)
9505 Gravois Rd.
Suite 201
St. Louis, MO 63123
(888) 45-BIRTH
http://nfnf.org

Sidelines
(For expectant mothers on bed rest)
P.O. Box 1808
Laguna Beach, CA 92652
(714) 497-2265
http://www.sidelines.org

First Candle/SIDS Alliance
1314 Bedford Ave.
Suite 210
Baltimore, MD 21208
(800) 638-SIDS
http://www.sidsalliance.org

Subsequent Pregnancy After a Loss
Support
http://www.spals.com
and **Parenting After Loss**
http://groups.yahoo.com/group/pal-parents/

TTT Helpline
The Toxoplasmosis Trust
61–67 Collier St.
London N1 9BE
UK

U.S. Department of Health and
Human Services
Office on Women's Health
200 Independence Ave. SW
Washington, DC 20201
(877) 696-6775
http://www.4woman.gov/pregnancy

Vaginal Birth After Cesarean
(VBAC)
c/o Center for Family
24050 Madison St.
Suite 200
Torrance, CA 90505
(310) 375-3141
http://www.vbac.com

GLOSSARY

Abdomen The part of the body containing the intestines, stomach, bowel, and uterus.

Abortion (Miscarriage) Either spontaneous or induced delivery of the fetus before the 28th week of development.

Abruption (Accidental hemorrhage) The peeling away of part of the placenta from the wall of the uterus during late pregnancy, which may result in bleeding.

Accelerated labor The artificial augmentation of contractions, after the cervix has started to dilate, by the injection of pitocin through an intravenous drip. Often used to speed up a long labor.

Active birth An approach to childbirth that entails practicing stretching positions and movements and being in "open" and upright positions in labor.

Active management of labor The constant monitoring and technical control of labor to limit its duration.

Alphafetoprotein (AFP) A substance produced by the embryonic yolk sac, and later by the fetal liver, that enters the mother's bloodstream during pregnancy.

Alveoli Milk glands in the breasts, which produce a flow of milk when they are stimulated by prolactin and the baby's sucking.

Amenorrhea The absence of menstrual periods.

Amino acids The main organic chemical constituents of proteins, found in all foods produced from animals but only in limited and varying combinations in vegetables.

Amnesia Loss of memory, usually short term, which can be a side effect of certain drugs, especially Valium.

Amniocentesis The surgical extraction of a small amount of amniotic fluid through the pregnant woman's abdomen. This procedure is usually carried out as a test for fetal defects or maturity.

Amnion The layer of membrane immediately enveloping the fetus and the amniotic fluid inside the uterus; it is also referred to as the amniotic sac, or bag of waters.

Amniotic fluid The fluid surrounding the fetus in the uterus. Ultrasound scans may be done in late pregnancy to ensure that enough is present.

Amniotic sac See *Amnion*.

Amniotomy The surgical rupture of the amniotic sac, often done to speed up labor. Referred to as ARM (artificial rupture of the membranes).

Analgesics Painkilling agents not inducing unconsciousness.

Anemia A condition in which there is an abnormally low proportion of red corpuscles in the blood, treated by iron (Fe) supplements.

Anencephaly The congenital absence of the upper parts of the brain.

Anesthetic Medication that produces partial or complete insensibility to pain.

Anesthetic, general Anesthetic that affects the whole body, with temporary loss of consciousness.

Anesthetic, local Anesthetic that affects a limited part of the body. See also *Caudal; Epidural*.

Antepartum cardiotography Test to check fetal heartbeat.

Anterior position See *Occipito anterior*.

Antibacterials Chemical agents that destroy or limit the growth of bacteria.

Antibiotics Substances capable of destroying or limiting the growth of microorganisms, especially bacteria.

Antibodies Proteins produced naturally by the body to combat any foreign bodies, germs or bacteria.

Anticholinergic drugs Used in the treatment of nausea and vomiting, partly by limiting the impulses through the nervous system and partly by restricting the secretion of stomach acids.

Anticoagulants Drugs that prevent the blood from clotting.

Anticonvulsants Drugs that combat convulsions, especially epilepsy.

Antihistamines Tranquilizers used in the treatment of nausea, vomiting, and certain allergies.

Apgar scale A general test of the baby's well-being given immediately after birth to ascertain the heart rate and tone, respiration, blood circulation, and nerve responses.

Apnea Interrupted breathing that may occur in preterm and low-birth-weight babies.

Areola The pigmented circle of skin surrounding the nipple.

ARM See *Amniotomy*.

Arrhythmic contractions Irregular contractions.

Aspirin (Salicylate) A mild analgesic.

Bag of waters See *Amnion*.

Barbiturates Powerful and highly addictive tranquilizers.

Bearing down The pushing movement made by the uterus in the second stage of labor.

Bile pigment See *Bilirubin*.

Bilirubin Broken-down hemoglobin, normally converted to nontoxic substances by the liver. Some newborn babies have levels of bilirubin too high for their livers to cope with. See also *Jaundice, neonatal*.

Birth canal See *Vagina*.

Blastocyst An early stage of the developing egg when it has segmented into a group of cells.

Blighted ovum An abnormal development of the egg in which the cells do not develop in the usual way to form a baby. It results in miscarriage.

Bradycardia A slow heart rate in the fetus and newborn baby. This is a rate of less than 120 beats a minute.

Braxton Hicks contractions (Rehearsal) Contractions of the uterus that occur throughout pregnancy, but which may not be noticed until toward the end.

Breast pump Apparatus for drawing milk from the breasts.

Breech presentation The position of a baby who is bottom down rather than head down in the uterus.

Brow presentation The position of a baby who is head down in the uterus, but with chin up, so that the brow comes through the cervix first.

Candida See *Thrush*.

Caput A small, temporary swelling on the crown of the baby's head caused by the head being pressed against an incompletely dilated cervix.

Carpal tunnel syndrome Numbness and tingling of the hands arising from pressure on the nerves of the wrist. In pregnancy it is caused by the body's accumulation of fluids.

Catecholamines Stress hormones produced by the mother and baby during labor that play an important part in preparing the baby for birth.

Catheter A thin plastic tube inserted into the body through a natural channel to withdraw fluid from, or introduce fluid into, a part of the body. It can be used to draw off urine from the bladder, or to maintain a constant input of fluids into a vein, or to introduce anesthetic into the epidural space.

Caudal (Caudal epidural block) An anesthetic injected into the base of the spine. See also *Epidural*.

Cephalhematoma A temporary swelling on the side of the baby's head caused by pressure during labor.

Cephalic presentation (Vertex presentation) The position of a baby who is head down in the uterus. The most common presentation.

Cephalopelvic disproportion A state in which the head of the fetus is larger than the cavity of the mother's pelvis. Delivery must therefore be by Cesarean section.

Cervical dilation See *Dilation*.

Cervical erosion Superficial inflammation of the cervix.

Cervical incompetence A disorder of the cervix, usually arising after a previous mid-pregnancy termination or damage to the cervix during a previous labor, in which the cervix opens up too soon, resulting in repeated mid-pregnancy miscarriages. It is sometimes treated by suturing to hold the cervix closed.

Cervix The lower entrance to the uterus, or neck of the womb.

Cesarean section Delivery of the baby through a cut in the abdominal and uterine walls.

Chloasma Skin discoloration during pregnancy, often facial.

Chloral drugs Nonbarbiturate hypnotic tranquilizers.

Chlorpromazine (Thorazine) A powerful sedative often used in conjunction with hypnotics, analgesics, and anesthetics.

Chorion The outer membranous tissue that envelops the fetus and placenta.

Chorionic gonadotrophin See *Human chorionic gonadotrophin (HCG)*.

Chorionic villi The tiny fronds around the fertile ovum that enable it to become embedded in the uterine wall.

Chorionic villus sampling A method of screening for genetic disability by analysis of tissue from the small protrusions on the outer membrane enveloping the embryo that later form the placenta.

Chromosomes Rodlike structures containing genes occurring in pairs within the nucleus of every cell. Human cells each contain 23 pairs. See also *Gene*.

Circumcision An operation to cut the foreskin from the penis.

Cleft palate A congenital abnormality of the roof of the mouth.

Clitoris Exquisitely sensitive small organ at the upper end of a woman's genitals, just under the pubic bone and between the folded external labia.

Clubfoot A congenital abnormality in which the foot is painlessly twisted out of shape.

Codeine An addictive painkilling agent derived from opium.

Colostrum A kind of milk, rich in proteins, formed and secreted by the breasts in late pregnancy and gradually changing to mature milk some days after delivery.

Conception The fertilization of the egg by the sperm and its implantation in the uterine wall.

Congenital abnormality An abnormality or deformity existing from birth, usually arising from a damaged gene, the adverse effect of certain drugs, or the effect of some diseases during pregnancy.

Contractions The regular tightening of the uterine muscles as they work to dilate the cervix in labor and press the baby down the birth canal.

Cordocentesis See *Umbilical vein sampling*.

Corpuscles Constituents of blood, divided into red and white varieties.

Corpus luteum A glandular mass that forms in the ovary after fertilization. It produces progesterone, which helps to form the placenta, and is active for the first 14 weeks of pregnancy.

Cortisone A steroid produced by the adrenal gland; it appears in the amniotic fluid immediately before labor.

Crowning The moment when the baby's head appears in the vagina and does not slip back again.

CVS See *Chorionic villus sampling*.

Cystitis An inflammation of the bladder and urinary tract, producing a painful stinging sensation when urine is passed.

D and C The surgical dilatation (opening) of the cervix and curettage (removal of the contents) of the uterus.

Dehydration A physical condition caused by the loss of an excessive amount of water from the body, often resulting from severe vomiting or diarrhea.

Depression, respiratory Breathing difficulties in the newborn baby.

Dextrose A solution of glucose used to supplement the level of blood sugar, usually introduced by intravenous drip.

Dextrostix A test to assess the level of sugar in the urine.

Diabetes Failure of the system to metabolize glucose, traced by excess sugar in the blood and urine.

Diastolic pressure The blood pressure between the heartbeats. See also *Systolic pressure*.

Diazepam (Valium) See *Tranquilizers*.

Dilation The progressive opening of the cervix caused by uterine contractions during labor.

Distress See *Fetal distress*.

Diuretics Drugs that increase the amount of urine excreted.

Dizygotic See *Twins*.

Doppler A method of using ultrasound vibrations to listen to the fetal heart.

Doula A supportive woman helper who provides physical and emotional support during childbirth.

Down's syndrome A severe congenital abnormality producing subnormal intelligence.

Drip See *Intravenous drip*.

Dura The outer membrane protecting the spinal cord.

Dyspareunia Painful intercourse.

Dystocia A diagnostic term for prolonged labor.

Dystocia, shoulder A state in which the baby's shoulders get stuck during delivery.

Eclampsia The severe form of preeclampsia, which is characterized by extremely high blood pressure, headaches, visual distortion, convulsions, and, in the worst cases, coma and death. The condition is now rare since the symptoms of preeclampsia are treated immediately. See also *Preeclampsia*.

Ectopic (tubal) **pregnancy** A pregnancy that develops outside the uterus, usually in one of the Fallopian tubes. The mother has severe pain low down on one side in her abdomen at any time from the 6th to 12th week of pregnancy. The pregnancy must be surgically terminated.

EDD The estimated date of delivery.

Edema Fluid retention, which causes the body tissues to be puffed out.

Elective induction Induction done for convenience rather than for medical reasons. See also *Induction*.

Electrode A small electrical conductor used obstetrically for monitoring the fetal heartbeat during labor.

Electronic fetal monitoring The continuous monitoring of the fetal heart by a transducer placed on the mother's abdomen over the area of the fetal heart, or by an electrode inserted through the cervix and clipped to the baby's scalp.

Embryo The developing organism in pregnancy, from about the 10th day after fertilization until about the 12th week of pregnancy, when it is termed a fetus.

Endocrinological changes Changes in the secretion of the endocrine glands that occur in pregnancy or the four weeks after delivery (the puerperium).

Endometrium The inner lining of the uterus.

Enema The injection of fluids through the rectum to expel its contents.

Engaged (Eng/E) The baby is engaged when it has settled with its presenting part deep in the pelvic cavity. This often happens in the last month of pregnancy.

Engorgement The overcongestion of the breasts with milk. If long periods are left between feedings or the baby is not well latched on, painful engorgement can occur. This can be relieved by putting the baby to the breast or expressing the excess milk.

Entonox A mixture of 50 percent oxygen and 50 percent nitrous oxygen, breathed in through a mask during labor, that gives pain relief as contractions peak.

Epidural (Lumbar epidural block) Regional anesthesia, used during labor and for Cesarean sections, in which an anesthetic is injected through a catheter into the epidural space in the lower spine.

Episiotomy A surgical cut in the perineum to enlarge the entrance to the vagina.

Estriol A form of estrogen.

Estrogen A hormone produced by the ovary.

External version (External cephalic version, or ECV) The manipulation by gentle pressure of the fetus into the cephalic position. This may be done by an obstetrician at the end of pregnancy if the baby is breech or transverse.

Face presentation The position of a baby coming through the cervix face first.

Fallopian tube (Oviduct) The tube into which a ripe egg is wafted after its expulsion from the ovary, along which it travels on its way to the uterus.

False labor Braxton Hicks (rehearsal) contractions which are so strong and regular that they may be mistaken for the contractions of the first stage of labor.

Fertilization The meeting of the sperm with the ovum, or egg, to form a new life. See also *Conception*.

Fetal distress A shortage in the flow of oxygen to the fetus, which can arise from numerous causes.

Fetus The developing child in the uterus, from the end of the embryonic stage at about the 12th week of pregnancy, until birth.

FH Fetal heart.

Fiber optics The transmission of light along flexible bundles of glass. Sometimes fiber-optic instruments are used to view the fetus inside the uterus; fiber-optic bands are used to treat neonatal jaundice.

Fluid retention See *Edema*.

FMF Fetal movement felt.

Folic acid A form of vitamin B essential for the production of blood cells and hemoglobin, the shortage of which may produce disabilities in the fetus.

Fontanels The soft spots between the unjoined sections of the fetal skull.

Foremilk Thirst-quenching milk that accumulates in the ducts behind the nipple. The baby takes foremilk at the beginning of a feeding.

Fraternal twins See *Twins*.

Fundal palpation Feeling through the abdominal wall for the top of the uterus to assess its height.

Fundus The upper part of the uterus.

Gamma globulin A protein-based antibody used to prevent or treat infections such as hepatitis.

Gene The part of every cell that stores genetic characteristics.

Genetic counseling Advice on the probability of recurrent hereditary abnormalities or diseases.

Gentle birth One term used for a method of delivery proposed by Frederick Leboyer in which the shock of birth upon the baby is minimized and the baby is welcomed by loving hands, skin contact, soft lights, and a warm bath.

German measles See *Rubella*.

Gestation The length of time between conception and delivery.

Glucose A natural sugar found in certain organic materials and in the blood: the main source of energy.

Glycogen The natural source of glucose; glycogen stores carbohydrate materials and is formed by the liver and muscles.

Gynecologist A doctor who specializes in the female reproductive system.

Hb See *Hemoglobin*.

HCG See *Human chorionic gonadotrophin*.

Hegar's sign The softening of the lower part of the uterus that gradually occurs during the first six weeks of pregnancy.

Hemoglobin (Hb) A constituent of the red blood cells that contains iron (Fe) and stores oxygen.

Hemorrhage Excessive bleeding.

Hemorrhoids (Piles) Swelling of the veins around the rectum.

Hormone A chemical messenger in the blood that stimulates various organs to action.

Hormone-accelerated labor See *Induction*.

Human chorionic gonadotrophin (HCG) A hormone released into the woman's bloodstream by the developing placenta from about six days after the last period was due. Its presence in the urine means that she is pregnant.

Hyaline membrane disease Respiratory distress affecting some preterm babies, resulting from a lack of surfactant that holds the lungs open.

Hydatidiform mole A rare abnormality in which the embryo fails to develop, so there is no baby, although the placenta and chorionic villi go on developing rapidly. If the woman does not miscarry, the growth must be removed.

Hydrocephalus A congenital abnormality in which the baby's head is swollen with fluid.

Hyperemesis gravidarum Almost continuous vomiting during pregnancy.

Hypertension (High blood pressure) In pregnancy this can reduce the fetal blood supply.

Hyperventilation Abnormally heavy breathing that flushes carbon dioxide out of the bloodstream, so that the normal chemical balance of the blood is lost.

Hypnosis A state of mental passivity with a special susceptibility to suggestion. This can be used as an anesthetic, and can be self-induced.

Hypnotics See *Tranquilizers*.

Hypoglycemia Low blood sugar, which is sometimes apparent in babies who have suffered a difficult delivery, preterm babies, or those of diabetic mothers. It can be artificially produced by giving the mother intravenous glucose in labor, since this increases the release of insulin, which breaks the sugar down. The baby may have to be given extra sugar.

Hypotension Low blood pressure.

Hypothermia A very low body temperature, which can be fatal.

Identical twins See *Twins*.

Implantation The embedding of the fertilized ovum or egg within the wall of the uterus.

Incoordinate uterine action See *Uterine action, incoordinate*.

Induction The process of artificially starting labor and keeping it going.

Insulin A hormone produced by the pancreas that regulates the level of carbohydrates and amino acids in the system. It may be used as a means of controlling the effects of diabetes. See also *Diabetes*.

Internal monitoring See *Electronic fetal monitoring*.

Intramuscular injection An injection into a muscle.

Intrauterine growth restriction (IUGR) A term used when a baby is "small for dates."

Intravenous drip The infusion of fluids directly into the bloodstream by means of a fine catheter introduced into a vein.

Intravenous injection An injection into a vein.

Invasive techniques Any medical technique that intrudes into the body.

Involution of the uterus The process by which the uterus returns to its normal state after pregnancy.

IUGR See *Intrauterine growth restriction*.

Jaundice, neonatal A common complaint in newborn babies, caused by inability of the liver to break down successfully an excess of red blood cells. See also *Bilirubin*.

Ketosis The accumulation of lactic acid in various body tissues and fluids, which is often indicated by acetone in the urine.

Labia The folds (or lips) of skin at the entrance of the vagina.

Lamaze approach See *Psychoprophylaxis*

Lanugo The fine, soft body hair of the fetus.

Lateral position Transverse lie or horizontal position of a fetus in the uterus (sometimes occurring if the mother has a large pelvis), where the presenting part is either a shoulder or the side of the head.

Laxatives Purgative drugs.

Leboyer approach See *Gentle birth*.

Let-down reflex See *Milk ejection reflex*.

Lie The position of the fetus in the uterus.

Ligament A fibrous tissue binding and connecting bones.

Lightening The engagement of the fetus in the pelvis, with its presenting part fitting securely in the pelvic inlet like an egg in an egg cup.

Linea nigra A line of dark skin that appears down the center of the abdomen over the rectus muscle in some women during pregnancy.

Lithotomy position A position for delivery, in which the mother lies flat on her back, with her legs wide apart and raised, fixed in stirrups.

Lochia Postnatal vaginal discharge.

Longitudinal lie The position of the fetus in the uterus in which the spines of the fetus and the mother are parallel.

Long l See *Longitudinal lie*.

Low-birth-weight baby A baby who weighs below 5½ lb (2.5 kg) at birth.

Meconium The first contents of the bowel, present in the fetus before birth and passed during the first few days after birth. The presence of meconium in the amniotic fluid before delivery is usually taken as a sign of fetal distress.

Milk ejection reflex (Let-down reflex) The flow of milk into the nipple.

Miscarriage See *Abortion*.

Molding The shaping of the bones of the baby's skull as it passes through the birth canal.

Mongolism See *Down's syndrome*.

Monilia See *Thrush*.

Monitoring See *Electronic fetal monitoring*.

Monozygotic See *Twins*.

Montgomery's tubercles Small bumps on the areola surrounding the nipple.

Morphine A narcotic opium derivative used as an analgesic.

Morula A stage in the growth of the fertilized egg when it has developed into 32 cells.

Mucus A sticky secretion.

Multigravida A woman in her second or subsequent pregnancy.

Multiple pregnancy The development of two or more babies. See also *Twins*.

Mutation A damaged genetic cell. This can occur naturally or, more commonly, as an effect of outside agents, such as radiation.

Nasogastric tube A pliable catheter that is passed through the nose into the stomach. Nasogastric tubes are used either for passing nourishment into the digestive tract or for draining digestive fluids.

Neural tube defects Abnormalities of the central nervous system. See also *Anencephaly; Hydrocephalus; Spina bifida*.

Nicotine A highly poisonous substance present in tobacco. During pregnancy it enters the bloodstream of a woman who smokes and may affect the efficiency of the placenta, often resulting in a low-birth-weight baby.

Notochord The cells that form the primitive nervous system.

Nucleus The central part or core of a cell, containing genetic information.

Occipito anterior The position of the baby in the uterus when the back of its head (the crown or occiput) is toward the mother's front (anterior).

Occipito posterior The position of the baby in the uterus when the back of its head (the crown or occiput) is toward the mother's back (posterior).

Opioids (Narcotics) Painkilling drugs that induce drowsiness and stupor.

Os The mouth of the cervix.

Ovary One of the two female glands, set at the entrance of the Fallopian tubes, which regularly produce eggs until menopause.

Oviduct See *Fallopian tube*.

Ovulation The production of a ripe ovum or egg by the ovary.

Oxygenate To saturate with oxygen.

Oxytocin A hormone secreted by the pituitary gland that stimulates uterine contractions during labor and stimulates milk glands in the breasts to produce milk.

Oxytocin challenge test A way of assessing the condition of the fetus and of the placenta, in which oxytocin is introduced into the mother's bloodstream and the reactions of the fetal heart to uterine contractions are recorded.

Palpation Feeling the parts of the baby through the mother's abdominal wall.

Pelvic floor The springy muscular structure set within the pelvis that supports the bladder and the uterus, and through which the baby descends during labor.

Pelvis The pelvis is a solid ring of bone at the base of the abdomen; it shields the bladder and portions of the genital tract.

Perinatal The period from the 24th week of gestation to one week following delivery.

Perineum The area of soft tissues surrounding the vagina and between the vagina and the rectum.

PET See *Preeclampsia*.

Pethidine See *Analgesics*.

Phenothiazine Strong tranquilizers used in the treatment of nausea and vomiting. See also *Tranquilizers*.

Phototherapy Treatment by exposure to light, which may be used when a baby has jaundice.

Pitocin A synthetic form of oxytocin, used to stimulate labor.

Pituitary gland A gland set just below the brain that, among other functions, secretes various hormones controlling the menstrual cycle. In late pregnancy it releases a hormone, oxytocin, into the bloodstream, which stimulates uterine contractions and also the milk glands.

Placenta The organ that develops on the inner wall of the uterus and supplies the fetus with all its life-supporting requirements and carries waste products to the mother's system.

Placental insufficiency A condition in which the placenta provides inadequate life support for the fetus, resulting in a baby at special risk.

Placenta previa A condition in which the placenta lies over the cervix at the end of pregnancy. This part of the uterus stretches in the last few weeks of pregnancy, but the placenta cannot stretch, so it may separate; the result is bleeding during late pregnancy. A woman with a complete placenta previa is delivered by Cesarean section.

Polyhydramnios An excess of amniotic fluid in the uterus.

Posterior See *Occipito posterior*.

Postmaturity The state of the fetus in an overdue pregnancy. The skin may be dry and peeling, and the fingernails may need cutting immediately after birth.

Postnatal After the birth.

Postpartum After delivery.

Post-traumatic stress disorder Panic and anxiety experienced by some women after traumatic and disempowering childbirth.

PP See *Presenting part*.

Preeclampsia (Preeclamptic toxemia or PET) An illness in which a woman has high blood pressure, edema, protein in the urine, and often sudden excessive weight gain. See also *Eclampsia*.

Premature See *Preterm*.

Prenatal Before delivery.

Prepping Procedures carried out to prepare the woman for labor.

Presentation The position of the fetus in the uterus before and during labor.

Presenting part The part of the fetus that is lying directly over the cervix.

Preterm A baby born before the 37th week of pregnancy and weighing less than 5½ lb (2.5 kg).

Primigravida A woman having her first pregnancy.

Progesterone A hormone produced by the corpus luteum and then by the placenta.

Progestogen A synthetic variety of the hormone progesterone used in oral contraceptives.

Prolactin A hormone that stimulates milk production for breast-feeding.

Prostaglandins Natural substances that stimulate the onset of labor contractions. Prostaglandin gel may be used to soften the cervix and induce labor.

Proteinuria The presence of protein in the urine, which may be a sign of preeclampsia. See also *Preeclampsia*.

Psychoprophylaxis A method of preparation for childbirth that is centered on techniques of distraction and breathing.

PTSD See *Post-traumatic stress disorder*

Pubis The bones forming the front of the lower pelvis.

Pudendal block Injection of anesthetic to numb the nerves in the perineum.

Puerperium The four weeks following birth.

Purse-string suture (Shirodkar or MacDonald) Stitches passed through and around the cervix and then drawn tight to support the uterus when the cervix is "incompetent."

Pyelonephritis An infection of the kidneys. It is treated by a course of antibiotics.

Pyridoxine Vitamin B_6.

Quickening The first noticeable movements of the fetus felt by the mother.

Rectus muscle The muscles running up the center of the abdomen.

REM Rapid eye movement in sleep, indicating mental activity.

Respiratory depression See *Depression, respiratory*.

Rh factor A distinguishing characteristic of the red blood corpuscles. All human beings have either Rh positive or Rh negative blood. If the mother is Rh negative and the fetus Rh positive, severe complications and Rh disease (the destruction of the red corpuscles by antibodies) may occur, unless prevented by anti-D gamma globulin.

Rooting The baby's instinctive searching for the breast.

Rubella (German measles) A mild virus that may cause congenital abnormalities in the fetus if it is contracted by a woman during the first 12 weeks of pregnancy.

Sacrum The big bone at the base of the spine, forming the back of the pelvis.

Salicylate See *Aspirin*.

Scan (Screen) A way of building up a picture of an object by bouncing high-frequency sound waves off it. The sonar or ultrasound scan is used during pregnancy to show the development of the fetus in the uterus. See also *Transducer*.

Senna Derivatives of the cassia plant, components of many laxatives.

Shirodkar See *Purse-string suture*.

Shoulder dystocia See *Dystocia, shoulder*.

Show A vaginal discharge of bloodstained mucus occurring before labor, resulting from the onset of cervical dilation. A sign that labor is starting.

Small-for-dates Babies who are born at the right time but for some reason have not flourished in the uterus. See also *Placental insufficiency*.

Sonogram See *Doppler*.

Sperm (Spermatozoon) The male reproductive cell that fertilizes the ovum, or egg.

Spina bifida A congenital neural tube defect in which the fetal spinal cord forms incorrectly, outside the spinal column.

Spinal anesthesia An injection of local anesthetic around the spinal cord.

Spontaneous abortion See *Abortion*.

Stanislavsky technique Sensory exercises that increase body awareness.

Stasis of milk A reduction in the flow of breast milk with blocking of ducts.

Steroids Drugs used in the treatment of skin disorders, asthma, hay fever, rheumatism, and arthritis. Because they alter the chemical balance of the metabolism they may, very rarely, cause fetal abnormalities if used extensively during pregnancy.

Stethoscope, fetal A trumpet-shaped instrument placed against the pregnant woman's abdomen for the fetal heart to be heard.

Stillbirth The delivery of a dead baby after the 24th week of pregnancy.

Stool bulk producers Drugs to treat constipation.

Streptomycin A broad-spectrum antibiotic that should not be taken in pregnancy. See also *Antibiotics*.

Stress tests Tests during pregnancy that cause stress to the fetus and note fetal reactions.

Stretch marks See *Striae*.

Striae Silvery lines that sometimes appear on the skin after it has been stretched during pregnancy.

Supplementary feeding Additional formula given to a breast-fed baby.

Surfactant A creamy fluid that reduces the surface tension of the lungs so that they do not stick together when deflated. Preterm babies may have breathing difficulties if surfactant has not developed sufficiently.

Suture The stitching together of a tear or a surgical incision.

Systolic pressure The blood pressure built up in the arteries when the heart beats. The upper figure on a blood pressure record. See also *Diastolic pressure*.

Telemetry A method of monitoring, using radio waves. See also *Electronic fetal monitoring*.

TENS machine See *Transcutaneous electronic nerve stimulation*.

Teratogenic A general term for drugs that cause physical defects in the embryo.

Term The end of pregnancy: 38–42 weeks from the last menstrual period.

Termination An artificially induced abortion before the end of the 28th week of pregnancy.

Test weighing A method of assessing how much breast milk the baby is taking by weighing it immediately before and after a feeding.

Tetracycline A wide-spectrum class of antibiotic that should be avoided during pregnancy, because it can affect the development of the fetal teeth and bones. See also *Antibiotics*.

Thrombosis A blood clot in the heart or blood vessels.

Thrush A yeast infection that can form in the mucus membranes of the mouth, genitals, or nipples.

Thyroid gland A gland in the throat that produces hormones to control the metabolic rate.

Tochodynamometer A pressure gauge attached by a belt to the mother's abdomen in order to record her contractions.

Touch relaxation A means of stimulating release of muscular tension by resting the hands on tense areas and gently drawing out the tension.

Toxemia See *Preeclampsia; Eclampsia*.

Toxoplasmosis, congenital A parasitic disease spread by cat feces. If it crosses the placenta during pregnancy, it can cause eye or central nervous system damage in the baby.

Tranquilizers Drugs used to calm a state of anxiety or tension without inducing unconsciousness. Mild tranquilizers, such as Valium, may be prescribed during pregnancy, but should be avoided during labor since they can cause fetal respiratory depression. Powerful tranquilizers (along with antihistamines and hypnotics, which are sometimes used for their tranquilizing properties) should be avoided during pregnancy. See also *Barbiturates*.

Transcutaneous electronic nerve stimulation A method of pain relief that uses electrical impulses to block pain messages to the brain.

Transducer An instrument that translates echoes of very high-frequency sound waves, bounced off the developing fetus in the uterus, to build up an ultrasound image on a monitor. See also *Scan*.

Transition A phase between the first and second stages of labor when the cervix is dilating to between 7 and 10 cm.

Trial of labor A situation in which, although a Cesarean section may be necessary, the mother labors in order to see if a vaginal delivery is possible.

Twins The simultaneous development of two babies in the uterus, either after two eggs are fertilized independently by two sperm—dizygotic or fraternal twins—or, more rarely, after one fertilized egg divides to produce monozygotic or identical twins.

Ultrasound See *Scan; Transducer*.

Umbilical cord The cord connecting the fetus to the placenta.

Umbilical vein sampling (Cordocentesis) A fine needle is passed through the mother's abdomen into the fetal vein in the umbilical cord. The technique allows fetal blood to be tested, facilitates intra-urine blood transfusions, and enables drugs to be injected directly into the baby.

Undescended testicle A testicle that has failed to drop naturally from the lower abdomen into the scrotum.

Uterine action, incoordinate Irregular uterine contractions.

Uterine inertia Weak and ineffective uterine contractions.

Uterus (Womb) The hollow muscular organ in which the fertilized egg becomes embedded, where it develops into the embryo and then the fetus.

Vacuum extractor An instrument, used as an alternative to forceps, that adheres to the baby's scalp by suction and, with the help of the mother's bearing down, can be used to guide the baby out of the vagina.

Vagina The canal between the uterus and the external genitals. It receives the penis during intercourse and is the passage through which the baby is delivered.

VE Vaginal examination.

Vernix A creamy substance that often covers the fetus in the uterus.

Vertex presentation (VX) See *Cephalic presentation*.

Vulva The external part of the female reproductive organs, including the labia and clitoris.

Water birth Birth of a baby under water.

XX/XY chromosomes The chromosomes that genetically distinguish the female and male, respectively.

Yolk sac The sac that stores the nutrients for the developing fertile egg.

RESEARCH REFERENCES

These research references relate to the asterisks in the text. Where there is more than one asterisk on a page, the references appear in order. A bold dot indicates where a new reference begins.

p. 26 Quoted by Pamela Nowicka, *Independent*, November 23, 1987.

p. 35 S. Golombok, C. Murray, V. Jadva, F. MacCallum, and E. Lycett, "Families created through a surrogacy arrangement: Parent-child relationships in the first year of life." Submitted to *Developmental Psychology*.
• Linda Cohen, quoted in *Independent*, July 1, 2002.

p. 41 S-Z. Chen, K. Aisaka, H. Mori, et al., "Effects of sitting position on uterine activity during labor," *Obstetrics and Gynecology*, 69, 1, 67–73, 1987.
• *Pregnancy and Childbirth*, Cochrane Database, Cochrane Institute, Oxford, *available from* BMJ Publishing Group, P.O. Box 295, London WC1H 9TE.

p. 45 U. Waldenström and K. Gottvall, "A randomized trial of birthing stool or conventional semirecumbent position for second-stage labor," *Birth*, 18, 1, 5–10, 1991.
• J. P. Rooks, N. L. Weatherby, and E. K. M. Burst, "The National Birth Center Study Part II, Intrapartum and immediate postpartum and neonatal care," *Journal of Nurse Midwifery*, 37, 5, 301–330, 1992.
• D. Saunders, M. Boulton, J. Chapple, et al., "Evaluation of the Edgware Birth Centre," Northwick Park Hospital (North Thames Perinatal Public Health 2000).

p. 46 M. Tew, *Safer Childbirth*, Chapman and Hall, London, 1990.
• Ole Olsen, "Meta-analysis of the safety of home birth," *Birth*, 24, 1, 4–13, 1997.

p. 48 Sheila Kitzinger, *Birth Your Way: Choosing Birth at Home or in a Birth Center,* DK Publishing, London, 2002.
• M. Enkin and I. Chalmers (eds.), *Effectiveness and Satisfaction in Antenatal Care*, Spastics International Medical Publications, London, 1982; Ann Oakley, *The Captured Womb*, Blackwell, Oxford, 1984.

p. 51 "Routine iron supplements in pregnancy are unnecessary," *Drug and Therapeutics Bulletin*, 32, 4, 30–31, 1994.
• Jon F. R. Barrett et al., "Absorption of non-heme iron from food during normal pregnancy," *British Medical Journal*, 309, 79–81, 1994.

p. 53 Sheila Kitzinger, *The New Good Birth Guide*, Penguin, London, 1983.

p. 56 Helen Stapleton, Mavis Kirkham, and Gwenan Thomas, "Qualitative study of evidence based leaflets in maternity care," *British Medical Journal,* 324, 639–643, 2002.
• Ibid.

p. 58 J. G. Thornton and R. J. Lilford, "Active management of labour: current knowledge and research issues," *British Medical Journal*, 309, 366–369, 1994.
• Ibid.

p. 81 A. Saari-Kemppainen, O. Karjalainen, P. Ylöstalo, et al., "Ultrasound screening and perinatal mortality: controlled trial of systematic one-stage screening in pregnancy: the Helsinki ultrasound trial," *Lancet*, 336, 8712, 387–391, 1990; J. P. Newnham, S. F. Evans, C. A. Michael, et al., "Effects of frequent ultrasound during pregnancy: a randomized controlled trial," *Lancet*, 342, 8876, 887–891, 1993.

p. 91 *Pregnancy and Childbirth*, Cochrane Database.

p. 96 R. W. Smithells et al., "Maternal nutrition in early pregnancy," *British Journal of Nutrition*, 38, 3, 497–506, 1977; *Nutrition and Fetal Development* (ed. M. Winick), John Wiley & Sons, New York, 1974; H. A. Kaminetzky and H. Baker, "Micronutrients in pregnancy," *Clinical Obstetrics and Gynecology*, 20, 2, 363–380, 1977; R. M. Pitkin, "Nutritional support in obstetrics and gynecology," *Clinical Obstetrics and Gynecology*, 19, 3, 489–513, 1976.
• P. J. Illingworth, R. T. Jung, P. W. Howie, and T. E. Isles, "Reduction in postprandial energy expenditure during pregnancy," *British Medical Journal,* 294, 1573–1576, 1987.

p. 98 Gary K. Oakes and Ronald A. Chez, "Nutrition in pregnancy," *Contemporary Obstetrics and Gynecology*, 4, 147–150, 1974.
• M. D. G. Gillmer, "Obesity in pregnancy—physical and metabolic effects," *Nutrition in Pregnancy: Proceedings of the Tenth Study Group of the Royal College of Obstetricians and Gynaecologists*, 213–230, RCOG, London, 1983.

p. 100 A. Malhotri and R. S. Sawers, *British Medical Journal*, 293, 465–466, 1986.
• M. Puig-Abuli et al., "Zinc and uterine muscle contractivity," Paper given at European Congress of Perinatal Medicine, Dublin, 1984.
• M. Robinson, "Salt in pregnancy," *Lancet*, 1,178–181, 1958.

p. 101 Peter C. Rubin, "Prescribing in pregnancy: general principles," *British*

Medical Journal, 293, 1415–1417, 1986; Martin J. Whittle and Kevin P. Hanretty, "Identifying abnormalities," *British Medical Journal*, 293, 1485–1486, 1986.

p. 102 *Federal Register,* 43, 114, U.S. Department of Health, Education and Welfare, 1978.

p. 103 N. R. Butler and E. D. Alberman (eds.), *Perinatal Problems,* Livingstone, 1969.

p. 104 M. B. Meyer, "How does maternal smoking affect birth weight and maternal weight gain?" *American Journal of Obstetrics and Gynecology*, 131, 888–893, 1978.
• J. Kline et al., "Smoking: a risk factor for spontaneous abortion," *New England Journal of Medicine*, 297, 793–795, 1977; R. L. Naeye, "Relationship of cigarette smoking to congenital anomalies and perinatal death," *American Journal of Pathology*, 90, 289–297, 1978; M. B. Meyer and J. A. Tonascia, "Maternal smoking, pregnancy complications and perinatal mortality," *American Journal of Obstetrics and Gynecology,* 128, 494–502, 1977.
• F. D. Martinez et al., "The effect of paternal smoking on the birth weight of newborns whose mothers did not smoke," *American Journal of Public Health*, 84, 9, 1489–1491, 1994.

p. 106 I. J. Chasnoff et al., "Cocaine use in pregnancy," *New England Journal of Medicine*, 313, 666–669, 1985.

p. 107 Peter Parish, *Medicines: A Guide for Everybody*, Penguin, London, 1976.

p. 108 J. Moore-Gillon, "Asthma in pregnancy," *British Journal of Obstetrics and Gynaecology*, 1018, 658–660, 1994.

p. 109 Roger Hoag, "Perinatal psychology," *Birth and the Family Journal*, 113, 1974.

p. 110 Studies of babies born in England and Wales between 1943 and 1965 revealed that the children of mothers who had had pelvic X-rays in pregnancy were almost twice as likely to develop leukemia before they were 10 years old as those whose mothers had had no X-rays. The greatest risk is in the earliest weeks, when the mother may not know she is pregnant. The risk of cancer was increased 15 times when X-rays were done in the first three months of pregnancy. *See* A. Stewart and G. W. Kneale, "Radiation dose effects in relation to obstetric X-rays and childhood cancers," *Lancet*, 1, 1495, 1970.

p. 111 David W. Smith, Sterling K. Clarren, and Mary Ann Sedgwick Harvey, "Hyperthermia as a possible teratogenic agent," *Journal of Pediatrics*, 92, 6, 878–883, June 1978; Peter Miller, David W. Smith, and Thomas H. Shepard, "Maternal hyperthermia as a possible cause of anencephaly," *Lancet*, 1, 8063, 519–521, 1978.

p. 112 D. Josefson, "Rubella vaccine may be safe in pregnancy," *British Medical Journal* 322, 7288, 695, 2001.

p. 115 *British Journal of Obstetrics and Gynaecology*, 91, 724–730, 1984.
• *Pregnancy and Childbirth*, Cochrane Database.

p. 119 Sarah Key, *Body in Action*, Penguin, London, 1995. I am grateful to Sarah Key for the information and imagery about the spine included in this section.

p. 124 Aidan MacFarlane, *The Psychology of Childbirth*, Fontana, London, 1977.

p. 125 E. Noble, *Essential Exercises for the Childbearing Year*, 3rd ed., Houghton Mifflin, Boston, 1988.

p. 134 *Pregnancy and Childbirth*, Cochrane Database.

p. 137 Ibid.

p. 139 Fraser R. Watson, "Bleeding during the later half of pregnancy," in I. Chalmers, M. Enkin, and M. J. N. C. Keirse (eds.), *Effective Care in Pregnancy and Childbirth,* Vol. 1, 594–611, Oxford University Press, 1989.

p. 141 *Pregnancy and Childbirth*, Cochrane Database.

p. 144 David J. S. Hunter and Marc J. N. C. Keirse, "Gestational Diabetes," in Chalmers et al. (eds.), *Effective Care*, 403–410.
• P. Steer, M. A. Alam, J. Wadsworth, et al., "Relation between maternal haemoglobin concentration and birth weight in different ethnic groups," *British Medical Journal*, 310, 489–491, 1995.
• Pregnant women often have "physiological" anemia. Because there is a greater volume of blood circulating in their bodies, the red blood cells are dilated. This is normal—these women are not suffering from anemia, and unnecessary iron supplements may do more harm than good. This is because excess iron makes red blood cells too big to pass through some of the capillaries in the mother's and the baby's circulatory systems (macrocytosis). This deprives the baby of essential nutrients and may cause its growth to be retarded. *See* T. Lind, *British Journal of Obstetrics and Gynaecology*, 83, 760, 1976.

p. 175 Sherry L. Jimenez, Linda C. Jones, and Ruth G. Jungman, "Prenatal classes for repeat parents," MCN, 4, 305–308, Sept./Oct. 1979.

p. 180 Penny Simkin, "Just another day in a woman's life? Part I: Women's long-term preconceptions of their first birth experiences," *Birth*, 18, 4, 203–210, 1991; Penny Simkin, "Just another day in a woman's life? Part II: Nature and consistency of women's long-term memories of their first birth experiences," *Birth*, 19, 2, 64–81, 1992.

p. 183 Grantly Dick-Read, *Childbirth Without Fear*, Pan, London, 1969.
• Erna Wright, *The New Childbirth*, Tandem, London, 1969.

p. 184 Janet Balaskas, *Active Birth*, Harvard Common Press, Cambridge, Mass., 1992.

p. 188 Marshall H. Klaus, John H. Kennel, and Phyllis H. Klaus, *Mothering the Mother—How a Doula Can Help You Have a Shorter, Easier and Healthier Birth*, Addison Wesley, New York, 1993.
• *Pregnancy and Childbirth*, Cochrane Database.
• Sheila Kitzinger, *Rediscovering Birth*, Pocket Books, New York, 2002.
• Kitzinger, *Birth Your Way*.

p. 205 Both poems from Rosemary Palmeira (ed.), *The Gold of Flesh: Poems of Birth and Motherhood*, The Women's Press, London, 1990.

p. 207 Kitzinger, *Rediscovering Birth*.

p. 226 Christine Gosden, Kypros Nicolaides, and Vanessa Whitting, *Is My Baby All Right? A Guide for Expectant Parents*, Oxford University Press, Oxford, 1994.

p. 230 *New England Journal of Medicine*, 326, 1504, 1992.

p. 232 CMO's Update 4: A communication to all doctors from the Chief Medical Officer, Department of Health, London, November 1994.

• B. G. Ewigman, J. P. Crane, F. D. Frigoletto, et al., and the Radius Study Group, "Effect of pre-natal ultrasound screening on perinatal outcome," *New Journal of Medicine* 329, 821–822, 1993.

p. 234 *Pregnancy and Childbirth*, Cochrane Database.

p. 235 Medical Research Council Working Party on the evaluation of chorionic villus sampling, "Medical Research Council European trial of chorionic villus sampling," *Lancet*, 3, 37, 1491–1499, 1991.
• G. Kolata, "Fetuses treated through umbilical cords," *New York Times*, March 29, 1988.

p. 241 F. Chenia, C. B. and C. A. Crowther, "Does advice to assume knee-chest position reduce the incidence of breech presentation at delivery? A randomized clinical trial," *Birth*, 14, 2, 75–78, June 1987.
• *Pregnancy and Childbirth*, Cochrane Database.

p. 243 J. P. VanDorsten, B. S. Schifrin, and R. L. Wallace, "Randomized controlled trial of external cephalic version with tocolysis in late pregnancy," *American Journal of Obstetrics and Gynecology*, 141, 417, 1981.

p. 251 S. L. B. Duncan and S. Beckley, "Prelabour rupture of membranes—why hurry?" *British Journal of Obstetrics and Gynaecology*, 99, 543–545, 1992.
• J. Grant and M. J. N. C. Keirse, "Prelabour rupture of membranes at term," in Chalmers et al. (eds.), *Effective Care*, 1112–1117.

p. 255 Professor Mendez-Bauer found that dilation of the cervix and the efficiency of contractions is far greater when a woman stands up than when she lies on her back. The uterus works nearly twice as well. [1]

Professor Caldeyro-Barcia found that whether a woman stood or lay down, contractions were of a similar frequency but were stronger when she stood. He concluded that for the uterus to work really effectively, the woman should be standing. [2,3]

Eleven hospitals in seven Latin-American countries joined in a study of the effects of the mother's position in labor. Half the mothers were told to lie in bed during the first stage and the other half to get up, or sit or lie in bed as they liked. Some 95 percent of the women did not want to lie down. First-time mothers who stayed upright had shorter first stages than those who were lying down. The majority were more comfortable when upright.

To find out whether an upright position could produce traumatic pressure on the baby's head, the researchers studied the incidence of caput and also the effect on the baby's heart rate. They found that, when the membranes had not ruptured, there was no increased rate of caput if the mother was upright, nor was there an increase in deceleration of the fetal heart. They concluded that in normal labor an upright position is fine for the baby, shortens labor, and reduces pain. [4]

Further research at the Queen Elizabeth Hospital, Birmingham, England, showed the same results. [5]

See 1. Peter M. Dunn, "Obstetric delivery today," *Lancet*, 1, 7963, 790–793, 1976.
2. R. Caldeyro-Barcia et al., "Effects of position changes on the intensity and frequency of uterine contractions during labor," *American Journal of Obstetric Gynecology*, 80, 284, 1960.
3. Yuen Chou-liu, "Effects of an upright position during labor," *American Journal of Nursing*, December 1974.
4. R. L. Schwarcz et al., "Fetal heart rate patterns in labors with intact and with ruptured membranes," *Journal of Perinatal Medicine*, 1, 153, 1973.

5. A. M. Flynn, J. Kelly, G. Hollins, and P. F. Lynch, "Ambulation in labour," *British Medical Journal*, 11, 591–593, August 26, 1978.

p. 260 *Pregnancy and Childbirth*, Cochrane Database.

p. 262 Ibid.

p. 272 C. M. Andrews and E. C. Andrews, "Nursing, maternal postures and foetal position," *Nursing Research*, 32, 336–341, 1983.

p. 275 M. E. Hannah, W. J. Hannah, S. A. Hewson, et al., "Planned Caesarean section versus planned vaginal birth for breech presentation at term: a randomised multi-centre trial," *Lancet*, 356, 1375–1831, 2000.
• A. Shennan and S. Bewley, "How to manage term breech deliveries," *British Medical Journal* 323, 244–245, 2001.

p. 282 J. G. B. Russell, "Moulding of the pelvic outlet," *Journal of Obstetrics and Gynaecology, British Commonwealth*, 76, 817, 1967.
• Michel Odent, *Birth Reborn*, Fontana, London, 1986.

p. 283 Emanuel A. Friedman, *Labor: Clinical Evaluation and Management*, 2nd ed., Appleton-Century-Crofts, New York, 1978.

p. 285 K. S. Olah and J. P. Neilson, "Failure to progress in the management of labour," *British Journal of Obstetrics and Gynaecology*, 101, 1, 1–3, 1994.
• L. Albers, "Rethinking Dystocia: patience please," *MIDIRS Midwifery Digest*, 11, 3, 351–353, 2002.

p. 286 Marshall H. Klaus, John H. Kennel, Steven S. Robertson, and Roberto Sosa, "Effects of social support during parturition and infant morbidity," *British Medical Journal*, 293, 585–587, 1986.

p. 304 Ronald Melzack, *The Puzzle of Pain*, Penguin, London, 1973.

p. 305 Ibid.
• Ibid.
• Ibid.

p. 310 Josephine A. Williamson, "Hypnosis in obstetrics," *Nursing Mirror*, November 27, 1975.

p. 311 Sharon Yellard, "Using acupuncture in midwifery care," *Modern Midwife*, 5, 1, 8–11, 1995.
• Song Meiyu, "Acupuncture anaesthesia for caesarean section," *Midwives' Chronicle*, April 1985.
• I. F. Skelton, "Acupuncture in labor," *Society of Bio-physical Medicine*, June 1985.

p. 312 E. Burns, C. Blaney, S. J. Ersser, et al., "The use of aromatherapy in intrapartum midwifery practice," Oxford Brookes University Centre for Health Care, Research and Development, Oxford, 1999.

p. 313 Peter Webb, *Homoeopathy for Midwives*, 30–31, British Homoeopathic Association, London, 1992.

p. 314 E. Burns and S. Kitzinger, "Midwifery guidelines for the use of water in labour," Oxford Brookes University Centre for Health Care, Research and Development, Oxford, 2000.
• E. Burns, "Waterbirth," *MIDIRS Midwifery Digest*, 11, 2, 310–513, 2001.
• F. Alderdice et al., "Labour and birth in water in England and Wales," *British Medical Journal*, 310, 837, 1995.

p. 315 R. E. Gilbert and P. A. Tookey, "Perinatal mortality and morbidity among babies delivered in water," *British Medical Journal,* 319, 7208, 483–487, 1999.
• Paul Johnson, "Birth under water: to breathe or not to breathe," *British Journal of Obstetrics and Gynaecology*, 103, 3, 202–208, 1995.

p. 317 M. Rosen, "Patient controlled analgesia," *British Medical Journal*, 289, 640–641, 1984.

p. 318 Bertil Jacobson et al., "Opiate addiction in adult offspring through possible imprinting after obstetric treatment," *British Medical Journal*, 301, 1067–1070, 1990.

p. 320 R. J. Webb and G. S. Kantor, "Obstetrical epidural anaesthesia in a rural Canadian hospital," *Canadian Journal of Anaesthetics*, 39, 390–393.
• *Pregnancy and Childbirth*, Cochrane Database.
• Andrew Doughty, *Journal of Royal Society of Medicine*, December 1978.

p. 321 J. A. Thorp et al., "The effect of intrapartum epidural analgesia on nulliparous labor: a randomized controlled prospective trial," *American Journal of Obstetrics and Gynecology*, 169, 851–858, 1993.
• M. Maresh, K. H. Choong, and R. W. Beard, "Delayed pushing with lumbar epidural analgesia in labour," *British Journal of Obstetrics and Gynaecology*, 90, 623–627, 1983.
• C. MacArthur, M. Lewis, E. G. Knox, and J. S. Crawford, "Epidural anaesthesia and long-term backache after childbirth," *British Medical Journal*, 301, 9–12, 1990; C. MacArthur, M. Lewis, and E. G. Knox, *Health After Childbirth: An Investigation of Long-term Health Problems Beginning After Childbirth in 11,701 Women*, HMSO, London, 1991.
• A. D. Noble et al., "Continuous lumbar epidural using bupivicaine," *Journal of Obstetrics and Gynaecology*, British Commonwealth, 78, 559, 1971.
• Kay Standley et al., "Local-regional anesthesia during childbirth: effect on newborn behaviors," *Science*, 186, November 15, 1974.

p. 322 R. Russell, F. Reynolds, et al., "Epidural infusion of low-dose bupivicaine and opioid in labour: Does reducing the motorblock increase

the spontaneous delivery rate?" *Anaesthesia*, 516, 5, 266–273, 1996.
• Sheila Kitzinger, *Some Women's Experiences of Epidurals*, National Childbirth Trust, London, 1987.

p. 323 Rosen, "Patient controlled analgesia."

p. 324 Josephine M. Green, Vanessa A. Coupland, and Jenny V. Kitzinger, "Expectations, experiences and psychological outcomes of childbirth: a prospective study of 825 women," *Birth*, 17, 1, 15–23, 1990.

p. 325 Kieran O'Driscoll and Declan Meagher, *Active Management of Labour*, 3rd ed., Mosby Yearbook, Times/Mirror, London, 1993.

p. 327 *Pregnancy and Childbirth*, Cochrane Database.
• R. Caldeyro-Barcia et al., "Adverse perinatal effects of early amniotomy during labor," in L. Gluck (ed.), *Modern Perinatal Medicine*, 431–439, Yearbook Medical Publishers, Chicago, 1974.

p. 328 A. Huch et al., "Continuous transcutaneous monitoring of fetal oxygen tension during labour," *British Journal of Obstetrics and Gynaecology*, 84, Suppl. 1, 1977.
• G. C. Gunn et al., "Premature rupture of the fetal membranes," *American Journal of Obstetrics and Gynecology*, 106, 469–477, 1970.
• P. J. Steer et al., "The effect of membrane rupture on fetal heart in induced labour," *British Journal of Obstetrics and Gynaecology*, 83, 454–459, June 1976.

p. 330 *Pregnancy and Childbirth*, Cochrane Database.

p. 332 Ibid.
• Ian D. Graham, *Episiotomy: Challenging Obstetric Interventions*, Blackwell Science, Oxford, 1997.
• M. S. Klein, R. C. Gaultier, J. Robbins, et al., "Relation of

episiotomy to perineal trauma and morbidity, sexual dysfunction and pelvic floor relaxation," *American Journal of Obstetrics and Gynecology*, 1, 71, 3, 591–598, 1994.
• Argentine Episiotomy Trial Collaborative Group, "Routine vs. selective episiotomy: a randomized controlled trial," *Lancet*, 342, 1, 517–518, 1993.
• R. F. Harrison et al., "Is routine episiotomy necessary?" *British Medical Journal*, 288, 1971–1975, 1984.
• J. Sleep et al., "West Berkshire perineal management trial," *British Medical Journal*, 289, 587–590, 1984.

p. 333 S. Kitzinger and R. Walters, *Some Women's Experiences of Episiotomy*, 2nd ed., National Childbirth Trust, London, 1993; S. Kitzinger and P. Simkin (eds.), *Episiotomy and the Second Stage of Labor*, ICEA, Minneapolis, 1984.

p. 336 S. M. Menticoglu and P. F. Hall, "Routine induction of labour at 41 weeks gestation: nonsensus consensus," *British Journal of Obstetrics and Gynaecology,* 109, 485–491, 2002.

p. 337 Linda Cardozo, "Is routine induction of labour at term ever justified?" *British Medical Journal*, 306, 840–841, 1993.
• "Caesarean Childbirth," Summary of a National Institute of Health statement, *British Medical Journal*, 1981.

p. 338 A. W. Linston and A. J. Campbell, "Danger of oxytocin-induced labour to fetuses," *British Medical Journal*, 3, 606–607, 1974.

p. 340 O'Driscoll and Meagher, *Management of Labour*.
• J. G. Thornton and R. J. Lilford, "Active management of labour: current knowledge and research issues," *British Medical Journal*, 309, 6951, 366–369, 1994.

p. 341 D. A. Luthy, K. K. Shy, G. van Belle, et al., "A randomized

trial of electronic fetal monitoring in preterm labor," *Obstetrics and Gynecology*, 69, 5, 687–695, 1987; D. MacDonald, A. Grant, M. Sheridan Pereira, et al., "The Dublin randomized controlled trial of intrapartum fetal heart rate monitoring," *American Journal of Obstetrics and Gynecology*, 152, 5, 524–539, 1985.
• K. J. Leveno, F. G. Cunningham, S. Nelson, et al., "A prospective comparison of selective and universal electronic fetal monitoring in 34,995 pregnancies," *New England Journal of Medicine*, 315, 10, 615–619, 1986.

p. 342 A. D. Haverkamp, M. Orleans, S. Langendoerfer, et al., "A controlled trial of the differential effects of intrapartum fetal monitoring," *American Journal of Obstetrics and Gynecology*, 134, 4, 399–412, 1979; I. M. Kelso, R. J. Parson, G. F. Lawrence, et al., "An assessment of continuous fetal heart rate monitoring in labor: a randomized trial," *American Journal of Obstetrics and Gynecology*, 131, 5, 526–532, 1978.
• S. Neldam, M. Osler, P. K. Hanse, et al., "Intrapartum fetal heart rate monitoring in a combined low- and high-risk population: a controlled risk trial," *European Journal of Obstetrics, Gynaecology and Reproductive Biology*, 23, 1–11, 1986.
• G. Mires, F. Williams, and P. Howie, "Randomised controlled trial of cardiotocography vs doppler auscultation of fetal heart at admission in labour in low risk obstetric population," *British Medical Journal,* 322, 1457–1462, 2001.

p. 344 D. M. Okada and A. W. Chow, "Neonatal scalp abscess following intrapartum fetal monitoring," *American Journal of Obstetrics and Gynecology*, 127, 875, 1977.

p. 345 G. S. Sykes et al., "Fetal distress and the condition of newborn infants," *British Medical Journal*, 287, 943–945, October 1983; P. W. Howe, "Fetal monitoring in labour," *British Medical Journal*, 292, 6518, 427–428, February 1986.

p. 346 *Pregnancy and Childbirth*, Cochrane Database.

p. 348 Ibid.
• T. Henriksen et al., "Caesarean section in twin pregnancies in two Danish counties and different section rates," *Acta Obstetrica Gynaecologica Scandinavica*, 73, 123–128, 1994.
• B. E. Chalmers, J. A. McIntyre, and D. Meyer, *South African Medical Journal*, 82, 161–163, 1992.
• G. M. Leung, T. H. Lam, T. Q. Thach, et al., "Rates of Caesarean births in Hong Kong 1987–1999," *Birth*, 28, 166–72, 2001.

p. 349 *Pregnancy and Childbirth*, Cochrane Database.
• Stuart Campbell, *Sharing*, Maternal Health Committee of Social Planning and Review Council of British Columbia, Summer 1979.
• A. H. MacLennan, A. W. Taylor, D. H. Wilson, et al., *International Journal of Obstetrics and Gynaecology*, 107, 12, 1460–1470, 2000.

p. 350 John Jolly, James Walker, Kalvinder Bhabra, "Subsequent obstetric performance related to primary mode of delivery," *British Journal of Obstetrics and Gynaecology*, 106, 227–232, 2002.
• *Observer*, April 21, 2002.

p. 352 *Pregnancy and Childbirth*, Cochrane Database.

p. 359 Frederick Leboyer, *Birth Without Violence*, Fontana, London, 1977.

p. 360 Hugo Lagercrantz and Theodore A. Slotkin, "The 'stress' of being born," *Scientific American*, 4, 86, 100–107, 1986.

p. 361 R. Gitau, A. Cameron, N. M. Fisk, et al., "Fetal exposure to maternal cortisol," *Lancet*, 352, 9129, 707–708, 1998.

p. 365 J. C. Mercer, "Current best evidence: a review of the literature on umbilical cord clamping," *Journal of Midwifery and Women's Health*, 466, 402–414, 2001.

p. 367 Odent, *Birth Reborn*, and *Entering the World: The Demedicalization of Childbirth*, Penguin, London, 1985.
• Johnson's Baby Newsline, Autumn 1978.

p. 371 Robert Hinde found that rhesus monkey babies separated from their mothers shortly after birth became distressed and withdrawn. He suggested that separation might also be bad for a newborn human baby. [1]
Other research has indicated that mothers who had greater contact with their babies, and continued this contact through early childhood, raised children whose IQ at five years, was significantly higher than average. [2]
Those concerned about bonding at birth also advocate skin-to-skin contact between mother and child. In response to concerns about babies becoming chilled, a study of heat loss in warmed cribs as compared with that in the mother's arms showed no significant difference. [3]
See 1. Robert Hinde, *Proceedings of the Royal Society*, 196, 29, 1977.
2. F. S. W. Brimblecombe, *Separation and Special Care Baby Units*, Heinemann, London, 1978.
3. C. N. Phillips, "Neonatal heat loss in heated cribs vs. mother's arms," *Journal of Obstetrical, Gynecological and Neonatal Nursing*, 6, 11–15, 1974.

p. 373 Marshall Klaus and John Kennel, *Maternal-Infant Bonding*, Mosby, St. Louis, 1976.

p. 378 Ibid.

p. 380 L. Silverman, W. A. Silverman, and J. C. Sinclair, *Pediatrics*, 41, 1033, 1969.

p. 382 E. Jones, "Breastfeeding in the premature infant," *Modern Midwife*, 4, 1, 22–26, 1994.

p. 383 P. A. and J. P. Davies, *Lancet*, 2, 1216, 1970.

p. 387 *Pregnancy and Childbirth*, Cochrane Database.
• Kevin Forbes, "Management of first trimester spontaneous abortions," *British Medical Journal*, 310, 1426, 1995.

p. 392 Harriet Sarnoff Schiff, *The Bereaved Parent*, G. K. Hall, London, 1977.

p. 398 H. Varendi et al., "Does the newborn baby find the nipple by smell?" *Lancet*, 344, 8, 989–990, 1994.

p. 403 A. Vogel, B. Hutchison, and E. A. Mitchell, *Birth*, 26, 4, 218–225, 1999.

p. 406 F. Cockburn et al., "Effect of diet on the fatty acid composition of the major phospholipids of the infant cerebral cortex," *Archives of Disease in Childhood*, 72, 198–203, 1995.

p. 408 Rudolph Schaffer, *Mothering*, Fontana, London, 1977.

p. 412 *Mother and Baby*, April 2002.

ACKNOWLEDGMENTS

Dorling Kindersley Limited would like to thank all the parents and the parents-to-be who allowed themselves and their children to be photographed for this book. Marcia May would especially like to thank those who so generously agreed to share the experience of the birth of their babies with her.

The publisher and photographer are also deeply grateful to the nurses, doctors, and midwives involved for their warm cooperation and advice. Special thanks go to the staff of the maternity ward at King's College Hospital, London. Thanks also to the Active Birth Centre and Blooming Marvellous Ltd., who kindly supplied props for studio photography. Thanks also to Georgia Rose.

Parents and children in this edition
Grace Andrade, Kasey Berhardsen, Shelley and Jez Groswell, Louise Hazell, Sheila Kitzinger, Mark and Lupia Noor with Sasha, Andrea Peters with Joel, David Picking, Anne Stenett with Ella, India Terras, and Shelley Zesturi.

Thanks, too, to the parents, children, and midwives in earlier editions who appear in this book.

FOR THE FOURTH EDITION
Project Editor Esther Ripley
Senior Art Editor Glenda Fisher
Senior Editor Julia North
DTP Designer Karen Constanti
Production Controller Heather Hughes
Managing Editor Anna Davidson
Managing Art Editor Emma Forge

FOR THE U.S. EDITION
Editor Jordan Pavlin
Consultant Georgia Rose

Additional color photography Andy Crawford, Ruth Jenkinson
Art direction Sally Smallwood
Illustrations Joanna Acty, Karen Cochrane, Deborah Maizels, Halli Verrinder

The publisher would like to thank the following for their kind permission to reproduce their photographs: (Abbreviations key: t = top, b = bottom, r = right, l = left, c = center)

37: Sally & Richard Greenhill/Sally Greenhill (b)
44: Science Photo Library/Faye Norman (bl)/Saturn Stills (tl)
66: Bubbles/Katie Van Dyck
70: Science Photo Library/Richard Rawlins/Custom Medical Stock Photo (bl)
94: Mother & Baby Picture Library/emap esprit/Indira Flack (b)
97: Bubbles/Lucy Tizard
137: Science Photo Library/Dr. P. Marazzi
154: Mother & Baby Picture Library/emap esprit/Paul Mitchell (tl)
174: Getty Images/Ian O'Leary
176: Getty Images/Barbara Peacock
178: Getty Images/V.C.L
206: Corbis/Jennie Woodcock/Reflections Photolibrary
228: Science Photo Library (bl)
231: Science Photo Library/Bernard Benoit (tl)
239: Getty Images/Ericka McConnell
246: Sally & Richard Greenhill/Sally Greenhill
288: Corbis/Jennie Woodcock/Reflections Photolibrary
316: Mother & Baby Picture Library/emap esprit/Rupert Jenkinson
333: Sally & Richard Greenhill/Sally Greenhill (bl)
341: Bubbles/Darren Curtis (b)
354: Science Photo Library/Ron Sutherland
374: Mother & Baby Picture Library/emap esprit/Mampta Kapoor (tr)
381: Science Photo Library/Aaron Haupt (b)
384: Getty Images/Vincent Oliver (b)
413: Corbis/Elizabeth Hathon (b)

All other pictures © Dorling Kindersley
For further information, see www.dkimages.com

INDEX

A

abdominal muscles 120–1, 123, 127, 192, 398
abdominal palpation 15, 51
abnormalities *see* disability
abortion *see* miscarriage; termination
accelerated (augmented) labor 339
accidental hemorrhage 139–40
acetaminophen 102, 106, 107
aches and pains 106–7, 130–5, 144
  backaches 130, 133, 198–9
active birth 184
active management of labor 58, 325, 340
acupressure 274–5
acupuncture 310–11
AFP (alphafetoprotein) test 142, 227
alcohol 11, 105
alphafetoprotein (AFP) test 142, 227
aminoglycosides 108
amniocentesis 232–4
amniotic sac 74, 75
amniotomy (ARM/artificial rupture of the membranes) 326, 327–30, 335
analgesics (painkillers) 106–7, 317–18
anemia 42, 51, 144
anesthesia 110, 318–23, 351
angry cat exercise 131
anomaly scans 229
antacids 15, 102
antibiotics 107–8, 136
antibody tests 16, 26, 49, 51, 113–14, 314
anticholinergic drugs 107
anticoagulants 109, 319, 388
anticonvulsants 110
antidepressants 108–9
Anti-D protection 113–14
anti-epileptic drugs 110
antihistamines 107
antiphospholid disorder (APA) 388
anti-psychotic drugs 109
anti-sickness drugs 107
anxieties *see* emotions
Apgar scale 370, 373
APH (antepartum hemorrhage) 139
apnea 380
appearance, newborns 375–8

APS (antiphospholipid syndrome) 388
ARM (artificial rupture of the membranes/amniotomy) 326, 327–30, 335
arms, touch relaxation 195
aromatherapy 311–12
artificial rupture of the membranes (amniotomy/ARM) 326, 327–30, 335
aspirin 107, 388
asthma 108
attractiveness 154, 171
augmented (accelerated) labor 339
autogenic method 184
autonomy and dependence 152–3

B

babies
  birth experience 356–61
  losing a baby *see* miscarriage; stillbirth
  postnatal exercises with 416–19
  reflexes 358, 366, 372
  sex determination 71–2
  solid foods 402
  special care 380–5
  worries about 156
  see also fetus; newborns
Bach flower remedies 313
back
  backaches 130, 133, 198–9
  back labor 270–5
  breathing down your back 208
back care 119–20, 133
  touch relaxation 198–200
balance, posture and movement 93, 125–9, 132
Balaskas method (active birth) 184
bathing babies 366–7, 409
bearing down (pushing) 223–5, 259, 260–3, 321
bending and lifting 132
bilirubin 382–3
birth
  baby's experience of 356–61
  children's presence at 46–7, 177, 298–9, 303
  choices in pregnancy and childbirth 47–8, 56, 324–5
  emotional challenges 150–7
  gentle birth 356–67

birth (cont.)
  home births 36–7, 45–7, 258, 264–9, 296–303
  in a hospital *see* hospital births
  journey through the pelvis 261, 356–9
  medical intervention *see* specific procedures, e.g., episiotomy
  preparation for *see* specific topics, e.g., relaxation
  stages *see* delivery; labor
  surprise births 294–5
birth centers 45
birth companions
  at Cesarean sections 353
  choosing 32, 58, 187–9, 286
  father's role 162, 287, 364
  role during labor 287–94
  surprise births 294–5
  see also specific activities, e.g., massage
birth dance 213–25, 252–3, 276–9, 309
birth plans 52, 57–9, 177
birth pools *see* water births and birth pools
birth rooms 41, 186, 289, 361–4
bladder problems 136, 414–15
blastocyst 73, 83
bleeding
  nosebleeds 138
  vaginal 138–40, 386–7
  see also miscarriage
blocks (local and regional anesthetics) 318–23, 351
blood
  blood tests 26, 49–51, 113–14, 227
  fetal circulation 76–7, 375
  pH levels, fetal blood 345
  Rh factor 16, 49, 113–14
blood pressure 42, 44, 320, 329
  high (hypertension) 42, 140
  and preeclampsia 141–2
blood sugar levels 142–4, 382
body shape changes 10–19
bonding
  with fetus 80–1, 149, 232
  with newborn 46, 364–5, 371–3, 378–9, 423–5
  with special care babies 384–5
bottle-feeding and formula milks 401, 405–8
Bradley method 183–4

bras 12, 137, 146
Braxton Hicks contractions 15, 19, 170, 254
breast-feeding 366, 398–405
  as contraceptive 421
  HIV transmission 26
  nipple problems 137, 402–3
  and oral contraceptives 423
  special care babies 383
breasts
  changes 10–19, 26–7, 167
  problems 137, 402–3
  stimulation 167, 171
breathing
  breathing difficulties, babies 380–2
  labor and contractions 205–13, 291, 309–10
  shortness of breath 145
  see also relaxation
breech presentation 90, 241–3, 275–82
bridging 127
bromocriptine 405
bupivacaine 322
burials and funeral arrangements 391–2
butterfly breathing 211, 212–13
buttocks, touch relaxation 200

C

calcium 100
candida 136–7
cannabis 106
caput 376
carbohydrates 99
carpal tunnel syndrome 134
catecholamines 360–1
cat exercise 131
caudals 323
centering down 189–90
cephalic presentation 43, 86, 90, 241
cephalopelvic disproportion 348
Cervidil 335
cervix 43, 118
  cervical cerclage 115
  during birth 191
  Hegar's sign 23–4
  incompetent cervix 115, 388
  mucous plug 118, 170, 250
  ripening 19, 118, 250, 337
  see also dilatation of the cervix

Cesarean section 348–55, 403
  breech presentation 275,
    280, 282
  rate increased by EFM 342,
    344–5
  twin births 90, 95
charts and records, medical
    42–3, 329
checkup, postnatal 412
childbirth *see* birth
children, other/older children
  in family 46–7, 173–7,
    298–9, 303, 378
chloasma 146
choices in pregnancy and
    childbirth, official policies
    47–8, 56, 324–5
chorionic villus sampling
    (CVS) 234–5
chromosomes 71–3
  prenatal tests 232–5
circulation
  fetal 76–7, 375
  newborn 375–6
circumcision 379
clary sage 312
classes, prenatal/childbirth 48,
    152, 163, 180–5
clinic, prenatal *see* prenatal care
clitoris 117
clothing
  newborns 411
  in pregnancy 145–6, 147,
    148
clozapine 109
co-amoxiclav 107
cocaine 106
coils (IUDs) 24–6, 422–3
coitus interruptus 421
colostrum 16, 398
color tests 23
comfort aids 242
communication with doctors
    52–8, 105–6, 153
co-mothering 34
companions *see* birth
    companions
complementary therapies, pain
    relief 310–13
conception 10, 22–3, 73, 82–3,
    89
condoms 422
confirming pregnancy 22–4,
    229
constipation 108, 135–6, 397
consultant units 39–40
contraception 24–6, 421–3
  see also types, e.g., IUDs
contractions
  Braxton Hicks 15, 19, 170,
    254
  breathing through 207–13,
    291

contractions (cont.)
  early stages of labor 254–5,
    305–6
  imagery and visualization
    191, 204–5, 224–5, 307
  induced labor 337–8
  partograms 329
  pushing (bearing down)
    223–5, 259, 260–3, 321
  simulating/rehearsing 210,
    222–3
  support from birth
    companion 289–94
  timing 254, 256
  see also labor; pain and pain
    relief
control, loss of 151–2
cord
  clamping and cutting 295,
    333–4, 365
  cord traction 333–4
  effect of amniotomy 328
cordocentesis (umbilical vein
    sampling) 235–6
corpus luteum 69, 70
cracked nipples 403
cramps, leg 134–5
crowning 261, 262, 362
crying, newborns 361, 371,
    408–9
CVS (chorionic villus
    sampling) 234–5
cystitis 136
Cytotec (misoprostol) 335–6

D

D and C (dilatation and
    curettage) 387
dairy products 99
dating pregnancy 24–5, 229,
    243–4
deceleration, fetal heart rate
    328, 344
deep transverse arrest 321
defective genes 73
delivery
  expected date of (EDD)
    24–5, 229, 243–4, 336
  forceps delivery 255, 346–7
  placenta 263, 295, 333–4
  positions 220–1, 225, 280–1
  vacuum extraction 346–7
Demerol 317–18
dental health and hygiene 11,
    15, 146
dependence and autonomy
    152–3
depression 108–9, 240, 394,
    414
development, fetal 10–19,
    68–87, 103
dextrose drips 330

diabetes 110, 142–4, 387–8
diagnosing pregnancy 22–4,
    229
diamorphine (heroin) 106, 318
diapers 409–11
diaphragm, contraceptive 422
diastolic pressure 42, 140
diet *see* food and diet
digestive disturbances 144–5
dilatation and curettage
    (D and C) 387
dilatation of the cervix
  early labor 250, 254, 284
  examining 326
  painful 306
  recording 329
  transition 258–9
disability
  mothers 411
  newborns 385
  screening for 226–7, 229
discussions with doctors 52–8,
    105–6, 153
disks, vertebral 119–20
disposable diapers 409–11
diuretics 108
dizygotic twins 89
doctors
  questions for and talking to
    52–8, 105–6, 153
  dominant genes 72–3
double-leg raising 121, 123
double screening 227
doulas 32, 58, 188–9
Down's syndrome 227, 232,
    385
dreams 28
drips, intravenous 330–1
driving 148
drugs and medication 101–10,
    317–23, 329, 334–6
dysfunctional labor 285
dyspareunia (painful
    intercourse) 420–1

E

early miscarriage 73, 102,
    387–8
eclampsia 142
EDD (expected date of
    delivery) 24–5, 229,
    243–4, 336
edema 43, 101
EFM (electronic fetal
    monitoring) 244, 257,
    329, 340–5
eggs 68–70, 71, 83, 89
elective induction 338–9
electroacupuncture 311
electronic fetal monitoring
    (EFM) 244, 257, 329,
    340–5

diabetes 110, 142–4, 387–8
embryos 10–12, 74–6, 103, 387
emotions
  Bach flower remedies 313
  birth disabilities 385
  emotional support in labor
    see birth companions
  gentle birth 356–67
  losing a baby 389–93
  postnatal 394–7, 423–4
  reactions to pregnancy
    28–31, 164–6, 172–5
  surrounding home births
    46–7
  worries and fears 150–7,
    167–8, 226, 240, 423
  see also bonding; fathers;
    relationships
engagement 18, 43, 80, 87
engorged breasts 402
Entonox (gas and oxygen) 318
epidural anesthesia 319–23,
    338, 351
episiotomy 59, 155, 280, 331–3
equipment, birth rooms 41,
    186, 289, 325–6
ergotamine 107
essential oils 311–12
estriol test 227
estrogen 69–70, 77, 406, 423
examinations, internal 23–4,
    49, 51, 326–7
exercises
  abdominal muscles 121,
    123, 127
  easing aches and pains
    130–2
  exercises to avoid 121, 123
  pelvic floor 93, 118–19, 155
  pelvic rocking 121, 122, 124,
    131, 416
  postnatal 416–19
  posture and movement
    127–9
  sports 147
  see also specific exercises e.g.
    leg sliding
expected date of delivery
    (EDD) 24–5, 229, 243–4,
    336
expressing milk 404–5
external monitors 340, 342,
    343
external version 241–3, 349
eye prophylaxis 373

F

face, touch relaxation 194
failure, fear of 152
Fallopian tubes 68, 70, 82–3
family practice physicians 40
FAS (fetal alcohol syndrome)
    105

fathers
  emotions during pregnancy 30–1, 33, 158–66, 172
  reactions to newborns 364, 375, 396, 425
  see also birth companions; relationships
fatigue 27, 91, 168, 173, 412–13
feeding
  bottle-feeding and formula milks 401, 405–8
  excitable/unsettled babies 403–4
  solid foods 402
  special care babies 382, 383
  test weighing 402
  water 401
  see also breast-feeding
feet
  fetal development 75
  foot acupressure and reflexology 274–5, 311
  foot exercises 130
  swollen feet and ankles 101
fertilization 10, 23, 68–70, 71–3, 82–3, 89
fetal alcohol syndrome (FAS) 105
fetal heart monitoring *see* electronic fetal monitoring
fetal heart rate (FHR) 328, 329, 344–5
fetal movement recording 244–5
fetoscopy 235
fetus
  blood pH levels 345
  circulation 76–7, 375
  development 10–19, 68–87, 103
  hearing 16, 79, 81
  hiccups 79, 238
  movements 13–19, 78–81, 85, 93–4, 238, 244–5
  screening for disability 226–7, 229
  sleeping during labor 344
  see also miscarriage
FHR (fetal heart rate) 328, 329, 344–5
financial planning 36
fluid retention 101, 108
folic acid 99, 110
fontanels 259
food and diet 11, 96–101
  anemia 144
  babies *see* feeding
  blood sugar level reduction 143, 144
  constipation 135, 397

food and diet (cont.)
  digestive disturbances 144–5
  food poisoning 111–12
  nausea prevention 27
  placental insufficiency 388
  preeclampsia 100, 141
  thrush 137
  twin pregnancies 94
forceps delivery 255, 346–7
foremilk 399
formula milks and bottle-feeding 401, 405–8
fraternal twins 89
full chest breathing 208–9, 211
fundal palpation 51
fundus 43, 78, 85–7
funeral arrangements 391–2

G

gas and oxygen (Entonox) 318
general anesthesia 110, 351
general practitioners 40
genetics 71–3
  genetic counseling 236–7
  genetic testing 51
genitals 116–19, 376–7, 379
gentle birth 356–67
German measles (rubella) 112
gestational diabetes 143–4
gestosis (preeclampsia) 141–2
getting up from lying down 129, 132–3
glucose challenge and glucose tolerance tests 143–4
grandparents 33, 160–1
grasp reflex 372
greeting breath 208
grieving and mourning 389–93
groin pain 134
gums *see* dental health and hygiene

H

hammock exercise 418
hammocks 218–19
handicaps *see* disability
hands, development 75, 85, 87
HCG (human chorionic gonadotrophin) test 22–3, 227
HDP (hypertensive disease of pregnancy/preeclampsia) 141–2
head, touch relaxation 194
headaches 144, 322
head-down presentation 43, 86, 90, 241
head molding 330, 376
hearing, fetal 16, 79, 81
heartburn 144–5
Hegar's sign 24

hematocrit 42
hemoglobin 42, 51, 144
hemorrhage 139–40
hemorrhoids (piles) 135
heparin 109, 388
heroin (diamorphine) 106, 318
hiccups, fetal 79, 238
high blood pressure (hypertension) 42, 140
  and preeclampsia 141–2
high temperature 111, 387
HIV infection 26, 314
home births 36–7, 45–8, 258, 264–9, 296–303
homeopathy 313
hormones
  factor in miscarriage 387–8
  menstrual cycle 69–70
  oral contraceptives 24, 26, 423
  start of labor 249, 254
  see also specific hormones, e.g., progesterone
hospital births
  admission procedures 255–7, 342
  birth companion's role 287–94
  experiences of 60–5, 187
  fears and anxieties 46, 153–4
  options and choices 38–45, 47, 324–5
  partograms 329
  safety 38–9, 46
  what to pack 242
  see also specific procedures, e.g., epidural anesthesia
human chorionic gonadotrophin (HCG) test 22–3, 227
hyperemesis 137–8
hypertension (high blood pressure) 42, 140
hypertensive disease of pregnancy (HDP/preeclampsia) 141–2
hyperventilation 205–7
hypnosis 310
hypoglycemia 382

I

ibuprofen 107
identical twins 89
imagery and visualization 191, 204–5, 224–5, 307
immunizations 112
implantation 10, 73, 83
incompetent cervix 115, 388
incontinence 414–15
indigestion 144–5
induced labor 238, 243–4, 251, 334–9, 342

inevitable abortion 387
infections *see* specific infections, e.g., mastitis
informed choice, official policies 47–8, 56, 324–5
inheritance *see* genetics
insulin 110, 142–3
insurance 38
intercourse *see* sex
internal examinations 23–4, 49, 51, 326–7
internal monitors 340, 342, 343, 344
intrauterine devices (IUDs) 24–6, 422–3
intravenous drip 330–1
inverted nipples 137
iron 51, 100, 144
itching 147
IUDs (intrauterine devices) 24–6, 422–3

J

jaundice 381, 382–3

K

Kitzinger psychosexual approach 184–5
kneeling positions, labor and delivery 215, 220–1, 253, 276–9

L

labia 116–17, 420
labor
  active management 58, 325, 340
  atmosphere and environment 361–4
  augmented/accelerated 339
  baby's experience of 356–61
  back labor 270–5
  birth rooms 41, 186, 289, 361–4
  breathing 205–13, 291
  breech presentation 275–82
  children's presence 46–7, 177, 298–9, 303
  companions *see* birth companions
  dysfunctional 285
  emotional challenges 150–5
  fetus sleeping during 344
  first signs 250–4
  first stage 254–9
  induced 238, 243–4, 251, 334–9, 342
  long-drawn-out 283–5, 347

labor (cont.)
  medical intervention *see*
    specific procedures, e.g.,
    amniotomy
  partograms 329
  positions for *see* positions
    and movement during
    labor
  posterior presentation 270–5
  preparation for *see* specific
    topics, e.g., relaxation
  preterm labor 115
  second stage 260–3, 280–2,
    293–4, 347
  sensations and feelings
    307–9
  sex as trigger 167, 170–1
  short sharp 282–3, 305
  start–stop 292–3
  third stage 263, 333–4
  transition 258–9
  see also contractions; pain
    and pain relief
Lamaze (psychoprophylaxis)
  7, 183
language 248–9
lanugo 13, 14, 78, 85–7, 376
last menstrual period (LMP)
  24
late miscarriage 388
lavender 312
laxatives 108
legs
  leg cramps 134–5
  leg-raising exercises 121,
    123
  leg sliding 123, 416
  swollen legs 101
  touch relaxation 196–7
libido 169, 170
lifting and bending 132
linea nigra 13
liquid paraffin 108
listeriosis 111
local anesthetics 318
lochia 263
loneliness 156
losing a baby 389–93
loss of control 151–2
low backaches 133, 199
low-birth-weight babies 380–5
lull (rest and be thankful
  phase) 260, 293
lung surfactant 79, 381
lying down, getting up from
  129, 132–3

M

magnesium 100, 142
mask of pregnancy 146
massage 155, 190–200, 272–5
mastitis 403

maternal serum screening
  227
meconium 19, 327
medical interventions and
  technology 324–6
  see also specific procedures,
    e.g., electronic fetal
    monitoring
medical records 42–3, 329
medication and drugs 101–10,
  317–23, 329, 334–6
membranes rupturing
  artificial (ARM/amniotomy)
    326, 327–30, 335
  natural (waters breaking)
    151, 251, 275
men *see* birth companions;
  fathers; relationships
menstrual cycle 68–70, 82
  and breast-feeding 421
  last menstrual period (LMP)
    24
  late/missed period 10, 22,
    74
mercury poisoning 112
metronidazole 108
midwives
  birth centers 45
  one-to-one care 47, 58
  see also prenatal care
migraine treatments 107
milk ejection reflex 398–400
minerals 100, 134
minipill 423
miscarriage 386–9
  early 73, 102, 387–8
  fears of, and sex 167–8
  risk factors 24, 102, 234
misopristol (Cytotec) 335–6
mobile epidurals 322
molding, head 330, 376
Mongolian spots 376
monilia 136–7
monitoring
  blood sugar levels 142–3
  electronic fetal (EFM) 244,
    257, 329, 340–5
  telemetry 343–4
monozygotic twins 89
mood-altering drugs 106
morning sickness *see* vomiting
  and nausea
Moro (startle) reflex 372
mourning and grieving 389–93
movement
  fetus 13–19, 78–81, 85,
    93–4, 238, 244–5
  posture and movement
    during pregnancy 93,
    125–9, 132
  see also exercises; positions
    and movement during
    labor

moxibustion 311
mucous plug 118, 170, 250
multiple pregnancy (twins) 39,
  88–95
muscles
  abdominal 120–1, 123, 127,
    192, 398
  pelvic floor 118–19, 197
  rectus muscle separation
    120–1, 124
  see also uterus

N

narcotics 317–18
nasal congestion 138
natural family planning 422
nausea *see* vomiting and
  nausea
neonatal jaundice 382–3
neural tube defects 99, 227
newborns
  appearance 375–8
  assessments and tests 370,
    373, 374
  bathing 366–7, 409
  circulation 375–6
  circumcision 379
  crying 361, 371, 408–9
  disabled 385
  jaundiced 381, 382–3
  practical care 409–11
  reflexes 358, 366, 372
  sleep 408
  special care babies 380–5
  see also bonding; feeding
nicotine, smoking and tobacco
  11, 103–5
nipples
  inverted 137
  sore/cracked 402–3
  stimulation 167, 171
  see also breast-feeding
nitrous oxide and oxygen
  (entonox) 318
nosebleeds 138
notochord 74
NSAIDs (nonsterodial anti-
  inflamatory drugs) 107
Nubain 318
nuchal fold 229
numbness and tingling 134
nutrition *see* food and diet

O

Odent approach 184
ophthalmia neonatorum 373
opioids 317–18, 322
oral contraceptives 24, 26,
  423
orgasm 167, 170
ovaries 69–70, 82–3

overbreathing
  (hyperventilation) 205–7
overdue 243–4, 336
  see also EDD; induced labor
ovulation 24
ovulation cycle 69
oxygen and gas (Entonox)
  318
oxytocin
  natural 255, 334, 398, 420
  synthetic drip (pitocin) 285,
    330, 335–39

P

packing, for hospital birth
  242
pain and pain relief
  back labor (posterior
    presentation) 270–5
  complementary therapies
    310–13
  cultural differences 306–7
  drugs and anesthesia 106–7,
    110, 317–23, 329, 351
  during pregnancy *see* aches
    and pains
  fear of pain 151
  induced labor 337
  perception and context
    304–9
  physical causes 305–36
  support from birth
    companion 291–2
  see also water births and
    birth pools
painkillers (analgesics) 106–7,
  317–18
palpation 15, 51
partners *see* birth companions;
  fathers; relationships
partograms 329
pathologic jaundice 383
pelvic floor and pelvic floor
  exercises 93, 118–19, 155,
  166–7, 197
pelvic infection 328, 388
pelvic rocking 121, 122, 124,
  131, 416
pelvis 121, 261, 306
penicillin and derivatives 107
perineum 116, 155, 257
  episiotomy 59, 155, 280,
    331–3
  perineal tears 59, 332–3
  postnatal care 397, 415,
    420
Phenergan 318
phenothiazines 107
pH levels, fetal blood 345
phototherapy 381, 383
physiological jaundice 383
pigmentation, skin 146

PIH (pregnancy-induced
    hypertension/
    preeclampsia) 141–2
piles (hemorrhoids) 135
pill, contraceptive 24, 26, 423
pitocin 285, 330, 335–39
placenta
    aging 244
    delivery 263, 295, 333–4
    functions 12, 76–7, 101
    placental abruption 139–40
    placental insufficiency 388
    placenta previa 139, 230
plans, birth 52, 57–9, 177
position in uterus *see*
    presentations for birth
positions and movement
    back labor 272, 275
    breech labor 280–2
    delivery positions 220–1,
        225, 280–1
    during labor 213–25, 252–3,
        255, 306, 309
    in water 41, 276–9, 300–1
    start–stop labor 292–3
positions, sexual 169–71, 415
posterior presentation (back
    labor) 240–1, 270–5
postpartum exercises 416–19
postpartum health and
    emotions 394–8, 412–15,
        423–4
postpartum sex 415, 420–3
post-traumatic stress disorder
    (PTSD) 413–14
posture and movement 93,
    125–9, 132
preeclampsia 141–2
pregnancy-induced
    hypertension (PIH/
    preeclampsia) 141–2
pregnancy tests 23
premature pushing urge 259,
    321
prenatal care 48–53
    classes 48, 152, 163, 180–5
    partner's role 162–3
    talking to doctors 52–8,
        105–6, 153
    timing 12, 15, 16, 17, 18, 49
prenatal risk profile 142
prepartum hemorrhage (PPH)
    139
Prepidil 335
presentations for birth 43, 51,
    90, 230, 271
    see also breech presentation
pressure
    as pain relief in labor 272–5
preterm babies 380–5
preterm labor 115
progesterone 12, 70, 77, 423
prostaglandins 171, 254, 335

protein 99
proteinuria 42, 141, 142
Prozac 109
psychoprophylaxis (Lamaze)
    7, 183
psychosexual approach 184–5
PTSD (post-traumatic stress
    disorder) 413–14
pubic pain 133
pudendal block 319
puppet-strings relaxation 201
pushing (bearing down) 223–5,
    259, 260–3, 321
pyelonephritis 136

Q

quickening 80–1

R

Read method 183
recessive genes 72–3
records, medical 42–3, 329
rectus muscle separation
    120–1, 124
reflexes 358, 366, 372
reflexology and foot
    acupressure 274–5, 311
regional anesthetics 318–23,
    351
relationships
    with new baby 425
    with own parents 33, 160–1
    with partner 28–31, 156,
        160–6, 172, 364, 392
    see also sex
relaxation 149, 182, 183,
    189–203
reproductive system 68, 82,
    116–19
respiratory distress, babies
    381–2
rest 27, 91–3, 149, 173,
    412–13
rest and be thankful phase
    (lull) 260, 293
resting breath 208
Rh factor 16, 49, 113–14
rhythm method 422
ribs, pain under 134
ring tests 23
ripening and unripe cervix 19,
    118, 250, 337
rocking exercises
    complete rock 419
    pelvic rocking 121, 122, 124,
        131, 416
    rocking chair 128
    rocking the baby 418
roll up exercise 419
rooting reflex 366
rubella 112

S

safety
    birth centers 45
    electronic fetal monitoring
        (EFM) 341–2
    hospital births 38–9, 46
    routine amniotomy/ARM
        328–9
    ultrasound 231–2
    water births 315–17
saline laxatives 108
salmonella 111
salt 100, 134
scans, ultrasound *see*
    ultrasound scans
screening and tests 49–53,
    142–3, 226–37
    see also specific tests, e.g.,
        urine tests
second and subsequent
    pregnancies 172–7,
        392–3
second stage labor 260–3,
    280–2, 293–4, 347
serum
    Anti-D protection 113–14
    serum screening 227
sex 117, 166–71, 415
    painful intercourse 420–1
    postnatal 415, 420–3
    sexual attractiveness 154,
        156
sex chromosomes 71–2
shaving, perineal 257
sheep's breathing 213
shiatsu 274–5
shoes 145
shortness of breath 145
shoulders
    shoulder roll 130
    touch relaxation 193, 198
show 139, 250
siblings 46–7, 173–7, 298–9,
    303, 378
sideways curl-up exercise 417
single motherhood 31–4
sinusitis 138
sitting 132
sit-ups 121
skin pigmentation 146
sleep 149, 344, 408
sleeping pills 106
small-for-dates babies 380–5
smoking and tobacco 11,
    103–5
social expectations 157
solid foods 402
sore nipples 402–3
soy milk 406
special care babies 380–5
sperm 70, 71, 83, 89, 421
spina bifida 99, 227, 234

spinal block 322, 351
spine and back care 119–20,
    133
sports 147
spotting 23
squatting positions, labor and
    delivery 216–17, 220–1,
        276–7, 281, 300
Stadol 318
stages, labor 249–63
standing, posture and
    movement 93, 125–9,
        132
standing positions, labor 214,
    252
Stanislavsky relaxation 201–3
startle (Moro) reflex 372
step reflex 372
steroids 108
stillbirth 389–93
stimulant laxatives 108
stitches *see* episiotomy; tears
stool bulk producers 108
stress 360–1
stretch and sweep 335
stretch marks 146–7
striae (stretch marks) 146–7
stripping the membranes 335
subsequent pregnancies 172–7,
    392–3
sucking 399–401
sugar levels, blood 142–4,
    382
suitcase, packing your 242
support networks 34
surfactant 79, 381
surprise births 294–5
surrogate motherhood 35
swollen ankles, feet 101
symptothermal method 422
systolic pressure 42

T

tail muscles, touch relaxation
    200
tailor sitting 127
talking to doctors 52–8, 153
tears, perineal 59, 332–3, 415,
    420
technology and medical
    intervention 324–6
    see also specific procedures,
        e.g., electronic fetal
        monitoring
teeth *see* dental health and
    hygiene
telemetry 343–4
temperature, high 111, 387
tenderness, breast 137, 403
TENS (transcutaneous
    electronic nerve
    stimulation) 311

teratogenic drugs 102
termination 386, 392–3
tests and screening 49–53,
    142–3, 226–37
    see also specific tests, e.g.,
    urine tests
test weighing 402
tetracyclines 108
thalidomide disaster 101–2
third stage labor 263, 333–4
threatened miscarriage 386–7
thrush 136–7
thyroid conditions 109
tingling and numbness 134
tiredness 27, 91, 168, 173,
    412–13
tobacco and smoking 11,
    103–5
touch relaxation 190–200
toxemia (preeclampsia)
    141–2
toxoplasmosis 111–12
tranquilizers 106, 107
transcutaneous electronic
    nerve stimulation (TENS)
    311
transition 258–9
transverse arrest 321
transverse presentation 90
travel 147–8
tricyclic antidepressants
    108–9
triple screening 227

tummy muscles 120–1, 123,
    127, 192
twins 39, 88–95

U

ultrasound scans 227–32, 244
    dating pregnancy 24, 51,
    229
    placenta assessment 139, 230
    role in bonding 80–1, 232
    women with diabetes 143
umbilical cord *see* cord
umbilical vein sampling
    (cordocentesis) 235–6
underbreathing 207
unfolding exercise 417
unripe and ripening cervix 19,
    118, 250, 337
upper backaches 130, 133
upper chest breathing 209,
    211
up, up, and away exercise 419
urinary problems 136, 414–15
urine tests 23, 42, 141, 142, 143
urologist 414
uterine cycle 69
uterus
    anatomy 68, 82
    during labor and birth 191,
        222, 263, 305–6, 336–7
    during menstrual cycle
        68–70

uterus (cont.)
    during pregnancy 10–19,
        43, 78, 84–7, 250
    effect of pregnancy
        hormones 77
    fetal positions *see*
        presentations for birth
    postnatal 398, 420
    see also cervix; contractions;
        placenta

V

vaccinations 112
vacuum extraction 346–7
vagina 116–18
vaginal bleeding 138–40,
    386–7
    see also miscarriage
vaginal discharges and
    infections 136–7, 388
vaginal examinations 23–4,
    49, 51, 326–7
varicose veins 135
vernix 14, 79, 85, 86, 262,
    376
vertebrae 119–20
vertex presentation 43, 86,
    90, 241
visualization and imagery
    191, 204–5, 224–5,
    307
vitamins 99, 406

vomiting and nausea 11, 12,
    27–8, 96
    anti-sickness drugs 107
    hyperemesis 137–8
    opioids side effect 317
vulva 116–17

W

walking 125, 398
walking epidurals 322
wall stretching 131
Warfarin 109
water, for breast-fed babies 401
water births and birth pools
    275, 276–9, 296–303,
    313–17
    availability 41, 45, 47
water loss, postnatal 397
waters breaking 151, 251, 275
week-by-week guide 10–19,
    73–87
weight 98, 397
wheelbarrow exercise 131
white coat hypertension 140
withdrawal method 421
working 148

X, Y, Z

X-rays 110
yeast growths 136–7
zinc 100

A NOTE ABOUT THE AUTHOR

Sheila Kitzinger is known and respected all over the world as a leading authority on women's experiences of pregnancy, childbirth, and motherhood. As a social anthropologist, she has studied prenatal care, birth plans, midwifery, induction of labor, episiotomy, epidural anesthesia, and crying babies in many different countries. She lectures in North and South America, Europe, Australia, and Japan on the social and psychological dimensions of birth, parenthood, and female sexuality. She has successfully campaigned to improve conditions for women prisoners, to give women the choice of water birth and birth at home, and to deepen the understanding of unhappiness after giving birth.

Her books include *Women's Experience of Sex, The Experience of Childbirth, Breastfeeding, Freedom and Choice in Childbirth, The Year After Childbirth, Ourselves as Mothers, Becoming a Grandmother, Tough Questions* (with Celia Kitzinger)*, Rediscovering Birth,* and *Birth Your Way.*

Sheila Kitzinger is married to Uwe Kitzinger, founding President of Templeton College, Oxford. They have five daughters and three grandchildren.

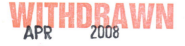